volumes in the series,

SAUNDERS MONOGRAPHS IN CLINICAL NURSING

1. Patient Care in Respiratory Problems
   by Jane Secor

2. The Cardiac Patient: A Comprehensive Approach
   by Richard G. Sanderson and others

3. The Newborn and the Nurse
   by Mary Lou Moore

4. Patient Care in Endocrine Problems
   by Roberta Spencer

5. Patient Care in Renal Failure
   by Joan Harrington and Etta Brener

PATIENT CARE IN RENAL FAILURE

JOAN DeLONG HARRINGTON, R.N., B.S.N., M.A.

Assistant Professor of Nursing, St. Louis University, St. Louis, Missouri
Formerly Staff Development Instructor, Barnes Hospital, St. Louis, Missouri; Clinical Nurse, Hemodialysis Unit, John Cochran Veterans Administration Hospital, St. Louis, Missouri; Clinical Nurse, St. Louis University Hospitals; Head Nurse, Open-Heart Team, Marymount Hospital, Cleveland, Ohio

ETTA RAE BRENER, R.N., B.S.N., M.Ed.

Clinical Nurse, Cardiac Intensive Care Unit, Columbia-Presbyterian Medical Center, New York City
Formerly Instructor in Nursing, Columbia University, New York City; Clinical Nurse, Intensive Care Unit, St. Luke's Hospital, New York City; Assistant Head Nurse, Medical Service, Barnes Hospital, and Clinical Nurse, Medical Service, Barnes Hospital, St. Louis, Missouri

Saunders Monographs in Clinical Nursing–5

W. B. SAUNDERS COMPANY
Philadelphia, London, Toronto

W. B. Saunders Company: West Washington Square
Philadelphia, PA 19105

1 St. Anne's Road
Eastbourne, East Sussex BN21 3UN, England

1 Goldthorne Avenue
Toronto, Ontario M8Z 5T9, Canada

Patient Care In Renal Failure ISBN 0–7216–4528–3

Print No: 9 8 7 6 5 4

Preface

This book is intended for the professional nurse, the nursing student, and the graduate student engaged in direct care of patients with renal failure. Although revolutionary changes have occurred in the treatment of renal failure since the early 1960's, until now little has been written specifically for nurses concerning these methods of treatment.

The goal of the book is to provide a clear, comprehensive, and practical guide to be used by nurses caring for patients with renal failure. With this in mind, we have devoted the first chapters to general background information concerning the kidney, its functioning and malfunctioning, and fluid and electrolyte regulation.

Chapter 1 gives a brief but complete review of the gross and microscopic anatomy of the kidney. The physiology of the kidney is presented in a concise manner in Chapter 2, followed by a review of fluids and electrolytes in Chapter 3. The emphasis throughout the text is on the application of physiological principles to the practice of nursing. Chapters 4 and 5 include information the nurse uses concerning the medical management of patients with renal failure. Chapters 6, 7, and 8, concerning peritoneal dialysis, hemodialysis, and transplantation, respectively, are the three major chapters of the book; they contain detailed descriptions of procedures, medications, and treatments and give concrete suggestions for nursing actions in routine situations and in cases with serious complications. Emphasis is on the nursing process, i.e., assessment, planning, intervention, and evaluation of nursing actions as they relate to patients with renal failure and transplants. Chapter 9, on prevention, suggests positive actions for the medical professions to take to decrease the number of patients contracting renal disease in the future, thereby decreasing the mortality from renal disease.

A list of references appears at the end of each chapter, both to acknowledge sources of information and to assist the student/practitioner in continuing his search for information concerning specific topics.

It is our conviction that the nurse's role in the management of patients is becoming an increasingly complex and crucial one, and that this is especially so for patients with renal failure. We hope that this book, written for nurses by nurses, will serve as a useful, readable guide to clinical practice in complex situations involving patients with renal failure.

JOAN DELONG HARRINGTON
ETTA RAE BRENER

Acknowledgments

The authors wish to thank the many people and institutions who have contributed information and encouragement in this project. We extend our gratitude to Dr. John J. Garrett, St. Louis, Missouri, whose patient teaching and guidance stimulated the authors' interest in renal patients; to Dr. Marie M. Seedor, Teachers' College, Columbia University, who guided the original study and carefully reviewed the first draft; to Brian Harrington, the first author's husband, who encouraged the authors to expand their study into a publishable manuscript; to Dr. Robert M. Levy, Dr. Robert G. Meny, and Dr. John J. Garrett for their helpful corrections and suggestions; to Robert E. Wright, our editor, who was most patient and encouraging; to the many librarians who aided us in researching this subject; to Mrs. Elizabeth Pelham, who assisted in proofreading; to our typists Ms. Dorothy Sherman, Mrs. Marion Sullivan and Mrs. Judith Toombs, who provided careful and dependable assistance.

We wish to thank the following hospitals for providing clinical experience, observational experience, and information: John Cochran V.A. Hospital, Barnes Hospital, and St. Louis University Hospital in St. Louis, Missouri; Downstate Medical Center in Brooklyn, New York; and St. Luke's Hospital Center, Columbia-Presbyterian Medical Center, Francis Delafield Hospital, and New York Hospital–Cornell Medical Center in New York City.

Most importantly, we wish to express our sincerest thanks to Brian and Susan Harrington, husband and daughter of Joan Harrington, to the Eldon Bush family, and to the dear friends of Etta Brener for their continued encouragement, support, and selflessness during the long and sometimes arduous task of writing this text.

J. D. H.

E. R. B.

Contents

CHAPTER 1

Anatomy

The kidneys are paired organs located in the dorsal part of the abdomen, one on either side of the vertebral column. Each kidney is about 11 cm long, 5–7 cm wide, and 2.5 cm thick, the left being slightly longer and narrower than the right. In the adult male each kidney weighs about 145 gm; in the adult female, 135 gm. The lower border of the kidneys is at the level of the third lumbar vertebra; the upper border, at the level of the twelfth thoracic vertebra. The left kidney is located slightly higher than the right.

To test for kidney pain and tenderness, the clinician gently hits the costovertebral angle—the angle made by the twelfth rib and the spinal column. The patient often describes pain from pyelonephritis or other kidney diseases as occurring in the back or side. Percutaneous kidney biopsy is performed through the back.

The kidneys are retroperitoneal—they are covered by peritoneum on portions of the anterior surface, but are not covered on all sides by this membrane. They are surrounded by fatty tissue and fascia, which help hold them in position. An adrenal gland is located on the upper part of each kidney.

The kidney is covered by a fibrous *capsule*. The outer portion of the kidney is called the *cortex*, the middle portion the *medulla*, and the inner portion the *sinus*. Portions of the cortex extend into the medulla and are called *renal columns*. The medulla contains *pyramids*—conical masses of tissue with radial striations; the pyramids, which are separated from each other by the renal columns, number 8 to 18 per kidney. The apices of the pyramids form small conical projections called *papillae*. The papillae empty into cup-shaped tubes in the renal sinus called *minor calyces*, which number 4 to 13. The minor calyces unite to form two or three larger tubes—the *major calyces*—which then unite to form a funnel-shaped sac—the *renal pelvis*. The volume of the calyces and pelvis together is about 8 ml. The renal pelvis diminishes rapidly in caliber and merges into the *ureter*. The ureter descends in the abdomen to the *bladder*. The *urethra* is the excretory duct from the bladder (Figs. 1 and 2).

Microscopic Anatomy

The *nephron* is the functional unit of the kidney. There are about 1,250,000 nephrons per kidney. The nephron begins with a *glomerulus*, a tuft of nonanastomosing capillaries located in the cortex and formed from an *afferent arteriole*. The glomerulus is drained by a slightly smaller *efferent* arteriole. It is surrounded by the *glomerular capsule* or *Bowman's capsule*, a membrane formed by the blind, dilated end of the renal tubule. The renal tubule continues from the glomerular capsule and forms the *neck*, a constricted section, and then forms the *proximal convoluted tubule*, a tortuous section in the cortex. The tubule enters the medulla, forms the *descending limb of the loop*

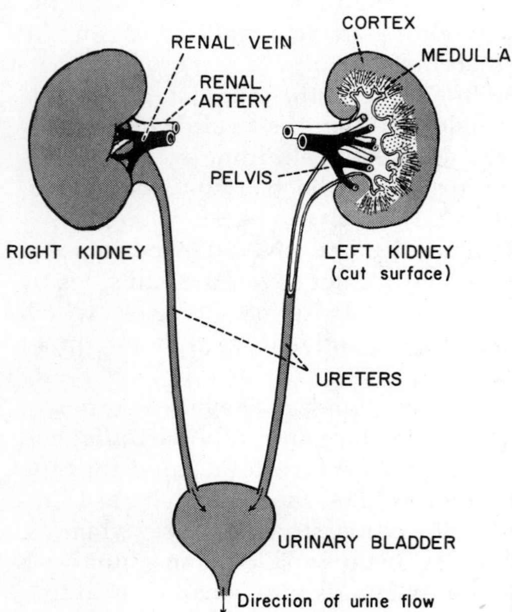

Figure 1. The kidneys, ureters, and bladder. (From Guyton, A. C.: *Textbook of Medical Physiology*. Fourth edition. Philadelphia, W. B. Saunders Co., 1971.)

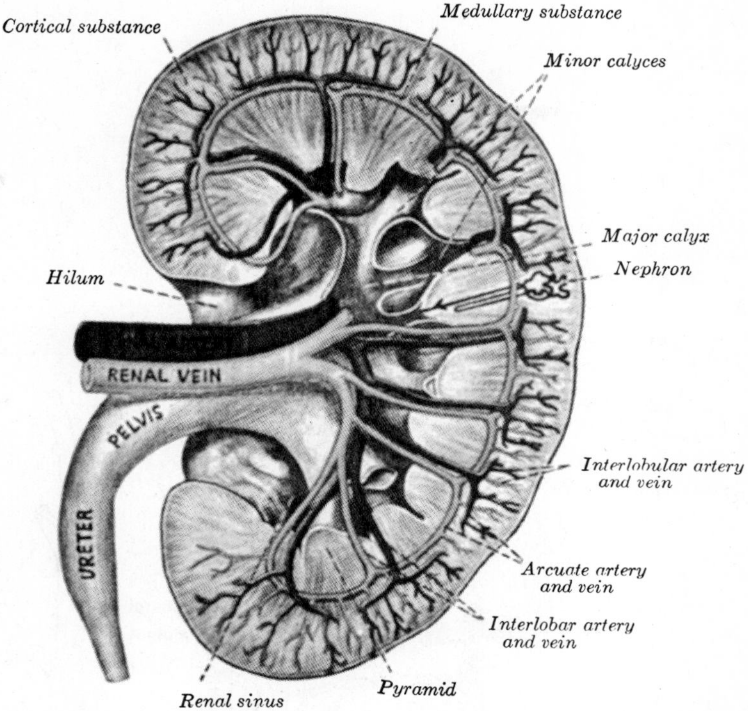

Figure 2. Diagram of a vertical section through the kidney. Nephron and blood vessels greatly enlarged. (From Goss, C. M. (Ed.): *Gray's Anatomy of the Human Body.* Twenty-ninth edition. Philadelphia, Lea & Febiger, 1973.)

of Henle and the *ascending limb of the loop of Henle*, and re-enters the cortex, where it becomes tortuous, forming the *distal convoluted tubule.* The end of the distal convoluted tubule marks the end of one nephron (Figs. 3 and 4).

The distal convoluted tubule empties into a *straight* or *collecting duct* in the cortex. Collecting ducts pass to the medulla, joining and increasing in size. The ducts of each pyramid coalesce to form a central duct—the *duct of Bellini*, which empties through the papilla into a minor calyx.

The *juxtaglomerular cells* are a group of special granulated cells found near the afferent arteriole before it enters the glomerular capsule. The *macula densa* is an area of granular, densely packed cells located near the afferent arteriole and the distal convoluted tubule where it passes close to the arteriole. The juxtaglomerular cells and the macula densa are together called the *juxtaglomerular apparatus.* This apparatus is thought to be a source of renin (Fig. 5).

The kidney is supplied by the *renal artery*, a large branch of the

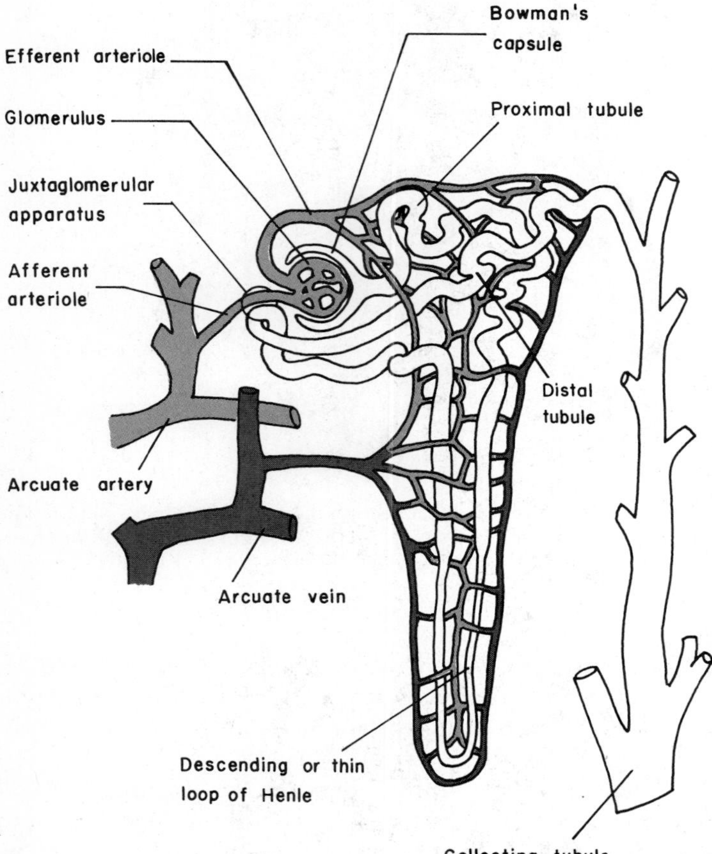

Figure 3. The nephron. (From Guyton, A. C.: *Textbook of Medical Physiology.* Fourth edition. Philadelphia, W. B. Saunders Co., 1971. Redrawn from Smith: *The Kidney.* Oxford University Press.)

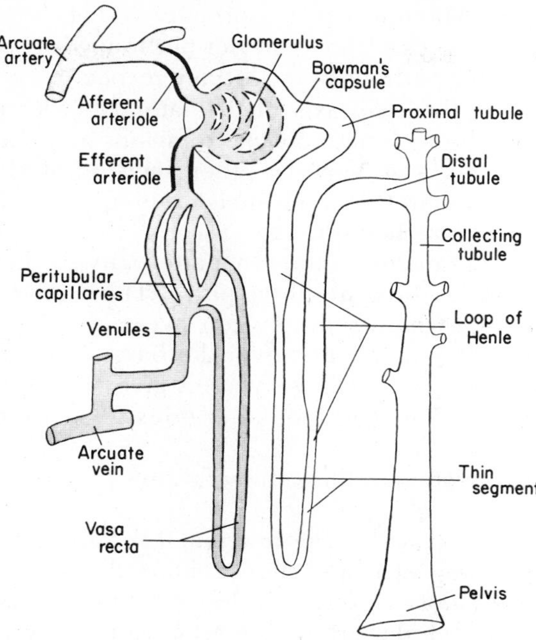

Figure 4. The functional nephron. (From Guyton, A. C.: *Textbook of Medical Physiology.* Fourth edition. Philadelphia, W. B. Saunders Co., 1971.)

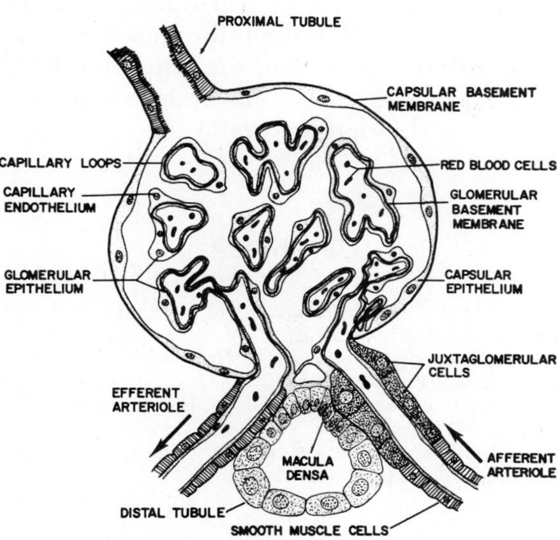

Figure 5. The juxtaglomerular apparatus. (Adapted from Ham, A. W.: *Histology.* Sixth edition. Philadelphia, J. B. Lippincott Co., 1969.)

abdominal aorta. The renal artery normally divides into two portions, a larger anterior and a smaller posterior portion, which supply the anterior and posterior portions of the kidney respectively. A line, called *Bröedel's line,* in the long axis of the lateral border of the kidney passes between the two main arterial divisions and marks an area in which there are no large vessels. When incision of kidney tissue is necessary, as in nephrotomy, the incision is often made along Bröedel's line to minimize hemorrhage.

The primary branches of the renal artery divide and subdivide to form *lobar arteries,* which supply papillae. These arteries divide into *interlobar arteries,* which run between pyramids. The arteries reach the corticomedullary zone, arch over the bases of the pyramids, and are called *arcuate arteries.* These vessels give off branches called *interlobular arteries.* The interlobular arteries give rise to the afferent arterioles (see Fig. 2).

The venous system of the kidney follows the basic pattern of the arterial system.

To correlate part of this information, it is helpful to trace the formation and pathway of urine. Blood enters the kidney through the renal artery and passes through the lobar artery, interlobar artery, arcuate artery, interlobular artery, afferent arteriole, and into the glomerulus. A portion of the blood, the glomerular filtrate, passes from the glomerulus into the glomerular capsule. The filtrate passes through the neck, the proximal convoluted tubule, the descending limb of the loop of Henle, the ascending limb of the loop of Henle, and the distal convoluted tubule. During this passage through the tubule, the filtrate is concentrated and transformed into urine. The urine passes into the collecting duct, through collecting ducts of increasing size to the duct of Bellini, through the duct of Bellini, the papilla, the minor calyx, the major calyx, the renal pelvis, the ureter, the bladder, and then through the urethra.

References

1. Ganong, W. F.: *Review of Medical Physiology,* Fifth edition. Los Altos, California, Lange Medical Publications, 1971.
2. Goss, C. M. (Ed.): *Gray's Anatomy of the Human Body.* Twenty-eighth edition. Philadelphia, Lea & Febiger, 1966.
3. Guyton, A. C.: *Textbook of Medical Physiology.* Fourth edition. Philadelphia, W. B. Saunders Co., 1971.
4. Romanes, G. J. (Ed.): *Cunningham's Manual of Practical Anatomy.* Thirteenth edition. New York, Oxford University Press, 1968.

CHAPTER 2

Physiology

The kidney is the chief regulator of all the substances of body fluids and is primarily responsible for maintaining homeostasis, i.e., an equilibrium of fluids and electrolytes in the body. The kidney has three main functions: the excretion of waste products of protein metabolism, the regulation of water and electrolytes and the regulation of arterial blood pressure.

The removal of potentially toxic waste products is the primary function of the kidney and is accomplished through the formation of urine. Urine is an aqueous solution of waste products of metabolism and foreign substances. The basic processes involved in its formation are: filtration, which occurs in the glomeruli, and reabsorption and secretion, which take place in the renal tubules. It is through these processes that the kidneys regulate the amounts of the various substances in the body and thus maintain the *milieu interieur* (internal environment) for the proper functioning of cells throughout the body. In healthy persons, the kidneys are sensitive to the wide daily fluctuation in diet and fluid intake and compensate by varying the volume and consistency of the urinary output.

The kidney plays a role in regulating the arterial blood pressure. Renin, an enzyme released from the renal cortex, affects the arterial blood pressure and the extracellular fluid volume. The process is as follows: a decrease in the blood flow to the kidneys, owing to shock, for example, triggers the release of renin from the renal cortex; renin, in turn, stimulates the production of angiotensin, which causes the secretion of aldosterone from the adrenal cortex. Aldosterone causes active reabsorption of sodium chloride and the consequent reabsorption of water. This increases the circulating blood volume and thus raises the blood pressure. The regulation of blood pressure, however, is complex and involves many factors in addition to the renin-angiotensin system of the kidney.

Erythropoietin secreted by the kidneys helps to regulate the amount of circulating hemoglobin by stimulating the bone marrow to produce hemoglobin. Diseased kidneys secrete very little erythropoietin, thus decreasing hemoglobin production and intensifying the anemia associated with chronic renal disease.

Glomerular Filtration

The nephron is the functional unit of the kidney. It is composed of the glomerulus, a tuft of capillaries that filters water and solutes, and the tubules, which selectively reabsorb substances needed by the body. Figure 6 schematically demonstrates its functions. The glomerulus is semipermeable, i.e., it is a porous membrane through which water and electrolytes pass freely but which is relatively impermeable to larger molecules, such as protein and glucose molecules. The glomeruli differ from other capillaries in the body in that the hydrostatic pressure (water pressure) within them is approximately three times as great as the pressure in other capillaries. Normal hydrostatic pressure in capillaries is 15–20 mm Hg, while that in the glomerulus is 70 mm Hg. The result of this high pressure is that fluid leaks out of the porous glomerular capillaries and into Bowman's capsule. Ultrafiltration is the term used to describe this event—"ultra" because it is filtration under exceedingly high pressure. The fluid that is filtered is known as glomerular filtrate and the amount of fluid filtered in a given length of time is the glomerular filtration rate (GFR).

Since pressure is a major factor in the formation of urine, any change in pressure within this system will alter the glomerular filtration rate. There is a direct relationship between the glomerular filtration pressure and the glomerular filtration rate, providing the colloidal osmotic pressure is constant. (Colloidal osmotic pressure or oncotic pressure is the force exerted by plasma proteins within the capillaries.) Therefore, an increase in the glomerular filtration pressure increases the GFR. On the other hand, an increase in the colloidal osmotic pressure (which enables the capillary to draw water in) or the pressure in Bowman's capsule will decrease the GFR. A decrease in cardiac output due to hemorrhage, congestive heart failure, or the like decreases the circulating blood volume and therefore the glomerular filtration pressure, which in turn decreases the GFR and ultimately decreases

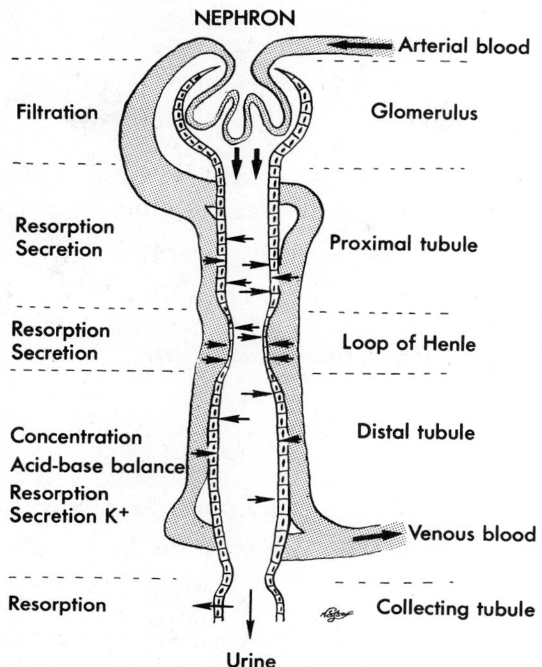

Figure 6. Schematic picture of the function of the nephron. (From Nosé, Y.: *Manual on Artificial Organs.* Vol. I. The Artificial Kidney. St. Louis, C. V. Mosby Co., 1969.)

the urinary output. Glomerular filtrate, then, is formed by the ultrafiltration of blood across a selective membrane that allows the passage of water and electrolytes but restricts proteins and red blood cells. Therefore, glomerular filtrate is essentially plasma without the proteins.

Approximately 25 per cent of the volume of blood pumped into the systemic circulation by each ventricular contraction is circulated through the kidneys. The normal cardiac output is 4–6 L/min. Thus 25 per cent, or 1000–1200 ml of blood, pass through the kidneys each minute. This fact emphasizes the tremendous role of the kidney in continually regulating the substances in the blood to maintain homeostasis. Approximately 12 times our total blood volume passes through the kidneys each hour; i.e., man's total volume of blood passes through the kidneys 12 times each hour. This is equal to 144 units of blood each hour. From this blood flow of 144 units per hour (1200 ml/min) only about 130 ml of filtrate is formed in a minute. Since there are 1440 minutes in one day and 130 ml is filtered per minute, 187,200 ml of filtrate is formed per day.

$$\begin{array}{r} 1440 \text{ min/day} \\ \times\ 130 \text{ ml/min} \\ \hline 187{,}200 \text{ ml/day} \end{array}$$

The obvious question is, "What happens to all this fluid?" Normal urinary output is 1500 ml per day, which is only about 1 per cent of the amount of filtrate formed; therefore, the other 99 per cent must be reabsorbed.

Tubular Reabsorption and Secretion

Reabsorption

Reabsorption takes place in the kidney tubules and is critical to the hydration and electrolyte balance of the body. The tubules reabsorb substances in two ways: by active reabsorption and by passive diffusion and osmosis.

Active reabsorption is the process whereby certain substances combine with a carrier and diffuse through the membrane from the tubules to the interstitial spaces where they are picked up by the capillaries. The most important substances reabsorbed in this way are glucose, amino acids, protein, uric acid, and most electrolytes. Active reabsorption is so effective for glucose, amino acids, and protein that they are practically absent in the urine. Electrolytes transported by this method include sodium, potassium, magnesium, calcium, chloride, and bicarbonate. The reabsorption of these substances is regulated by the kidney according to their levels in the blood and the body's needs. Specifically, the renal tubules are responsible for maintaining the balance of electrolytes in the body. Sodium chloride is the electrolyte most actively reabsorbed. Aldosterone, secreted by the adrenal cortex, determines the reabsorption of sodium chloride.

Reabsorption by diffusion and osmosis occurs passively and rather simply. A review of the principles of osmosis and diffusion is found in Chapter 3. Renal tubules are semipermeable membranes through which certain substances, whose particles are small enough, diffuse from the area of greater concentration to the area of lesser concentration. This diffusion takes place in both directions across the tubular membrane until an equilibrium is reached. Osmosis occurs when the concentration of solutes is high in the interstitial spaces, owing to active reabsorption. The concentration gradient causes water to move from the area of lesser solute concentration, the tubules in this case, to the area of greater concentration, the interstitial space.

Some substances are poorly reabsorbed by the tubules. Urea is an example of a waste product whose molecules are too large to diffuse easily through the pores of the tubular membrane. As water is reabsorbed by osmosis, the concentration of urea in the tubules increases and sets up a concentration gradient between the tubules and the interstitial spaces. This gradient then is totally responsible for the reabsorption of urea. The process is somewhat inefficient, producing the beneficial effect of poor urea reabsorption. Other poorly absorbed substances that are concentrated in the urine are phosphates, sulfates, nitrates, uric acid, and phenols. These are all waste products that would be harmful in large concentrations within the body.

A few substances, creatinine, inulin, mannitol, and sucrose, are not reabsorbed at all by the tubules. Therefore, their concentration is identical in the glomerular filtrate and in the urine. This is particularly helpful in testing kidney function.

SECRETION

In addition to reabsorption, the function of the tubular cells also includes secretion of certain substances. Secretion is a chemical activity that occurs in the opposite direction from reabsorption; substances are transported from the blood to the tubules and excreted in the urine. Potassium and hydrogen are the principal substances actively secreted, but some drugs including penicillin, iodopyracet (Diodrast), sodium *o*-iodohippurate (Hippuran), and phenolsulfonphthalein (PSP) are removed from the blood by active secretion. Diodrast, Hippuran, and PSP can therefore be used to test secretion by the renal tubules.

Regulation of Electrolytes[*]

The hormone aldosterone is thought to be sensitive to the concentration of sodium in the blood. For example, if the concentration of sodium ion in the blood is low, aldosterone is secreted to cause the reabsorption of sodium. If the secretion of aldosterone is decreased, more sodium is lost in the urine and the extracellular concentration of sodium is decreased. This typical feedback mechanism is illustrated in Figure 7.

---

[*]For more detailed information about electrolytes and their regulation by the kidneys, see Chapter 3.

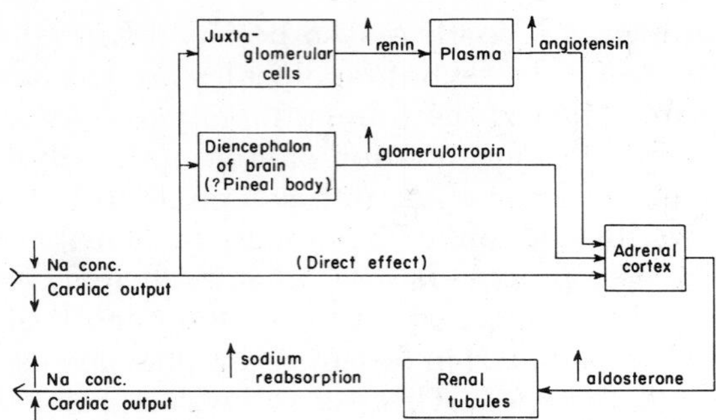

Figure 7. Three feedback mechanisms controlling sodium concentration and cardiac output. Note the relationship between sodium and aldosterone. (From Guyton, A. C.: *Textbook of Medical Physiology.* Fourth edition. Philadelphia, W. B. Saunders Co., 1971.)

Sodium reabsorption is very important because it affects the regulation of several other electrolytes. Active reabsorption of sodium ion results in passive transport of chloride and bicarbonate, which aid in maintaining the acid-base balance and the osmotic equilibrium of the body. It is the active reabsorption of sodium, accompanied by the passive reabsorption of water, that is responsible for the reabsorption of 99 per cent of the glomerular filtrate each day.

The concentration of potassium is regulated by the sodium concentration. As the reabsorption of sodium is increased by aldosterone, the reabsorption of potassium is concurrently decreased. An increased potassium concentration stimulates the production of aldosterone as does a low sodium concentration. Therefore the proper functioning of the sodium feedback mechanism is necessary for the excretion of potassium. The kidneys, however, have a second mechanism for maintaining normal potassium levels in the blood. That is secretion of potassium by the renal tubules as was described earlier. When the extracellular fluid level of potassium becomes too high, the renal tubules secrete the excess potassium into the urine.

Concentrating and Diluting Mechanisms

Urine is not concentrated by adding solute but by reabsorbing water without solute. Urine is diluted by reabsorbing solute without water. The counter-current mechanism of the kidney is responsible for its ability to concentrate or dilute urine.

The anatomical arrangement of the nephron and the capillaries is described in Chapter 1. The counter-current mechanism, illustrated in Figure 8, functions as follows: as the fluid flows through the loop of

Henle in the medulla, sodium chloride is actively reabsorbed from the loop into the interstitial fluid until the sodium chloride concentration in the medulla becomes several times greater than that of normal interstitial fluid. The sodium chloride concentration remains high owing to the sluggish blood flow in the area and the counter-current flow of blood and tubular fluid.

As the fluid descends the loop of Henle, sodium chloride readily diffuses from the interstitial fluid to the tubule; as the blood descends the vasa recta, sodium chloride diffuses into the blood until the concentration in the blood is several times that of normal blood. As the blood ascends the vasa recta, sodium chloride diffuses from the blood into the interstitial fluid; as the fluid ascends the loop of Henle, sodium chloride is actively transported out of the tubule into the interstitial fluid of the medulla. Thus the sodium chloride concentration remains high in the medulla and only a small amount of sodium chloride is removed from the blood.

The kidney, therefore, produces very dilute urine when the counter-current mechanism is functioning. However, under normal circumstances antidiuretic hormone (ADH) is secreted by a hypothal-

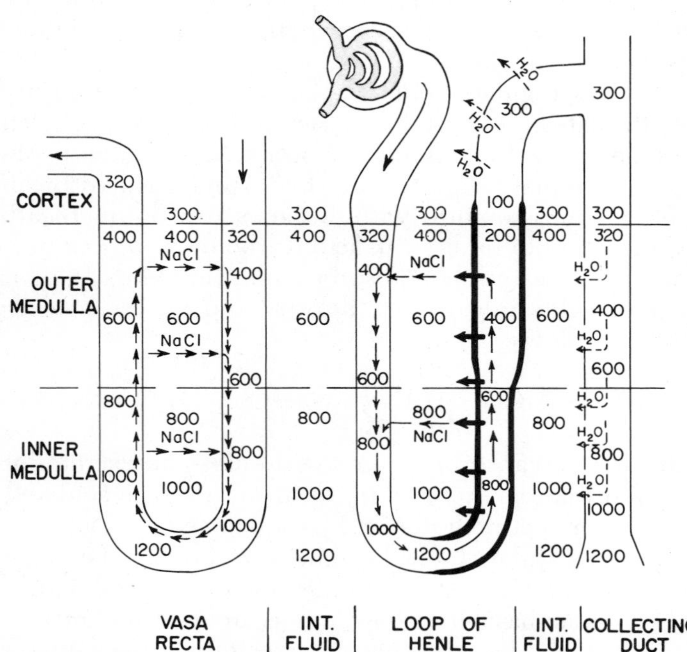

Figure 8. The "counter-current" mechanism for concentrating the urine. (From Guyton, A. C.: *Textbook of Medical Physiology.* Fourth edition. Philadelphia, W. B. Saunders Co., 1971.)

amic-neurohypophyseal mechanism, causing the pores of the distal tubule and collecting duct to become extremely permeable to water and to reabsorb it in large quantities. As water is reabsorbed the urine becomes more concentrated. Conversely, in the absence of ADH, the tubules will remain fairly impermeable to water and the urine excreted will be dilute. The secretion of antidiuretic hormone functions by an osmotic feedback mechanism. When the colloidal osmotic pressure of intracellular fluids is too great, osmoreceptors in the hypothalamus stimulate secretion of antidiuretic hormone. This causes the kidneys to reabsorb greater amounts of water until the body fluid concentrations become normal. When the body fluids are too dilute, the osmoreceptors do not stimulate and antidiuretic hormone is not released. Therefore excess water is excreted in the urine.

Acid-Base Regulation

The kidney is the chief regulator of the pH of the body. Normal blood pH is 7.35–7.45 and even in disease conditions it almost never becomes more acidic than 6.8 or more basic than 7.8. The kidneys normally excrete metabolic acids (phosphoric, sulfuric, uric, and keto acids) as they are formed, thus preventing excessive hydrogen ion concentration, i.e., acidosis.

The kidneys regulate acid-base balance by excreting hydrogen ions when the extracellular fluids are acidic and excreting bicarbonate ions when the extracellular fluids are too alkaline. Ordinarily the renal tubules secrete equal proportions of hydrogen ions and bicarbonate ions. Hydrogen ions combine with sodium salts (sodium bicarbonate) in the tubular fluid to form weak acid (carbonic acid) and to free the sodium ion. The sodium is reabsorbed into the body fluids and the carbonic acid splits into carbon dioxide and water. The chemical equation is as follows:

$$H^+ + NaHCO_3 \rightarrow H_2CO_3 + Na \rightarrow CO_2 + H_2O + Na^+$$

Carbon dioxide is reabsorbed from the tubules and excreted through the lungs, and water is excreted in the urine. Thus an acid and a base are destroyed, maintaining the acid-base balance.

If the extracellular fluids become very acidic, the quantity of bicarbonate in the glomerular filtrate decreases and more acidic hydrogen ions than basic bicarbonate ions are excreted, returning the fluids to normal acid-base balance. Conversely, if extracellular fluids become too alkaline, more bicarbonate ions than hydrogen ions are excreted, returning the acid-base balance to normal. In renal disease, the ability to excrete acid is reduced, and bicarbonate and other buffers are ineffective; thus the patient develops acidosis.

Blood Pressure Regulation

A decrease in the effective blood volume or ischemia in the kidney causes the renal cortex to secrete renin. It is believed that renin elevates the arterial blood pressure and corrects the ischemia by increasing the blood flow to the kidney. Figure 7 illustrates this mechanism. Renin is an enzyme that catalyzes the conversion of a plasma protein into angiotensin I, which is rapidly converted to angiotensin II by another enzyme.

Angiotensin, as described by Guyton, has two effects that can increase the arterial blood pressure.

1. Angiotensin causes vasoconstriction of the systemic arterioles; arteriolar constriction increases peripheral resistance and thus increases the arterial pressure.

2. Angiotensin stimulates an increased production of aldosterone by the adrenal cortex; aldosterone causes the kidneys to actively reabsorb sodium chloride and thus retain water, which elevates the arterial blood pressure because of the increased extracellular fluid volume.[6] Research demonstrates that in most types of hypertension the renin-angiotensin system is not responsible for the continued hypertension. Most renal hypertension is probably caused by salt and water retention due to other causes or other factors, as discussed in Chapter 4.

Kidney Function Tests

The kidney is an organ with many unique and complex functions. For this reason it is difficult to devise a test that measures all the renal functions. Renal function tests are used chiefly to determine the nature and extent of existing renal disease. They are also used to detect early renal disease since functional impairment often precedes symptoms. Since the tests do not ordinarily provide specific information concerning the underlying disease, no one test is used to arrive at a conclusive diagnosis. A comparative study of several tests is essential to evaluate renal function accurately. Renal tests currently being used evaluate filtration or secretion or reabsorption. The most frequently used tests of filtration are the clearance tests; urea and creatinine clearances are the ones most often measured. The phenolsulfonphthalein (PSP) test is commonly used to test secretion, while concentration tests are used to test reabsorption.

Tests of filtration

In order to evaluate the function of the kidneys, the glomerular filtration rate (GFR) is determined. Since it is not possible to measure the GFR directly, tests are used that measure the rate at which specific substances are cleared from the plasma. The term "plasma clearance" is used in reference to the ability of the kidney to remove various substances from the blood. If a true picture of the GFR is to be obtained, the substances must be freely filtered by the glomerulus and neither reabsorbed nor secreted by the renal tubules. If the blood plasma contains 0.1 gm of a substance in each 100 ml, and 0.1 gm of this substance passes into the urine each minute, then 100 ml of plasma is cleared of this substance each minute. The normal GFR is 105–135 ml/min. The formula for calculating clearances follows:[6]

$$\text{Plasma clearance (ml/min)} = \frac{\text{Quantity of urine (ml/min)} \times \text{Concentration in urine}}{\text{Concentration in plasma}}$$

Inulin clearance test. Inulin is a polysaccharide that is neither reabsorbed nor secreted and is therefore an ideal substance for measuring plasma clearance. The inulin clearance test shows the volume of plasma that is cleared of inulin in one minute. The normal clearance rate for the average man (1.73 sq. m of body surface area) is 120 ml/min, which is 70 ml/sq m/min.[8] Interpretation of the inulin clearance requires a knowledge of the renal blood flow. Primary glomerular diseases manifest a decrease in glomerular filtration rate with normal or moderately reduced renal blood flow. On the other hand, vascular renal diseases show an early decrease in renal plasma flow with a relatively normal GFR. In far-advanced chronic renal disease, regardless of the cause, there is a parallel reduction in blood flow, glomerular filtration, and tubular function.

The disadvantages of the inulin clearance test are, first, that a foreign substance is injected into the patient intravenously, which necessarily carries risks, and second, that exact timing of collection of specimens is required for an accurate result. The advantage is that inulin is the substance most completely cleared by the kidney and therefore provides the most exact test of GFR.

Creatinine clearance test. The creatinine clearance is frequently used as an index of the GFR. Like inulin, creatinine is neither reabsorbed nor secreted by the tubules. Unlike inulin, creatinine is an endogenous waste product. The quantity produced and excreted depends on the muscle mass and remains constant in an individual from day to day. Creatinine is unaffected by the rate of protein catabolism and the variation of protein in the diet. Since creatinine is excreted primarily by glomerular filtration, the serum creatinine concentration rises when the GFR falls. Measurement of creatinine clearance is an accurate method of detecting renal disease and of following the progress of existing disease.

Normal creatinine clearance is:

Men 110–150 ml/min 1.73 sq m body surface area
Women 105–132 ml/min 1.73 sq m body surface area[1]

The test is relatively simple to execute. A 24-hour urine specimen is collected and blood for a serum creatinine determination is drawn during the 24-hour period. The test can also be performed with urine collections for shorter periods such as two or four hours. Creatinine clearance is interpreted as equal to the glomerular filtration rate. A low creatinine clearance rate then indicates depressed renal function. This may be due primarily to renal disease or to prerenal disease such as circulatory impairment.

Urea clearance test. The urea clearance, also a measure of renal function, is one of the most widely used indicators of glomerular filtration. Urea is freely filtered at the glomerulus; unlike inulin and creatinine, however, a certain percentage (approximately 40 per cent) of urea is reabsorbed in the tubules by passive diffusion as water is reabsorbed. It has been found that at urine excretion rates of 2 ml/min the urea clearance is consistently 50–60 per cent of the inulin clearance; therefore, urea can be used as a valid index of the GFR, given a urine flow rate of 2 ml/min. The normal urea clearance rate at maximum urine flow of 2 ml/min is 75 ml/min, which is approximately half the rate of inulin clearance. Urea clearance is not the test of choice in severe renal disease since it is influenced by tubular reabsorption as well as by glomerular filtration. Because the work load per functioning nephron increases as nephrons are destroyed by renal disease, urea clearance, which remains constant, represents a greater fraction of the GFR as diuresis occurs in the various stages of renal failure. Also, at the lower urine flow rates typical of severe renal disease, the diffusion of urea decreases because of limited water reabsorption in the tubules, thus increasing the amount of urea in the urine. Hence, the urea clearance may not show the exact degree of depression of the GFR in severely diseased patients. For general clinical use, however, this is not always considered a disadvantage.

There are several disadvantages to the urea clearance test. First, a urine flow of 2 ml/min is desired to measure the maximum urea clearance. Often, to achieve this the patient must drink several glasses of fluid prior to the test. Patients with advanced renal disease may require large amounts of fluid to obtain a 2 ml/min output and may suffer acute water intoxication if hydrated too rapidly. Second, collection of urine and blood specimens must be accurately performed. Last, diet and activity must be controlled so that normal urea production occurs. For these reasons the creatinine clearance rate is a more convenient and reliable measure of the glomerular filtration.

The test is usually begun in the morning following a light breakfast in which protein foods, coffee, and tea are omitted. The patient is given water and fruit juices in large amounts – approximately 1000 ml in the hour prior to the test and 240 ml every half hour during the test. At the start of the test, the patient is instructed to void and discard this specimen, noting the exact time. If the patient has a catheter, specimens are obtained from the sterile collecting bag. One hour later the patient is asked to void into a clean specimen bottle or clean dry bed pan, or the collecting bag is emptied into a clean bottle. The bottle is labeled with the time and number of the specimen. At the end of the second hour a second urine specimen is obtained in the same manner. Midway through the test a blood sample is drawn for blood urea nitrogen determination.

Interpretation of the urea clearance test requires an understanding of the physiology of filtration and tubular reabsorption of urea. In general, it is used to detect renal disease and to monitor the progress of disease. The urea clearance will be decreased in renal diseases that affect the GFR and in prerenal diseases that decrease the plasma flow rate. The degree of depression will depend on the stage of disease.

TESTS OF TUBULAR FUNCTION

Secretion. The secretion of phenolsulphonphthalein (PSP) is frequently used as an indicator of the kidney's ability to eliminate foreign substances and end products of metabolism from the blood. Since secretion occurs in the tubules, the PSP test measures tubular function. This test is of greatest value in evaluating chronic kidney disease. PSP excretion is low in diseases that decrease the GFR and is generally proportional to it. If the GFR is reduced to less than 10–20 per cent of normal, PSP excretion is minimal and further changes are too small to evaluate. The disadvantage of the PSP test is that it requires that the patient be rapidly loaded with water and overhydration may occur in patients with severe renal disease who have grossly abnormal excretion patterns.

The test is performed in the following manner: The patient is given a light breakfast but no coffee or tea. He is instructed to void completely and then drink one to two glasses of water before the dye is injected. During the test the patient is to be resting. One milliliter of PSP (a red dye) is injected intravenously. Urine specimens are collected at 15, 30, and 120 minutes following injection. The percentages of dye in the urine are compared colorimetrically with a standard solution. Normal values are:

25–45 per cent at 15 min.
50–65 per cent at 60 min.
60–80 per cent at 120 min.

Elimination of less than 25 per cent in the first 15 minutes indicates impairment in ability of the kidneys to eliminate foreign substances from the blood. Reduction in total dye excretion indicates more serious impairment, and excretion of less than 10 per cent shows severe renal damage.

Concentration and dilution tests. Normal kidneys vary greatly in the amount of urine and the specific gravity of the urine excreted from hour to hour and day to day. In disease the kidney loses the ability to regulate water and electrolytes and thus loses its ability to maintain homeostasis. Since these functions occur in the renal tubules, tests of concentration and dilution measure tubular function. There are many tests of concentration and dilution, most of which involve intake of a prescribed amount of fluid, a period of collecting specimens, and examination of the amount and quality of the urine. The disadvantages of most of these tests are numerous. Water intoxication or dehydration may occur if the patient has severe functional loss. The patient must be cooperative and able to follow directions exactly. Discarding any specimen in a series will invalidate the test. The patient and the nurse must be well informed regarding the procedure. Timing may be a problem if samples are to be collected at exact intervals.

The concentration test is usually performed first. The procedure for the Fishberg concentration test is as follows: The evening before the test, the patient has a high protein meal with only 200 ml of fluid. Following this he receives nothing further and remains at bed rest until the test is completed. In the morning the patient empties his bladder and the specimen is saved. Second and third specimens are collected one and two hours later. The specific gravity of each is measured; normally, that of at least one specimen is greater than 1.025. If all the specific gravities are below 1.025, some impairment exists in the ability of the kidney to concentrate and eliminate solid substances. Values considerably lower indicate severe renal disease.

An example of a dilution test procedure is as follows: After the evening meal the night prior to the test, fluids are withheld and the patient is kept at bed rest. The first morning specimen is collected and discarded. Next the patient is asked to drink approximately 1000 ml of water in 30–45 minutes. Voided specimens are obtained hourly for four hours. Specific gravity is measured on each specimen and the total excretion is recorded. Normally the specific gravity of at least one specimen will fall below 1.003. The usual output is 1200 ml in four hours. Abnormal results include low rate of excretion and specific gravity of 1.010 or higher, indicating impaired water elimination and possible renal disease such as nephritis or the nephrotic syndrome.

SPECIFIC GRAVITY. Measurement of specific gravity is a test of concentration and dilution that is relatively simple and inexpensive. The specific gravity of urine is its weight compared with the weight of an equal volume of distilled water. It measures the density of the urine and is an indicator of renal tubular function. The specific gravity of distilled water is 1.000; that of urine ranges from 1.003–1.030. The higher the solute concentration of urine the higher the specific gravity.

A consistently low specific gravity indicates that the renal tubules have lost their ability to reabsorb water and concentrate urine. In diseases such as early pyelonephritis, the GFR is normal while the specific gravity is low, indicating normal glomerular function but disturbed tubular function.

The procedure is as follows: A small cylinder (approximately 25 ml) is filled three fourths full with urine and a urinometer is floated in the fluid. The urinometer must not be touching the sides of the cylinder when the reading is taken. The specific gravity is read where the meniscus crosses the scale on the urinometer.

ADDITIONAL TESTS

Urinalysis. Although urinalysis is not primarily a test of kidney function, it is an important diagnostic tool used in evaluating renal disease. A routine urinalysis provides general information concerning renal function. The normal constituents of the urine are the waste products of protein metabolism and excess electrolytes. The most abundant of these are:

Metabolic wastes	*Electrolytes*
Urea	Chloride
Creatinine	Calcium
Ammonia	Sodium
Uric acid	Potassium
Nitrogen	Magnesium
	Phosphates
	Sulfates

A table of normal laboratory values for urine is given in Appendix A.

Substances not normally present in the urine in significant amounts include: protein, glucose, erythrocytes, leukocytes, pus cells, and casts.

The presence of any one of these substances in a significant amount signals malfunction of some type. Although urinalysis alone is not specific enough to pinpoint the actual problem, it may be the earliest evidence of disease. The presence of measureable protein, for example, may be the result of severely diseased glomeruli or merely the result of vigorous exercise, restriction of fluids, or a high-protein diet immediately preceding the test. Erythrocytes in the urine may be indicative of disease or trauma of the nephron, the tubules, the ureters, or the bladder. Therefore, the urinalysis may be used as a preliminary screening device, but further testing and examination are required to follow up any abnormalities adequately.

Proteinuria. Measurement of proteinuria is an important laboratory technique for diagnosing glomerular disease.

The protein in the plasma is not ordinarily filtered through the glomerulus in measureable amounts because the pores of the glomerular membrane are too small for protein molecules to pass through easily. In disease, however, the glomerular membrane is frequently damaged or destroyed and measureable protein is filtered through.

Degrees of proteinuria are expressed as follows:

30 mg/100 ml = 1+
100 mg/100 ml = 2+
300 mg/100 ml = 3+
1000 mg/100 ml = 4+

False proteinuria can occur following dehydration, strenuous exercise, or ingestion of a high-protein diet.

References

1. Beeson, P. B., and McDermott, W. (Eds.): *Cecil-Loeb Textbook of Medicine.* Thirteenth edition. Philadelphia, W. B. Saunders Co., 1971.
2. Bernstein, L. M., et al.: *Renal Function and Renal Failure.* Baltimore, Williams & Wilkins Co., 1965.
3. Black, D. A. K. (Ed.): *Renal Disease.* Second edition. Philadelphia, F. A. Davis Co., 1967.
4. Brest, A. N., and Moyer, J. H. (Eds.): *Renal Failure.* Philadelphia, J. B. Lippincott Co., 1968.
5. De Wardener, H. E.: *The Kidney. An Outline of Normal and Abnormal Structure and Function.* Third edition. Baltimore, Williams & Wilkins Co., 1968.
6. Guyton, A. C.: *Textbook of Medical Physiology.* Fourth edition. Philadelphia, W. B. Saunders Co., 1971.
7. Hamburger, J., Ricket, G., Crosnier, J., Funck-Brentano, J. L., Antoine, B., Ducrot, H., Mery, J. P., and DeMontera, H.: *Nephrology.* Vol. I. Translated by A. Walsh. Philadelphia, W. B. Saunders Co., 1968.

8. Levinson, S. A., and MacFate, R. P.: *Clinical Laboratory Diagnosis.* Seventh edition. Philadelphia, Lea & Febiger, 1969.
9. Merrill, J. P.: *The Treatment of Renal Failure.* Second edition. New York, Grune & Stratton, 1965.
10. Nosé, Y.: *Manual on Artificial Organs.* Vol. I. The Artificial Kidney. St. Louis, C. V. Mosby Co., 1969.
11. Page, L. B., and Culver, R. J. (Eds.): *A Syllabus of Laboratory Examinations in Clinical Diagnosis.* Cambridge, Harvard University Press, 1960.
12. Pitts, R. F.: *Physiology of the Kidney and Body Fluids.* Second edition. Chicago, Year Book Medical Publishers, 1968.
13. Rouiller, C., and Muller, A. (Eds.): *The Kidney. Morphology, Biochemistry, Physiology.* New York, Academic Press, 1971.
14. Schreiner, G. E., and Maher, J. F.: *Uremia: Biochemistry, Pathogenesis and Treatment.* Springfield, Ill., Charles C Thomas, 1961.
15. Strauss, M. B., and Welt, L. G. (Eds.): *Diseases of the Kidney.* Second edition. Boston, Little, Brown and Co., 1971.
16. Wesson, L. G.: *Physiology of the Human Kidney.* New York, Grune & Stratton, 1969.

CHAPTER 3

Fluids and Electrolytes

Body Fluids

WATER

Water is the most abundant component of the human body, constituting approximately 40–70 per cent of the body weight. Body water and therefore body weight, remain fairly constant from day to day in normal adults despite marked fluctuation in water intake. If several extra liters of water is consumed it will be eliminated by the kidneys within three hours by diuresis. In males, characteristically, water accounts for 60 per cent of body weight, while in females it accounts for only 50 per cent. The difference is attributed to difference in adipose tissue. Leanness is associated with high body water content and obesity with low. Women normally have more subcutaneous adipose tissue than men and thus a lower body water content. Infants have the highest proportion of water in relation to body weight. Body water provides a stable environment for optimal cellular activity. Any variations in volume or in solute concentrations, outside certain limits, result in cellular dysfunction.

DISTRIBUTION OF BODY WATER

The total body water is divided into two basic compartments; the intracellular compartment, inside the cells, and the extracellular com-

<table>
<tr><td colspan="3">TOTAL BODY WATER
70% OF TOTAL WEIGHT</td></tr>
<tr><td rowspan="2">INTRACELLULAR FLUID</td><td colspan="2">EXTRACELLULAR</td></tr>
<tr><td>INTERSTITIAL FLUID</td><td>PLASMA</td></tr>
<tr><td>50% BODY WEIGHT</td><td colspan="2">20% BODY WEIGHT</td></tr>
</table>

***Figure* 9.** The distribution of body water. (From Pendras, J. P., and Stinson, G. W. (Eds.): *The Hemodialysis Manual.* Seattle, Wash., Edmark Corp., 1970.)

partment, outside the cells. Fluid in the extracellular compartment is further divided into plasma and interstitial fluid. Plasma circulates rapidly in the blood vessels while interstitial fluid seeps more slowly between the cells. Figure 9 depicts the distribution of body water by weight.

FUNCTION OF BODY FLUIDS

Body fluids have two main functions; they provide a stable environment for cellular metabolic activity and a transport medium for bringing nourishment to the cells and taking waste products away from the cells. Ingested substances are absorbed from the gut, pass into the blood stream, then diffuse through the interstitial fluids and into the cell. Waste products of cellular metabolism diffuse in the opposite direction. Protein wastes, such as urea and creatinine, diffuse from the cells through the interstitial fluid and into the blood, where they are filtered by the kidney and excreted in the urine.

ELECTROLYTE COMPOSITION OF BODY FLUIDS

Body fluids are composed of water and electrolytes. Electrolytes are substances that, when dissolved in water, separate into charged particles (ions) capable of conducting electricity. The most important electrolytes physiologically are listed in Table 1. The electrolyte composition of body fluids is expressed in milliequivalents per liter (mEq/L).* When concentrations of ions in body fluids are expressed

*In this context "equivalent," or "equivalent weight," is the atomic or formula weight of an element or ion divided by its valence. It is also called the "combining weight," for elements or ions entering into combination do so in quantities proportional to their equivalent weights. A "normal" solution contains 1 gram equivalent (equivalent weight expressed in grams) of solute per liter. A milliequivalent is the number of grams of solute contained in 1 ml of a normal solution.

TABLE 1. Most Important Electrolytes

Cations		Anions	
Sodium	Na^+	Chloride	Cl^-
Potassium	K^+	Bicarbonate	HCO_3^-
Calcium	Ca^{++}	Phosphate	PO_4^-
Magnesium	Mg^{++}	Sulfate	SO_4^-
		Protein	

in that manner, the sum of the concentrations of positive ions (cations) equals the sum of the concentrations of negative ions (anions). This balance is essential for normal body functioning.

The difference between extracellular and intracellular fluids lies, not in their function, but in the electrolytes they contain. Figure 10 illustrates this difference in electrolyte composition. Note that the extracellular fluid contains large amounts of sodium, chloride, and bicarbonate, and small quantities of potassium, phosphates, and magnesium. In contrast, the intracellular fluid contains large quantities of potassium, magnesium, and phosphates, and little sodium and chloride. These differences between intracellular and extracellular fluid composition are important to the life of the cell. Substances are transported through the cell membrane by two major processes, diffusion and active transport.

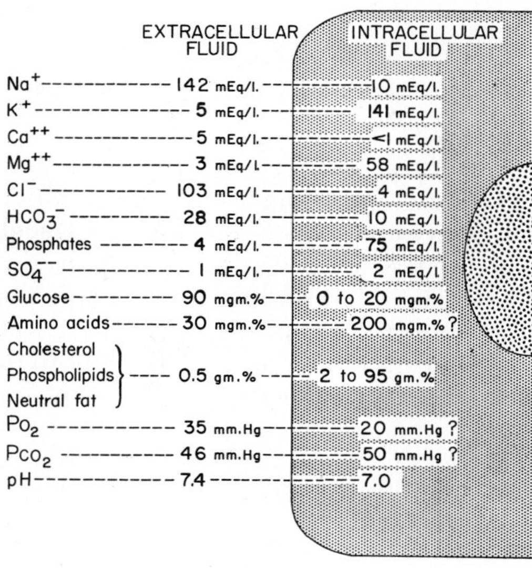

Figure 10. Chemical composition of extracellular and intracellular fluids. (From Guyton, A. C.: *Textbook of Medical Physiology.* Fourth edition. Philadelphia, W. B. Saunders Co., 1971.)

Diffusion of Water and Electrolytes

Diffusion is the continual movement of molecules, ions, or other particles in liquids or in gases. The diffusion of substances through the cell membrane or the permeability of the membrane is dependent on the solubility of the substances in the lipid portion of the cell membrane, the membrane pore size, and the electrical charge of the substance. For example, the pore size of the membrane will cause it to be selectively permeable to various molecules. Small molecules, such as urea and water, pass easily through the pore while larger protein molecules do not. In addition, three factors determine the net rate of diffusion of a substance across the cell membrane. They are the concentration gradient, the electrical gradient, and the pressure gradient. The concentration gradient causes molecules to diffuse from an area of greater to an area of lesser concentration of molecules. The electrical gradient causes charged particles (ions) to move toward the opposite electrical pole, i.e., a negatively charged ion moves toward the positively charged side of the membrane and vice versa. The pressure gradient causes movement of molecules from an area of high pressure across the membrane to an area of low pressure.

Water diffuses constantly through the cell wall in both directions. Normally the intracellular water volume remains constant. Under certain circumstances, however, a concentration gradient for water can occur, causing water to diffuse across the cell membrane from the area of lesser solute (particle) concentration to an area of greater solute concentration. This process of diffusion of water across a semipermeable membrane in the presence of a concentration gradient is called osmosis.

Active Transport of Electrolytes

Some substances, such as sodium and potassium, obviously do not diffuse according to the concentration gradient since they are not found in equal concentrations in intracellular and extracellular fluid. The process of active transport keeps the intracellular potassium and the extracellular sodium levels high. The basic mechanism of active transport involves energy and an enzyme to carry substances against the concentration gradient. In addition to sodium and potassium ions, the ions of iron, hydrogen, chloride, iodide, and urate, as well as sugars and amino acids, are actively transported through the cell membrane. Active transport of sodium is so essential to the maintenance of normal body function that the process is designated as the sodium pump.

Shifts in Body Fluids

Osmotic equilibrium

Osmosis of water molecules across a semipermeable membrane can be halted by applying pressure across the membrane in the opposite direction to the osmosis. The exact amount of pressure necessary to halt the osmosis is known as osmotic pressure. Osmotic pressure can be created by adding undiffusible or poorly diffusible solutes, such as glucose, to the solution on one side of a semipermeable membrane until an equilibrium is reached. Osmotic pressure is sometimes used to rid the body of excess fluid.

Isotonicity, hypotonicity, and hypertonicity

A solution that has the same concentration as normal body fluid is said to be isotonic. A saline solution of 0.9 per cent is isotonic. A normal cell placed in this solution will be in osmotic equilibrium with it. A hypotonic solution is one whose concentration is far less than that of the normal cell. When a cell is placed in a hypotonic solution, water moves by osmosis from the solution into the cell until equilibrium is reached. As a result the cell swells and the intracellular fluid is diluted. A hypertonic solution is one whose concentration is greater than that of the normal cell. When a cell is placed in a hypertonic solution water moves out of the cell by osmosis, causing the cell to shrink. Figure 11 shows the cell's reaction to the various solutions.

Clinical situations

When a large amount of water is added to extracellular fluid either through ingestion or infusion, the extracellular fluid becomes hypotonic. The water then moves by osmosis to the intracellular compartment until an equilibrium is reached. The whole process occurs in minutes. Ultimately, excess water is excreted in the urine or lost through the skin, lungs, or gastrointestinal tract. Water then leaves the intracellular compartment by osmosis, causing relative dehydration of the cells.

Hypertonic solutions of glucose, mannitol, or sucrose are used therapeutically to decrease intracellular fluid volume rapidly in patients with cerebral edema or congestive heart failure.

Isotonic intravenous solutions administered to patients to supplement or replace oral intake do not cause fluid shifts unless the pa-

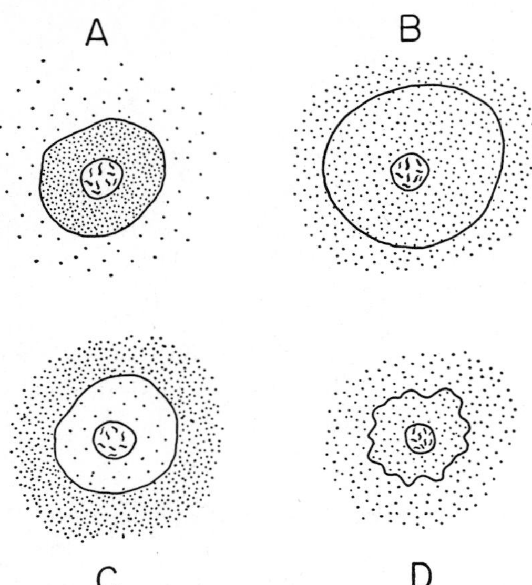

Figure 11. Establishment of osmotic equilibrium when cells are placed in a hypotonic or hypertonic solution. A. A cell is placed in a solution that has an osmolality far less than that of the intracellular fluid. As a result, osmosis of water begins immediately from the extracellular fluid to the intracellular fluid, causing the cell to swell and diluting the intracellular fluid, while concentrating the extracellular fluid. When the fluid inside the cell becomes diluted sufficiently to equal the concentration of the fluid on the outside, further osmosis then ceases. This condition is shown in B. In C, a cell is placed in a solution having a much higher concentration outside the cell than inside. This time, water passes by osmosis to the exterior, diluting the extracellular fluid while concentrating the intracellular fluid. In this process the cell shrinks until the two concentrations become equal, as shown in D. (From Guyton, A. C.: *Textbook of Medical Physiology.* Fourth edition. Philadelphia, W. B. Saunders Co., 1971.)

tient's kidneys are not functioning, in which case circulatory overload and water intoxication may occur.

Regulation of Body Fluids

The normal daily intake of fluid, including water ingested orally and water synthesized from the metabolism of foods, is about 2400 ml. Normal body water losses also equal 2400 ml/day. Of this total output 1400 ml is in urine, 100 ml is in sweat, 200 ml is in feces, and the remaining 700 ml is in insensible water loss, i.e., water lost through the skin and lungs. The factors affecting the regulation of extracellular fluids include antidiuretic hormone, aldosterone, thirst, increased arterial pressure, and nervous reflexes. The mechanisms of fluid volume regulation by antidiuretic hormone and aldosterone are discussed in Chapter 2.

Extracellular dehydration and circulatory failure stimulate the thirst center located in the hypothalamus, and the individual seeks fluids to relieve his thirst. Increased arterial pressure regulates extracellular fluid volume in the following manner: When the extracellular fluid volume becomes too great, the blood volume increases, which in turn increases the venous return and cardiac output. The rise in cardiac output increases arterial pressure, which causes the kidney to excrete the excess fluid.

Many nervous system reflexes play a role in regulating body fluids. The baroreceptor reflex responds to low arterial pressure, causing arterial constriction in the kidney and thus retention of extracellular fluid and gradual increase in arterial pressure. The ischemic response of the central nervous system can decrease the urinary output to almost zero. More important, however, are the stretch receptors or volume receptors in the walls of the left atrium, which, when stimulated by increased fluid volume, cause increased excretion of urine. The effect is only temporary, however, since the stretch receptors adapt in a few days.

Abnormalities in Extracellular Fluid Volume

VOLUME DEFICIT

Decreased extracellular volume represents a deficit of both water and electrolytes in the same concentration as they exist in extracellular fluid. It is not the same as dehydration, which means loss of water alone. Extracellular fluid volume deficit is caused by one or more of the following: decreased water intake, vomiting, diarrhea, fever, burns, intestinal obstruction, and bowel fistulas. In severe losses circulatory collapse ensues. In renal disease volume deficits occur in patients with (1) chronic renal failure when salt replacements are not given during salt wasting phases, (2) acute tubular necrosis during the diuretic phase, (3) postoperative nephropathy, (4) adrenal insufficiency, (5) osmotic diuresis, and (6) with diuretic therapy.

Clinical symptoms include dry skin and mucous membranes, loss of skin turgor, oliguria or anuria due to decreased renal perfusion, lassitude, and acute weight loss. Postural hypotension and a rapid resting pulse may also occur. Laboratory tests show a higher than normal hemoglobin level and packed cell count due to the decreased plasma volume. Treatment consists of restoring adequate blood volume and blood pressure by infusing blood plasma or isotonic saline. Once shock has been corrected, electrolyte derangements can be corrected by administering proper IV solutions.

Volume excess

Excess extracellular fluid volume is caused by an increase in both water and electrolytes in the same concentration as they exist in extracellular fluid. This is not the same as overhydration, which represents an increase in water only. Extracellular fluid volume excess is commonly seen in chronic renal disease. It is also caused by congestive heart failure, excessive infusion of isotonic saline solution, and hyperaldosteronism.

Clinical symptoms include edema, particularly periocular and dependent edema, acute weight gain, and moist rales in the lungs. Laboratory tests show abnormally low hemoglobin level, red blood cell count, and packed cell volume due to increased plasma volume. Treatment consists of decreasing the fluid overload by administering diuretic drugs or, in the case of renal failure, by drastically decreasing fluid intake and, if necessary, by dialysis.

Abnormalities in Extracellular Electrolytes

It must be kept in mind that changes in the concentration of serum electrolytes may be due either to a change in the quantity of the electrolyte or in the quantity of water in the extracellular fluid. For example, a sodium deficit can be the result of either a decreased sodium intake or increased loss of sodium or it can be the result of an increased intake or decreased loss of water.

Sodium

Regulation. Sodium is the main cation found in extracellular fluid. It represents about 90 per cent of the total cations. Therefore, it is the single most important ion that needs to be regulated. The normal level of serum sodium is 136–145 mEq/L. Sodium is filtered through the glomerulus and actively reabsorbed by the tubules of the nephron. In the preceding chapter it was explained that aldosterone, a hormone excreted by the adrenal cortex, regulates the precise amount of sodium reabsorbed.

Sodium deficit. Hyponatremia can be caused by excessive fluid loss through sweating or gastrointestinal suction followed by drinking plain (non-saline) water, by repeated tap water enemas, by potent diuretics, or by administration of electrolyte-free IV solutions. In chronic renal disease sodium deficit may result from fluid retention after ingestion of large quantities of water to promote urea excretion. The patient in acute renal failure with oliguria may display dilutional hyponatremia if fluids are not limited. Clinical symptoms include abdominal cramps, apprehension, irritability, confusion, oliguria, or anuria. In severe cases peripheral edema, hypotension, and convulsions may occur owing to the osmotic shift of hypotonic extracellular fluid to the intracellular compartment. Laboratory tests show low levels of plasma chloride, usually below 98 mEq/L, and plasma sodium, below 137 mEq/L, and a urine specific gravity of less than 1.010. Treatment of hyponatremia is usually accomplished by simply limiting intake of plain water until the sodium level is normal. Only in severe cases is a hypertonic (5 per cent) solution of sodium chloride administered.

Sodium excess. Hypernatremia occurs in patients whose water intake is decreased, such as the unconscious patient or the elderly patient who does not drink an adequate amount of liquids. It also occurs following excessive water loss due to watery diarrhea or excessive loss of water through the lungs. The most common cause of hypernatremia is a fluid intake inadequate to replace urinary and insensible losses. In renal disease, sodium excess may occur during the diuretic phase of acute renal failure or, in chronic renal failure, when the patient fails to follow his low-sodium diet.

Clinically the patient has flushed skin, a dry tongue and mucous membranes, and oliguria or anuria. He typically has an elevated temperature and complains of thirst. Laboratory findings include a serum sodium level above 147 mEq/L, chloride above 106 mEq/L, and a urine specific gravity over 1.030. Treatment consists simply of administering enough water to restore the serum sodium to normal.

Chloride

The concentration of chloride parallels that of sodium and therefore is influenced by the same factors. Chloride imbalances occur concurrently with sodium imbalances and thus each plays a role indistinguishable from the other's in producing the signs, symptoms, and laboratory results seen in hypernatremia and hyponatremia.

Potassium

Regulation. Potassium is one of the most important of all the body electrolytes. Although it is present in both the intracellular and extracellular compartments, it is the chief cation of intracellular fluid. Maintenance of a normal potassium level is essential to the life of the cells. There is no simple laboratory test to measure intracellular potassium; therefore the serum potassium level is measured and evaluated as a reflection of total body potassium. The normal serum potassium value is 3.5–5.0 mEq/L. Potassium ion concentration is regulated in two ways: by an aldosterone feedback mechanism and by direct secretion of potassium into the tubules when the serum potassium level is high. Both these mechanisms are discussed in Chapter 2.

Potassium deficit. Hypokalemia results from many different medical problems but it is most frequently seen in patients who are vomiting, have diarrhea, colitis, intestinal fistulas, or diabetic acidosis, and those who are receiving potent diuretics, adrenal steroid therapy, or potassium-free IV fluids. In renal disease acute tubular acidosis and the diuretic phase of acute tubular necrosis may cause hypokalemia.

The most observable effects of hypokalemia are those that affect the muscular function of the body. Clinically the patient complains of malaise and exhibits symptoms of skeletal, cardiac, and respiratory muscular weakness including generalized weakness, faint heart sounds, weak pulse, and shallow respirations. Gastrointestinal symptoms include vomiting and paralytic ileus. Laboratory tests show serum potassium less than 3.5 mEq/L, and a low serum chloride level.

Abnormalities in the EKG commonly occur in hypokalemia. Characteristically it shows depression of the ST segment, depression of the T wave, and appearance and elevation of the U wave (Fig. 12). Hypokalemia does not usually cause serious cardiac excitation; however, in digitalized patients it may precipitate dangerous arrhythmias. Potassium also plays an important role in acid-base regulation, and it is believed that loss of potassium is a factor in metabolic alkalosis. This is discussed later in this chapter. Treatment usually consists of

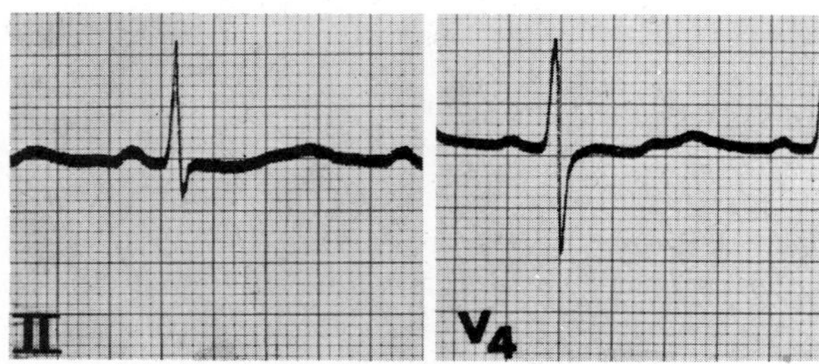

Figure 12. Typical electrocardiographic abnormalities induced by hypokalemia. (Serum potassium concentration 2.8 mEq. per liter.) Note the sagging ST segment, depression of the T wave, and elevation of the U wave. (From Beeson, P. B., and McDermott, W.: *Cecil-Loeb Textbook of Medicine.* Thirteenth edition. Philadelphia, W. B. Saunders Co., 1971.)

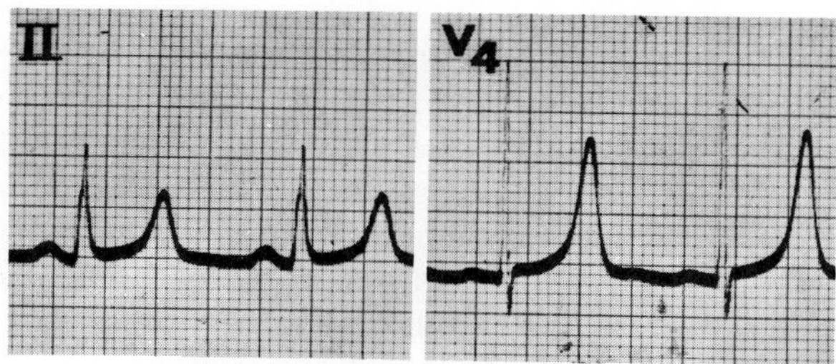

Figure 13. Typical electrocardiographic abnormalities induced by a moderate degree of hyperkalemia. (Serum potassium concentration 6.5 mEq. per liter.) Note the typical "tent-shaped" T waves. (From Beeson, P. B., and McDermott, W. (Eds.): *Cecil-Loeb Textbook of Medicine.* Thirteenth edition. Philadelphia, W. B. Saunders Co., 1971.)

oral administration of potassium salts. When IV replacement is required, potassium is administered at a rate not exceeding 20 mEq/hr since absorption into intracellular spaces is slow and high serum concentrations may be lethal.

Potassium excess. Hyperkalemia is most frequently seen in patients with advanced kidney disease. It is also seen with anuria or oliguria resulting from acute renal failure or adrenal insufficiency. Massive crushing injuries, severe burns, and large intravenous doses of potassium may also lead to hyperkalemia. Clinically the patient with a mild serum potassium increase, approximately 6 mEq/L, is irritable and nauseated and complains of abdominal cramps and diarrhea. Serum levels above 7 mEq/L are associated with anuria, weakness, flaccid paralysis, dyspnea, and cardiac arrhythmias followed by cardiac standstill if the level continues to rise to 9 or 10 mEq/L. Laboratory tests show a serum potassium concentration above 5.6 mEq/L and in most cases decreased renal function. The EKG reveals a peaked T wave, a depressed ST segment, decreased amplitude of P waves, and later atrial asystole (Fig. 13). Intraventricular block with a widening QRS complex may lead to ventricular standstill. Serum potassium levels may be high even though total body potassium levels are normal. Clinical signs and symptoms as well as laboratory findings are reviewed before the mode of treatment is decided.

The treatment of severe potassium intoxication is directed toward promoting rapid transfer of potassium into cells in order to reduce potassium in the serum. Two methods are frequently employed: the infusion of glucose and insulin, which induces a cellular deposition of glycogen and a shift of potassium into intracellular spaces, or the administration of hypertonic sodium bicarbonate to the acidotic patient, which causes a shift of potassium into the cell. These, however, are temporary treatments since they do not remove potassium from the body. Longer-term therapy is aimed at promoting gastrointestinal losses of potassium. A frequently employed treatment combines oral Kayexalate, a cation exchange resin, which binds protein, with sorbitol, which promotes diarrhea. If the patient is unable to take medications by mouth, Kayexalate can be given as a retention enema. Hemodialysis provides an efficient method of reducing potassium in several hours; however, it is used only in severe cases or in patients with chronic renal failure who are being maintained by dialysis.

Calcium

Regulation. Calcium is essential for teeth and bones and is also important in muscle metabolism and cardiac function. Calcium ions are located in both intracellular and extracellular spaces and a normal serum level is 4.5–5.5 mEq/L or 9–11 mg/100 ml. Parathyroid hormone is the body's chief regulator of the calcium ion. Although calcium is poorly absorbed from the gastrointestinal tract, parathyroid hormone has a direct effect on the gastrointestinal mucosa to increase the rate of calcium absorption. In addition, a feedback mechanism operates whereby a decrease in serum calcium stimulates increased production of parathyroid hormone, which in turn causes increased calcium absorption from the gut. Most of the daily intake of calcium is excreted in the feces, but a fraction is excreted in the urine. One of the factors that help to regulate this excretion is parathyroid hormone. When calcium ion concentration is low, parathyroid hormone is excreted and increases the rate of calcium reabsorption from the renal tubules.

Calcium deficit. Hypocalcemia results from excessive loss of calcium, as in certain types of diarrhea and subcutaneous infections. Calcium deficit also occurs following correction of acidosis because calcium ionizes readily in acidic conditions and, as acidosis is corrected, reduced ionization creates a deficit. Administration of a large amount of citrated blood can also cause hypocalcemia because citrate binds serum calcium, thus reducing its ionic concentration. Severe acute hypocalcemia triggers spontaneous depolarization of nerve tissue which leads to cardiac arrhythmias, decreased strength of contraction, and respiratory failure due to tetany. In uremia, urinary output of calcium is reduced but fecal excretion is increased, causing hypocalcemia. The low level of serum calcium triggers the release of parathyroid hormone, which in turn releases calcium from the bone to help supply the internal needs. When too much calcium is removed from bone, the bone becomes weakened and painful. This condition is known as azotemic osteodystrophy.

Clinically hypocalcemic patients have tingling of the finger tips, tetany, abdominal cramps, and convulsions. Only rarely are pathological fractures and deformities seen. The most serious effect of hypocalcemia clinically is respiratory arrest in tetany. Laboratory tests reveal serum calcium levels below 4.5 mEq/L. The Sulkowitch test for urine calcium reveals no precipitation. X-rays of long bones show areas of decalcification. Treatment varies with the cause, which is eliminated whenever possible. In the case of renal osteodystrophy, the bone disease rarely is severe enough to warrant treatment.

Calcium excess. Hypercalcemia occurs with hyperparathyroidism, parathyroid tumor, excessive administration of vitamin D, and multiple myeloma. In renal disease secondary hyperparathyroidism and retention of calcium result in hypercalcemia. Clinically patients exhibit hypotonicity of the muscles, pathological fractures, kidney stones, flank and bone pain, and bone cavitation.

Laboratory tests reveal serum calcium levels above 5.8 mEq/L, and the Sulkowitch urine test for calcium shows heavy precipitation. X-rays of long bones show bony decalcification. Treatment usually involves surgery for removal of a portion of the parathyroid gland.

Acid-Base Balance

The term "acid-base balance" refers to the regulation of hydrogen ion concentration in the body fluids. Changes in the hydrogen ion concentration may have serious effects on cellular metabolism. The actual hydrogen ion concentration, which is normally maintained in body fluids at about 4×10^{-8} Eq/L, is awkward to express. Therefore, a logarithmic notation has come into use together with the symbol pH to express the concentration. The formula for determining hydrogen ion concentration is:

$$\text{pH} = \log \frac{1}{\text{H}^+ \text{ conc}} = -\log \text{H}^+ \text{ conc}$$

A low pH indicates a high hydrogen ion concentration, which is acidosis. A high pH indicates a low hydrogen ion concentration, which is alkalosis. (A pH of 7.0 is neutral.) Normally, the pH of extracellular fluid is 7.35–7.45. When the pH of the blood rises above 7.8 or falls below 7.0 death is imminent unless the imbalance is corrected immediately.

Regulating mechanism

The control of the pH of the body is shared by three systems: acid-base buffers, the lungs, and the kidneys.

Acid-Base Buffers

Acid-base buffer systems are made up of chemical compounds that react with either acids or bases to prevent marked changes in the pH. The three major buffer systems of body fluids are the bicarbonate buffer, the phosphate buffer, and the protein buffer. All three operate in a nearly identical manner. Since the carbonic acid–bicarbonate system is the most important, it is described here in detail.

As food is oxidized both carbon dioxide (carbonic acid) and non-volatile acids, such as sulfuric acid, are added to the body fluids. Immediately bicarbonate compounds react with strong acids, reducing them to weaker acids that can be eliminated by the kidneys and lungs. The relationship between the pH and the bicarbonate and carbonic acid concentrations is expressed in the Henderson-Hasselbalch equation:

$$pH = 6.1 + \log \frac{HCO_3^-}{H_2CO_3}$$

From this equation it is evident that an increase in bicarbonate will cause an increase in pH, while an increase in carbonic acid will result in a decrease in pH. With a normal pH the ratio of bicarbonate to carbonic acid is 20 to 1.

The Lungs

Carbonic acid is simply dissolved carbon dioxide, which is normally excreted through the lungs. In addition to respiratory excretion of carbon dioxide there is also renal excretion of free hydrogen; both processes assist in maintaining the acid-base balance. This is visualized in the equation:

$$\overset{\text{Lungs}}{H_2O + CO_2 \uparrow} \rightleftarrows H_2CO_3 \rightleftarrows \underset{\text{Kidneys}}{H^+ \downarrow} + HCO_3^-$$

Note that the reaction occurs in both directions.

Since carbon dioxide excretion depends on alveolar ventilation, changes in the respiratory rate or functioning or both have a direct effect on acid-base balance. For example, an increase in carbon dioxide in the blood due to decreased ventilation results in retention of carbon dioxide and respiratory acidosis. On the other hand, an increase in ventilation due to increased respiration eliminates large amounts of carbon dioxide and results in respiratory alkalosis.

Not only do the lungs affect hydrogen ion concentration, but the hydrogen ion concentration has a direct effect on ventilation. It operates as a feedback mechanism, i.e., a decrease in pH causes an increase in respirations, which in turn eliminates carbon dioxide (carbonic acid) and increases the pH. Conversely, if there is a decrease in hydrogen ion concentration, respirations become depressed, carbon dioxide is retained, and the pH falls. The respiratory defense, however, is never strong enough to reverse metabolic acidosis and alkalosis. The foregoing formula makes it apparent that a reduction in bicarbonate (metabolic acidosis) results in an increased hydrogen ion concentration and, conversely, that an increase in bicarbonate concentration (metabolic alkalosis) results in a decreased hydrogen ion concentration.

The Kidneys

The kidneys regulate hydrogen ion concentration principally by increasing or decreasing the bicarbonate ion concentration in the body fluid. In order to accomplish this a series of reactions occurs in the nephron resulting in secretion of hydrogen ions and ammonia, reabsorption of sodium ions, and excretion of bicarbonate ions in the urine. These events occur in the following manner: Carbon dioxide, with the aid of the enzyme carbonic anhydrase, combines with water to form carbonic acid. Carbonic acid dissociates into bicarbonate ion and hydrogen ion. The hydrogen ion is then secreted through the cell membrane into the renal tubule.

The equation is the same as that used to describe respiratory control:

$$H_2O + CO_2 \uparrow \rightarrow H_2CO_3 \rightarrow H^+ \downarrow + HCO_3^-$$

Hydrogen ions can be secreted in the tubules until the concentration is 900 times that of the extracellular fluid, or at a pH of 4.5. The greater the carbon dioxide concentration, the greater will be the rate of hydrogen ion secretion. Each time a hydrogen ion is excreted into the tubules a bicarbonate ion is formed, i.e., $H_2CO_3 \rightarrow H^+ + HCO_3^-$. Sodium ions are reabsorbed in exchange for the secreted hydrogen ions. At the same time hydrogen ions in the tubules combine with bicarbonate ions to form carbonic acid (H_2CO_3). Carbonic acid dissociates into carbon dioxide and water. The water is excreted, thus ridding the body of hydrogen ions, and the carbon dioxide is reabsorbed to form a bicarbonate ion. The bicarbonate ion combines with a sodium ion that has been reabsorbed and diffuses into the peritubular fluid (Fig. 14). If plenty of hydrogen ions are available, the bicarbonate ions are almost completely reabsorbed.

In metabolic alkalosis an increase in the ratio of bicarbonate to carbonic acid causes a rise in pH. The kidney attempts to compensate

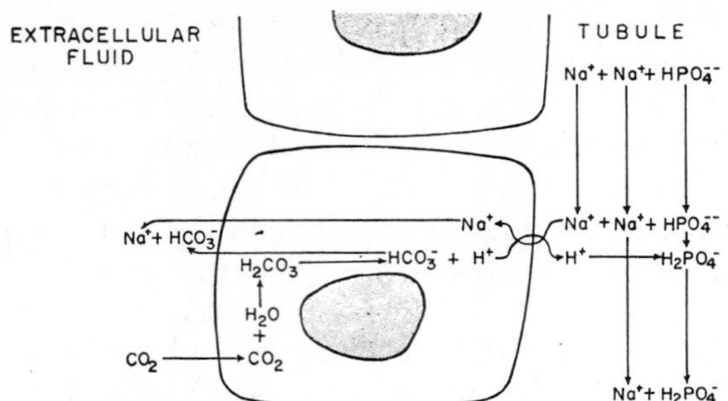

Figure 14. Chemical reactions for (1) hydrogen ion secretion, (2) sodium ion absorption in exchange for a hydrogen ion, and (3) combination of hydrogen ions with bicarbonate ions in the tubules. (From Guyton, A. C.: *Basic Human Physiology. Normal Function and Mechanisms of Disease.* Philadelphia, W. B. Saunders Co., 1971.)

by excreting excess bicarbonate ions into the urine in the form of sodium bicarbonate. The net effect is a decrease in the extracellular bicarbonate and a decrease in the pH with a correction of alkalosis.

In acidosis the kidneys compensate by increasing the rate of hydrogen ion secretion, thus removing hydrogen from the extracellular fluid and correcting acidosis. Increased secretion of hydrogen ions takes place without decreasing the urine pH below 4.5 because hydrogen ions combine with ammonia secreted by tubular epithelium to form ammonium chloride, a neutral salt. Renal compensation in acid-base imbalance takes place slowly but continues to function until the pH is in normal range.

Clinical abnormalities

Respiratory Acidosis

As just described, anything that causes a decrease in pulmonary ventilation increases the concentration of dissolved carbon dioxide in the extracellular fluid, which consequently increases the concentration of carbonic acid and hydrogen ions. This lowers the pH and results in acidosis. Since the cause of the imbalance is poor ventilation, it is called respiratory acidosis. Causes of respiratory acidosis include:

Morphine poisoning
Splinting
Atelectasis
Pneumonia

Asthma
Emphysema
Metabolic alkalosis

In metabolic alkalosis the lungs attempt to compensate for the bicarbonate overload by retaining carbon dioxide, thus increasing the acid content of extracellular fluid. This results in respiratory acidosis.

Clinically the patient in respiratory acidosis is confused, disoriented, exhibits respiratory embarrassment, weakness, and coma. Laboratory findings reveal arterial carbon dioxide tension (pCO_2) above 40 mm Hg, a plasma bicarbonate level above 29 mEq/L in adults and above 25 mEq/L in children, and a plasma pH below 7.35. Urine pH is below 6.0. The elevated bicarbonate level indicates renal compensation that conserves base to balance the acid-base ratio. Treatment consists of improving the basic disease condition and may include use of blow-bottles, ventilators, and breathing exercises to decrease the pCO_2.

Respiratory Alkalosis

Respiratory alkalosis results whenever there is excessive pulmonary ventilation with resultant blowing off of carbon dioxide, as in hyperventilation due to fever, anxiety, hysteria, or lack of oxygen, and in metabolic acidosis. In metabolic acidosis the lungs attempt to compensate for the carbonic acid overload by blowing off large amounts of carbon dioxide, thus reducing the acid content of the body.

Clinical symptoms include tetany, convulsions, and unconsciousness. Laboratory findings reveal an arterial pCO_2 below 40 mm Hg, a high plasma pH above 7.45, a urine pH above 7.0, and a low plasma bicarbonate level, below 25 mEq/L in adults and below 20 mEq/L in children. Low bicarbonate levels indicate compensatory renal excretion of base to restore normal balance. Treatment consists of assisting the patient to control his breathing if hyperventilation is voluntary. Rebreathing techniques using a paper bag, or adding dead space if a respirator is being used, will aid in increasing the pCO_2.

Metabolic Acidosis

Metabolic acidosis results whenever acid is added to or produced by the body, alkali is lost from the body, or impaired renal function prevents excretion of the normal acid load.

Excess acid. In *diabetes mellitus* normal glucose metabolism is inhibited and stored fats are split to form acetoacetic acid, which is used for energy. There is an imbalance between the production and utilization of the acid, resulting in its accumulation in the extracellular fluid and thus in acidosis. *Cellular anoxia*, such as may occur in dehydration, hemorrhage, or excessive exercise, results in anaerobic metabolism with production of excess lactic acid, thus acidosis. *Salicylate intoxication* also leads to accumulation of strong acid and reduction in the base reserve, thus acidosis.

Renal dysfunction. The diseased kidney is unable to excrete the normal acid waste load, which results in accumulation of nonvolatile acids, thus acidosis. In acute renal failure acidosis can be mild and transient, but in chronic renal failure metabolic acidosis is nearly always present and may be severe. In most patients with chronic renal failure the problem is an inability to excrete normal quantities of ammonium. In addition there may be a dysfunction in bicarbonate reabsorption that complicates the problem.

Clinically metabolic acidosis is difficult to diagnose since the only observable symptom may be hyperventilation and even this is not evident in patients with long-standing acidosis. However, dyspnea is often observed in patients with renal acidosis. Lethargy and coma and signs of central nervous system depression are seen in severe acidosis but may also be caused by uremia or diabetic acidosis. Fatigue, anorexia, and nausea are common in renal acidosis. In most cases both the history and the laboratory results are necessary for an accurate diagnosis.

Laboratory tests indicate a low plasma pH below 7.35 and a normal to low level of plasma bicarbonate (CO_2). Less than 25 mEq/L of CO_2 in adults and less than 20 mEq/L in children indicates respiratory compensation, which begins immediately in response to metabolic acidosis in patients with normal pulmonary function. If kidney function is assumed to be normal, the pH of the urine below 6.0 indicates renal compensation. In renal acidosis the pH of the urine may be normal or slightly more acidic but achieves maximal acidity of 4.5 only when the plasma bicarbonate level is very low.

Treatment consists of correction of the underlying cause or disease. In diabetic acidosis, restoring proper glucose metabolism by administering insulin will eliminate excess acetoacetic acid and correct acidosis, whereas in renal acidosis, a restricted protein diet will decrease the acid waste load. In addition sodium bicarbonate tablets are administered to restore or maintain the base level. Correction of metabolic acidosis may precipitate tetany or convulsions due to a decrease in serum calcium that accompanies an increase in pH. Only ionized calcium in the blood is effective and the degree of ionization is directly proportionate to the acidity of the blood. That is to say that a specific amount of calcium in an acid solution affords more free calcium than the same amount of calcium in an alkaline solution. Therefore an acidotic patient may have a calcium deficit but not manifest any symptoms until his acidosis is corrected. At this time less calcium will be free to ionize, and the symptoms of hypocalcemia, i.e., hyperirritability, tetany, and convulsions, will appear. This situation occurs frequently in patients with chronic renal failure who are being treated with hemodialysis. These patients are characteristically in chronic acidosis, which, if corrected too rapidly by dialysis, causes leg cramps and muscle irritability.

Metabolic Alkalosis

Metabolic alkalosis occurs whenever there is an abnormal loss of acid or an excessive retention of alkali. In either situation there is an increase in bicarbonate concentration and a decrease in hydrogen ion concentration with a resultant increase in pH. In metabolic acidosis the imbalance is corrected by buffers, while in metabolic alkalosis hydrogen ions diffuse from the cells into the extracellular fluid to correct the imbalance.

The lungs attempt to compensate by retaining carbon dioxide, which results in respiratory acidosis. However, this is inefficient. The kidneys, on the other hand, are responsible for correcting alkalosis by excreting excess bicarbonate.

Metabolic alkalosis is caused by excessive losses of acid from the gastrointestinal tract, administration of excessive sodium bicarbonate, diuretic therapy, and hyperadrenocorticism. There is also a close association between potassium deficiency and metabolic alkalosis. Potassium deficiency and hypokalemia occur in nearly all cases of metabolic alkalosis. The reason is that the potassium level has an effect on the hydrogen secretory mechanism of the kidney; potassium and hydrogen compete for exchange with sodium in the renal tubules, and a deficiency in potassium is believed to enhance the rate of hydrogen secretion and bicarbonate reabsorption. Chloride depletion and hypochloremia also lead to metabolic alkalosis since they cause a high rate of hydrogen and potassium secretion. In diuretic therapy and in hyperadrenocorticism large amounts of potassium are lost; this loss is believed to cause retention of bicarbonate as just described.

Clinically there are no specific symptoms of metabolic alkalosis. It is suspected when there is a history of vomiting, gastric drainage, or diuretic or adrenal steroid therapy.

Laboratory studies show a high serum pH above 7.45, a high urine pH above 7.0, a serum bicarbonate value above 29 mEq/L in adults and above 25 mEq/L in children. The serum potassium level is usually below 4 mEq/L and the chloride may be below 98 mEq/L.

Treatment consists of correction of dehydration and the various electrolyte deficits. Sodium chloride and water may be administered by mouth or vein, depending on the patient's condition. Potassium replacements are given by mouth or vein but must be given in conjunction with chloride replacement; neither the rate of hydrogen secretion nor that of potassium secretion can be reduced until the chloride deficit is corrected. In cases of alkalosis caused by sodium bicarbonate injection, diuretic therapy, and hyperadrenocorticism due to drugs, the treatment consists of reducing the dosage of the drug to a level that allows normal acid-base balance. In addition, with diuretic therapy it may be necessary to administer acidifying salts by mouth, and with steroid therapy supplemental potassium chloride may be required to prevent alkalosis. In patients with primary adrenal disease, surgical removal of the adrenal tissue is the treatment.

References

1. Beeson, P. B., and McDermott, W. (Eds.): *Cecil-Loeb Textbook of Medicine.* Thirteenth edition. Philadelphia, W. B. Saunders Co., 1971.
2. Black, D. A. K.: *Essentials of Fluid Balance.* Fourth edition. Philadelphia, F. A. Davis Co., 1968.
3. Black, D. A. K.: *Renal Disease.* Second edition. Philadelphia, F. A. Davis Co., 1967.
4. Bland, J. H. (Ed.): *Clinical Metabolism of Body Water and Electrolytes.* Philadelphia, W. B. Saunders Co., 1963.
5. Brest, A. N., and Moyer, J. H. (Eds.): *Renal Failure.* Philadelphia, J. B. Lippincott Co., 1968.
6. Burgess, R. E.: Fluids and electrolytes. *Amer. J. Nurs., 65:*90, 1965.
7. Christensen, H. N.: *Body Fluids and the Acid-Base Balance.* Philadelphia, W. B. Saunders Co., 1964.
8. Davenport, H. W.: *The ABC of Acid-Base Chemistry.* Fifth edition. Chicago, University of Chicago Press, 1969.
9. De Wardener, H. E.: *The Kidney.* Third edition. Baltimore, Williams & Wilkins Co., 1968.
10. Forster, R. P.: Kidney, water and electrolytes. *Ann. Rev. Physiol., 27:*183, 1965.
11. Goldberger, E.: *A Primer of Water, Electrolyte and Acid-Base Syndromes.* Fourth edition. Philadelphia, Lea & Febiger, 1970.
12. Guyton, A. C.: *Basic Human Physiology. Normal Functions and Mechanisms of Disease.* Philadelphia, W. B. Saunders Co., 1971.
13. Guyton, A. C.: *Textbook of Medical Physiology.* Fourth edition. Philadelphia, W. B. Saunders Co., 1971.
14. Hepinstall, R. H.: *Pathology of the Kidney.* Boston, Little, Brown and Co., 1966.
15. Maxwell, M. H., and Kleeman, C. R.: *Clinical Disorders of Fluid and Electrolyte Metabolism.* New York, McGraw-Hill Book Co., 1962.
16. Merrill, J. P.: *The Treatment of Renal Failure.* Second edition, New York, Grune & Stratton, 1965.
17. Pendras, J. E., and Stinson, G. W. (Eds.): *The Hemodialysis Manual.* Seattle, Wash., Edmark Corp., 1970.
18. Pitts, R.: *Physiology of the Kidney and Body Fluids.* Second edition. Chicago, Year Book Medical Publishers, 1968.
19. Ray, C. T.: Water and electrolyte balance. In Sodeman, W. A., and Sodeman, W. A., Jr. (Eds.): *Pathologic Physiology.* Fourth edition. Philadelphia, W. B. Saunders Co., 1967.
20. Reed, G. M., and Sheppard, V. F.: *Regulation of Fluid and Electrolyte Balance.* A programed instruction in physiology for nurses. Philadelphia, W. B. Saunders Co., 1971.

21. Relman, A. S.: Renal acidosis and renal excretion of acid in health and disease. *Advances Intern. Med., 12:*295, 1964.
22. Relman, A. S.: The acidosis of renal disease. *Amer. J. Med., 44:*706, 1968.
23. Robinson, J. R.: *Fundamentals of Acid-Base Regulation.* Third edition. Philadelphia, F. A. Davis Co., 1967.
24. Schwartz, W. B.: Disorders of fluids, electrolyte and acid-balance. In Beeson, P. B., and McDermott, W. (Eds.): *Cecil-Loeb Textbook of Medicine.* Thirteenth edition. Philadelphia, W. B. Saunders Co., 1971.
25. Strauss, M. B., and Welt, L. G. (Eds.): *Diseases of the Kidney.* Second edition. Boston, Little, Brown and Co., 1971.
26. Welt, L. G.: Water balance in health and disease. In Duncan, G. G. (Ed.): *Diseases of Metabolism.* Fifth edition. Philadelphia, W. B. Saunders Co., 1964.
27. Welt, L. G.: Acidosis and alkalosis. In Wintrobe, M. M., Thorn, G. W., Adams, R. D., Bennett, I. L., Braunwald, E., Isselbacker, K. J., and Petersdorf, R. G. (Eds.): *Harrison's Principles of Internal Medicine.* Sixth edition. New York, McGraw-Hill Book Co., 1970.
28. Welt, L. G.: Disorders of fluids and electrolytes. In Wintrobe, M. M., Thorn, G. W., Adams, R. D., Bennett, I. L., Braunwald, E., Isselbacker, K. J., and Petersdorf, R. G. (Eds.): *Harrison's Principles of Internal Medicine.* Sixth edition. New York, McGraw-Hill Book Co., 1970.
29. Wesson, L. G., Jr.: *Physiology of the Human Kidney.* New York, Grune & Stratton, 1969.
30. Wintrobe, M. M., Thorn, G. W., Adams, R. D., Bennett, I. L., Braunwald, E., Isselbacker, K. J., and Petersdorf, R. G. (Eds.): *Harrison's Principles of Internal Medicine.* Sixth edition. New York, McGraw-Hill Book Co., 1970.
31. Wolf, A. V., and Crowder, N. A.: *Introduction to Body Fluid Metabolism.* Baltimore, Williams & Wilkins Co., 1964.

CHAPTER 4

Pathology of Renal Failure

Acute renal failure and chronic renal failure are the forms that renal failure takes and are caused by many different diseases and conditions. Uremia is the syndrome resulting from renal failure and is characterized by derangements of body biochemistry and organ systems.

Acute Renal Failure

Acute renal failure is loss of renal function that develops rapidly—over a period of days or a few weeks. Acute renal failure can be reversible or irreversible. With reversible renal failure, kidney function returns and the patient can be expected to recover. With irreversible renal failure, kidney function does not return and the patient develops uremia.

The patient with reversible acute renal failure typically passes through two phases—the oliguric phase and the diuretic phase. During the oliguric phase, the urine output is less than 400 ml/day. (Even a patient with a bilateral nephrectomy will put out 30–40 ml of "urine" per day. This "urine" is not true urine, but is fluid secreted by the bladder, sometimes called "bladder sweat.") The oliguric phase usually lasts 10–14 days, although it may last as long as three weeks.

The second phase is the diuretic phase, during which the urine output increases. In some patients the urine output increases dramatically and can reach 3 L or more per day; in other patients the diuresis is less brisk. In the early part of the diuretic phase, metabolic wastes may continue to accumulate in the blood. In the later part of the diuretic phase, these wastes are cleared. Gradually, urine output, blood chemistry, and renal function return to normal.

The causes of acute renal failure are numerous. A partial list of these causes is as follows:

- Shock
  - Hypovolemic—due to
    - hemorrhage
    - burns
  - Septic
  - Cardiogenic
  - Neurogenic
- Complications of pregnancy
  - Placenta previa
  - Septic abortion
  - Postpartum hemorrhage
  - Eclampsia
- Hemolysis, as with mismatched blood transfusions
- Crush injuries with resulting myoglobinuria
- Surgery of the heart, aorta, and great vessels, during which renal circulation is interrupted
- Renal vasoconstriction due to drugs such as levarterenol (Levophed)
- Nephrotoxins (see Appendix C, for list of nephrotoxins)
- Infection
  - Pyelonephritis
- Disease due to abnormal antigen-antibody reactions
  - Glomerulonephritis
  - Systemic lupus erythematosus
  - Polyarteritis nodosa
- Obstruction of the urinary tract
  - Renal calculi
  - Fibrosis
  - Carcinoma

The prognosis for patients with acute renal failure is variable. It is excellent for those with little underlying disease, low urea production rate, and oliguria for less than 10 days, but worsens for older patients and those with severe underlying disease, high rates of urea production, and prolonged oliguria. In one series, the survival rate of patients with acute tubular necrosis who were treated by dialysis was 44 per cent.[9]

Chronic Renal Failure

Chronic renal failure is loss of renal function that occurs gradually—over months or years. The loss can be partial or complete.

Chronic renal failure can be divided into three stages—diminished renal reserve, renal insufficiency, and uremia—although there is no sharp division between the stages. During the stage of diminished renal reserve, renal function is impaired but metabolic wastes do not accumulate in the blood and the blood urea nitrogen (BUN) remains normal. During this stage, the patient may develop symptoms of polyuria, nocturia, and polydipsia. During the stage of renal insufficiency, metabolic wastes begin to accumulate in the blood, and there is a slight increase in BUN. Sudden changes in food and fluid intake, altered metabolic activity, and stress are tolerated poorly, and the consequent chemical abnormalities are corrected slowly. During the stage of uremia, the kidney loses the ability to maintain homeostasis; the urine output is usually scanty, electrolyte balance is severely disturbed, and nitrogenous wastes accumulate in the blood in high concentrations.

The relationship between renal function (glomerular filtration rate) and plasma urea is shown in Figure 15. The graph indicates that the plasma concentration of urea does not rise above normal until the GFR falls to about 50 per cent of normal. The graph also indicates that when the GFR is low, small fluctuations in GFR (such as those caused by infection) produce large changes in plasma urea.

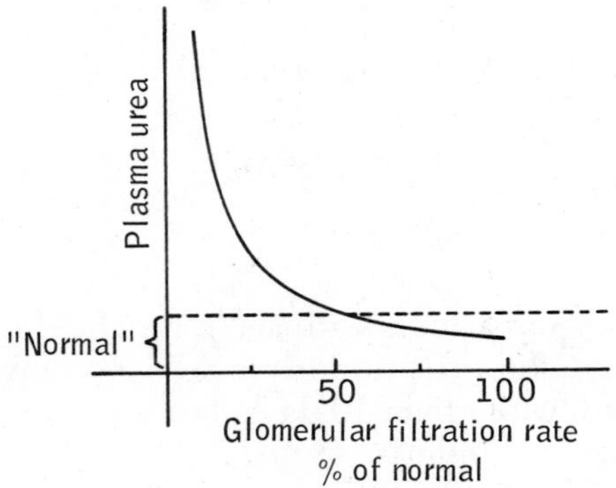

Figure 15. The relation between the plasma level of urea and the rate of glomerular filtration. (From Wintrobe, M. M., et al. (Eds.): *Harrison's Principles of Internal Medicine.* New York, McGraw-Hill Book Company, 1970. Used with permission.)

The causes of chronic renal failure are numerous. A partial list of these causes is as follows:

- Disease due to abnormal antigen-antibody reactions
  - Glomerulonephritis
  - Disseminated lupus erythematosus
  - Polyarteritis nodosa
  - Subacute bacterial endocarditis
- Infection
  - Pyelonephritis
  - Tuberculosis
- Obstruction of the urinary tract
  - Bilateral calculi
  - Prostatic obstruction
  - Urethral valves
- Congenital lesions
  - Polycystic disease
- Hypertension
  - Malignant
  - Nonmalignant
- Other diseases
  - Amyloidosis
  - Gout
  - Diabetes mellitus
  - Hypercalcemia
  - Chronic intermittent hemoglobinuria
    - sickle cell
    - nocturnal
  - Renal vein thrombosis
  - Radiation nephritis

The prognosis for patients with chronic renal failure is variable. If the failure is due to correctable, extrarenal factors such as obstruction, the outlook is more favorable. If the failure is due to loss of kidney parenchyma produced by progressive and irreversible lesions such as chronic pyelonephritis, the prognosis is less favorable. The patient can often survive in relative comfort until about 90 per cent of his glomerular filtration is lost. Death occurs when 97–99 per cent of glomerular filtration is lost. Overall prognosis is difficult to state because of individual response to illness and because of new modes of therapy—dialysis and transplantation.

The Uremic Syndrome

Uremia is the syndrome resulting from acute or chronic renal failure. It is caused by an imbalance between the patient's metabolism and the ability of his kidneys to excrete waste and regulate fluid and electrolyte concentration. Harrison and Mason present a poignant description of uremia. "The uremic death of the most highly integrated organism is strictly comparable to the dissolution of the most simple organism in an aging bacterial culture—both are destroyed in an environment poisoned by the product of their own metabolism."[7]

Numerous body alterations occur in the uremic syndrome. These involve the effects of uremia on body biochemistry, the effects of uremia on organ systems, and other effects of uremia.

Uremia and Body Biochemistry

Many changes in body biochemistry occur in uremia. Substances derived from protein metabolism, electrolytes, pH and acid-base balance, and water metabolism are altered. To facilitate understanding of these alterations, a list of pertinent laboratory values for blood and urine is given in Appendix A.

Substances Derived from Protein Metabolism

Urea. Urea is the principal end product of nitrogen metabolism; it is formed in the liver and excreted by the kidneys. Blood urea levels rise in uremia. Urea is commonly measured as blood urea nitrogen (BUN); the BUN can increase to 200 mg/100 ml or more. An elevated BUN value is not, however, diagnostic of renal failure. Blood urea nitrogen concentration is influenced by many factors including renal function, dietary intake of protein, rate of protein catabolism, rate of urea synthesis, and state of hydration. Therefore, serial BUN measurements, with influencing factors controlled, are of more value in assessing renal function than is one isolated measurement.

Creatinine. Creatinine is the end product of the metabolism of creatine, an amino acid present in body tissues and especially concentrated in muscle. Serum creatinine levels rise in uremia. Creatinine is related to muscle mass and is fairly constant for an individual; it is less affected by external factors than is BUN. Serum creatinine is, therefore, a more reliable index of renal function than is BUN.

Uric acid. Uric acid is the end product of the metabolism of purine, a nitrogenous base. Serum uric acid is increased in uremia. Uric acid is also increased in gout; it may precipitate out in body tissues and cause arthritis and other symptoms. Usually, however, it does not precipitate out when the patient is in the uremic state.

Cations (Positively Charged Ions)

Potassium. Serum potassium is usually increased in uremia. Several mechanisms can cause this hyperkalemia. The dietary intake of potassium may be high. Protein breakdown, which releases intracellular potassium into the blood, can occur at a high rate, as in the postpartum patient, the patient with an elevated temperature, and the patient whose carbohydrate intake is inadequate. Acidosis can cause hyperkalemia. In acidosis, hydrogen ions are buffered by intracellular proteins; this results in release of intracellular potassium. Lack of sodium can cause hyperkalemia. Potassium is secreted by the distal tubules of the nephron; a high sodium level enhances this tubular secretion, while a low sodium level reduces it. When the urine output is low, as usually occurs in severe renal failure, hyperkalemia is due primarily to failure of the distal tubules to secrete potassium. When the urine output is less than 500–1000 ml/24 hr, the distal tubules do not secrete adequate potassium, and the potassium concentration in the blood rises to dangerous levels.

Decreased serum potassium sometimes occurs in renal failure. The main causes of hypokalemia are diuresis, as in the diuretic phase of acute renal failure or diuresis induced by drugs, and gastrointestinal loss from vomiting or diarrhea accompanying uremia.

Sodium. Serum sodium can be increased or decreased in renal failure. Increased serum sodium usually occurs when urine output is reduced. In severe renal failure, the glomerular filtration rate is reduced, urine output is reduced, and the kidney is unable to excrete sufficient sodium. Hypernatremia can be further increased by high dietary intake of salt. Sodium retention usually leads to water retention.

Decreased serum sodium sometimes occurs in renal failure. It occurs when the urine output is great, as in the diuretic phase of acute renal failure. It occurs in specific diseases such as "salt-wasting" nephritis. And it occurs because of excessive sweating and gastrointestinal loss—vomiting and diarrhea.

Calcium. Serum calcium is reduced in uremia. A low calcium level occurs in association with an elevated phosphate level. There is a general relationship between calcium and phosphorus such that an increase in one results in a decrease in the other; an increase in phosphate results in a decrease in calcium. Hypocalcemia is also associated with decreased absorption of calcium from the gut, which occurs in uremia.

Hypocalcemia can cause parathyroid dysfunction. The lack of calcium stimulates the parathyroid gland, causing hyperplasia and secretion of additional parathyroid hormone; the serum calcium then returns to normal. This is called secondary hyperparathyroidism and is different from primary hyperparathyroidism in which the serum calcium is increased. Occasionally, however, the parathyroid gland further enlarges and secretes parathyroid hormone beyond physiological levels; the level of serum calcium then becomes elevated. This is called tertiary hyperparathyroidism.

These disturbances of calcium, phosphorus, and parathyroid gland metabolism can result in bone disease which is discussed later in this chapter.

Lack of calcium, less than 2.0 mEq/L, causes tetany under usual circumstances, but this low-calcium tetany rarely occurs in uremia. The patient in uremia is acidotic, and the acidosis protects him from tetany.

Magnesium. An increase in serum magnesium occurs in acute and chronic renal failure when the urine output is low. It is caused by decreased excretion of magnesium by the kidneys. Hypermagnesemia can be increased by the use of drugs containing magnesium, such as milk of magnesia, magnesium sulfate, Gelusil, Gelusil M, Maalox, and Mylanta.

A decrease in serum magnesium occasionally occurs in uremia because of diuresis or loss from vomiting or diarrhea.

Anions (Negatively Charged Ions)

Chloride. Serum chloride is usually decreased in uremia; the chloride level may fall as low as 36 mEq/L. Chloride is decreased because of loss from vomiting and diarrhea and because of replacement by sulfate and phosphate. Sulfate and phosphate increase in uremia and replace chloride as the negatively charged ion in various body solutions.

Phosphate. Serum phosphate increases in uremia and is usually associated with decreased serum calcium; this can adversely affect parathyroid function and bone metabolism (see under Skeletal System later in this chapter).

Sulfate. Serum sulfate is increased in uremia.

Acidosis

The concept of metabolic acidosis as a derangement of acid-base balance is discussed in Chapter 3. The metabolic acidosis that occurs in uremia is basically due to two mechanisms: decreased ability of the kidney to excrete acid and decreased ability of the kidney to reabsorb bicarbonate. The kidney normally excretes acid (H^+) as ammonium

(NH_4^+); in renal failure it fails to excrete sufficient ammonium. Bicarbonate neutralizes body acids. The kidney normally reabsorbs bicarbonate from the glomerular filtrate, but in uremia it fails to reabsorb adequate amounts. The severity of acidosis in uremia varies, but a pH below 6.8 is usually incompatible with life.

Water Metabolism

The patient in uremia has decreased ability to concentrate urine. This decreased ability to concentrate occurs early in renal failure and is responsible for some of the early signs of renal impairment: nocturia, polyuria, and polydipsia. As renal failure advances, there is a tendency for the urine to remain at about the same osmolality as plasma (1.010); this is called isosthenuria.

The patient in uremia also has decreased ability to dilute urine—he cannot excrete a large water load rapidly and adequately.

UREMIA AND ORGAN SYSTEMS

Cardiovascular and Pulmonary Systems

The cardiovascular and pulmonary complications of uremia are hypertension, congestive heart failure, edema, and pericarditis.

Hypertension. Hypertension occurs in more than 80 per cent of patients with chronic renal failure. The relationship between the kidneys and blood pressure is imperfectly understood. Some facts, however, seem clear: hypertension can lead to kidney disease, and kidney disease can lead to hypertension. Hypertension can cause both benign and malignant nephrosclerosis and can precipitate congestive heart failure. The kidney can cause elevated blood pressure, called renal hypertension. Renal hypertension accounts for less than 10 per cent of the cases of hypertension.

The mechanisms causing renal hypertension are not well understood. Decreased blood flow to the kidney, caused, for example, by renal artery stenosis, stimulates the juxtaglomerular apparatus to release renin. Renin causes the elaboration of angiotensinogen, angiotensin I, and angiotensin II. Angiotensin II stimulates the adrenal medulla to release aldosterone. Aldosterone causes sodium retention, which results in water retention and a rise in blood pressure, which should physiologically increase renal blood flow. This mechanism may be operative in some cases of renal hypertension. However, some investigators have failed to find elevated levels of renin and angiotensin in patients with chronic hypertension.

The kidney contains several vasodepressor substances, and decreased secretion of these may contribute to the hypertension, called "renoprival" hypertension.

Congestive heart failure. Congestive heart failure is a common complication in uremia and is usually associated with hypertension, anemia, and sodium and water retention. Symptoms of congestive heart failure include pulmonary edema, systemic edema, and decreased systemic perfusion, including decreased renal perfusion.

Pulmonary edema. The pulmonary edema that can occur in uremia is usually secondary to hypertension and congestive heart failure. The accumulation of fluid is more marked in the central portions of the lung, while the peripheral portions are relatively clear. This produces a "butterfly" picture on x-ray.

Systemic edema. The systemic edema that may occur in uremia can be caused by sodium and water retention, congestive heart failure, or a decrease in serum protein. Hypoproteinemia, which occurs in the nephrotic syndrome and other conditions, results in a decrease in serum oncotic pressure and movement of fluid out of the capillaries and into body tissue.

Pericarditis. Pericarditis, or inflammation of the pericardium, occurs in uremia. It develops more often when chemical control is poor; it rarely develops if the BUN is less than 100 mg/100 ml. The cause of uremic pericarditis is not clear. Sometimes the pericarditis causes pericardial effusion and cardiac tamponade—a condition in which the pericardial sac fills with fluid and exerts pressure on the heart, thus making cardiac contraction ineffective.

Hematopoietic System

Almost all patients with chronic renal failure are anemic. The anemia is characterized by red blood cells that are normal in shape and hemoglobin content but are present in inadequate numbers—normocytic, normochromic anemia. The anemia is roughly proportional to the severity of the uremia; i.e., the anemia is more pronounced in patients with more advanced uremia. Even in the most severe cases, however, the hemoglobin level rarely goes below 6 gm/100 ml.

The anemia seems to be caused by lack of erythropoiesis, or production of red blood cells by the bone marrow. The kidney normally secretes erythropoietin, a substance that physiologically stimulates the marrow to produce red blood cells; in renal failure it seems to secrete inadequate erythropoietin. The function of the bone marrow may also be depressed because of the azotemic milieu.

Another factor contributing to the anemia is the shortened life span of red blood cells. The red cell life span is reduced to about half of normal when the BUN exceeds 200 mg/100 ml.

Patients in uremia have a tendency to bleed. Easy bruising and oozing from the mucous membranes are common. This bleeding is probably related to quantitative and qualitative platelet defects. The platelet count is often low, and prothrombin consumption and thromboplastin generation are sometimes abnormal.

Gastrointestinal System

Gastrointestinal bleeding is common in uremia, can occur anywhere along the GI tract, and can be diffuse or focal. Mouth ulcers and bloody diarrhea occur frequently and can be quite distressing to the patient. The bleeding may be caused by defective clotting mechanisms due to decreased numbers of and defects in platelets.

Anorexia, nausea, and vomiting may be so severe in uremia that the patient is unable to maintain adequate nutrition. These symptoms may be caused by ammonia intoxication, acidosis, and dehydration. Electrolyte imbalance can also be a cause; one of the early signs of serum sodium deficiency is anorexia.

The patient may have parotitis or stomatitis. These can be caused by decreased salivary flow, dehydration, mouth breathing, which occurs in acidosis, and *Candida albicans* infections. The patient may complain of a metallic taste in the mouth. In advanced uremia, the patient's breath has an odor similar to urine; this is due to the high concentration of nitrogenous wastes in the blood.

Skeletal System

Bone disease occurs in about half the adult patients with uremia and is even more common among children and adolescents. The bone disease, called renal osteodystrophy, is not usually severe enough to produce overt clinical symptoms; it is diagnosed, rather, by x-ray and examination of bone tissue at autopsy.

Three pathological processes have been identified in renal osteodystrophy: osteomalacia, osteitis fibrosa, and osteosclerosis.

Osteomalacia. Osteomalacia is a softening of the bones owing to failure of calcium salts to be deposited in newly formed osteoid tissue. In children osteomalacia can cause renal rickets, a condition characterized by deformities of the epiphyses of the long bones. The mechanism causing osteomalacia is not completely understood. It may be due to increased serum phosphorus and decreased serum calcium, vitamin D resistance, acidosis, or high blood concentrations of nitrogenous wastes.

Osteitis fibrosa. Osteitis fibrosa is reabsorption of calcium salts from the bone and replacement of these salts by fibrous tissue. The mechanism causing osteitis fibrosa is thought to be as follows: the hypocalcemia that usually accompanies renal failure causes stimulation of the parathyroid gland. The additional parathyroid hormone thus released causes calcium to be reabsorbed from the bones in order to raise the blood calcium level back to normal.

Osteosclerosis. Osteosclerosis is an abnormal hardening of the bone characterized by areas of increased bone density. The disease occurs only rarely, and its cause is not known.

Endocrine System

In the child with renal failure, the onset of puberty is often delayed by several years. In the adult male, libido and potency are often depressed. In the adult female, libido is often depressed and ovulation and menstruation are suppressed. However, pregnancy can occur, so contraception is advisable. In general, pregnancy can be safely undertaken if the woman's renal disease is static or slowly progressive, and her BUN and blood pressure are normal at the start of pregnancy. Pregnancy is hazardous and unlikely to produce a live child if the woman's BUN increases on a normal diet and hypertension is present in the first trimester.

Psychological and Neuromuscular Systems

The patient with uremia often manifests psychological changes. He is frequently lethargic, less mentally acute, and less able to concentrate. He may have periods of confusion that alternate with periods of lucidity. He may become depressed, and, in severe uremia, exhibit psychotic behavior with paranoid delusions and hallucinations. The severity of the psychological disturbances is usually proportional to the severity of the azotemia.

Grand mal seizures can occur, especially if the patient is hypertensive.

Involuntary muscular twitching often occurs in uremia. Involuntary movement of the legs, which is particularly pronounced at night, is called the "restless foot" syndrome.

Peripheral neuropathy develops in some patients. It usually affects the legs, and occasionally, the arms. Early symptoms of neuropathy are pain, numbness, burning, and slowing of nerve conduction velocity. The condition may progress to involve loss of reflex, motor weakness, muscle atrophy, and paralysis, but in most cases the neuropathy does not incapacitate the patient.

Skin

Uremia has several effects on the skin. Uremic dermatitis—dryness, scaliness, and pruritus—occurs frequently and can be severe. The etiology of the dermatitis is not completely understood. In some cases, it is due to disturbances of calcium, phosphorus, and parathyroid gland metabolism.

Patients with uremia have a characteristic coloration. The nailbeds and mucous membranes are pale, reflecting the anemia that is usually present. The skin has a sallow, yellow-brown cast due to a combination of anemia and melanin deposits. The uremic coloration is most evident on exposed areas such as the face and hands, for light tends to accentuate it. Bruises and petechiae are evident, owing to the bleeding tendency in uremia. In patients with advanced untreated uremia, urea crystalizes out of the sweat as "uremic frost," and appears as a white, powdery material clinging to the skin and hair of the face, chest, and abdomen.

OTHER EFFECTS OF UREMIA

Infection. The uremic patient is particularly susceptible to infection for reasons that are not understood. Infection is becoming a leading cause of death among uremic patients, now that dialysis is available for treating the renal failure itself. Infection is sometimes difficult to treat, because of altered antibiotic metabolism in uremia (see Appendix B). In addition to other deleterious effects, infection increases metabolism and protein breakdown, and thus increases the severity of the azotemia.

Hypothermia. Hypothermia occurs in many patients with renal failure and is related to the degree of uremia—patients with more severe uremia tend to have lower temperatures. Some have a usual rectal temperature of 95°F or lower.

Wound healing. Wound healing occurs more slowly in the uremic patient than in the normal patient. The reasons for this are not understood.

Major Diseases and Conditions Causing Renal Failure

Some of the major diseases and conditions that cause acute and chronic renal failure and that can result in the uremic syndrome are described briefly in this section. The reader who desires further information about specific renal diseases is referred to any standard nursing or medical textbook.

PYELONEPHRITIS

Pyelonephritis is an infection of the kidney and its pelvis. The organisms that most commonly cause the infection are the gram-negative enteric bacilli, which are present in the lower gastrointestinal tract and enter the urinary system via the urethra. Other organisms causing the disease include gram-positive cocci, enterococcus, staphylococcus, and yeasts. Beta-hemolytic streptococcus is seldom the causative organism. Pyelonephritis and other urinary tract infections occur somewhat more commonly in females than in males.

Symptoms of pyelonephritis include pain over the area of the kidneys, fever, chills, and gastrointestinal upset. The urine contains bacteria (bacteriuria) and often pus (pyuria). The overt symptoms of pyelonephritis disappear in a few days, with or without treatment, although the urine still evidences infection.

The treatment for pyelonephritis is antibiotic therapy. The prescribed antibiotic should be effective against the specific infecting organism and be administered for one to two weeks, even though symptoms of the disease have disappeared. The acute symptoms of pyelonephritis can usually be readily treated. The danger from this disease is the persistence of a relatively asymptomatic infection that gradually destroys the kidney. It is most important that the patient be given adequate antibiotic therapy and be examined at intervals for quiescent disease.

GLOMERULONEPHRITIS AND OTHER AUTOIMMUNE DISEASES

Glomerulonephritis. Acute glomerulonephritis is an immunological disorder of the glomeruli of the kidneys The patient forms antibodies against circulating antigens or against his own renal tissue. Antigen-antibody complexes are formed and lodge in the kidneys, causing renal damage.

Acute glomerulonephritis occurs most frequently following infections with group A beta-hemolytic streptococcus. The streptococcal infection can be of the upper respiratory tract, skin, or other tissues. Glomerulonephritis can occur with other acute infections and in other autoimmune diseases, such as systemic lupus erythematosus.

Symptoms of acute glomerulonephritis typically appear one to two weeks after the streptococcal infection. These symptoms include fatigue, anorexia, pain in the area of the kidneys, edema, congestive heart failure, hypertension, mild anemia, and oliguria. Changes in renal function characteristic of acute glomerulonephritis are high BUN level, high urinary specific gravity, and almost normal phenolsulfonphthalein excretion.

The treatment for acute glomerulonephritis is bed rest; dietary restriction of protein, sodium, potassium, and fluid; and penicillin to eradicate any residual streptococcal infection. Symptoms such as congestive heart failure, hypertension, and anemia are treated as described in Chapter 5.

The prognosis for patients with acute glomerulonephritis varies. The recovery rate among children and young adults is about 95–98 per cent. Approximately 50 per cent of adults hospitalized with acute glomerulonephritis die during the acute episode or develop chronic glomerulonephritis.

Chronic glomerulonephritis is similar to acute glomerulonephritis, but chronic in nature. Although some cases are the result of streptococcal infection, most are due to other causes—autoimmune diseases such as polyarteritis nodosa, quartan malaria, and other factors. No known treatment will definitely alter the course of the disease. Cytotoxic drugs such as azathioprine (Imuran) and corticosteroids have been tried, and, in some cases, appear to be beneficial.

Systemic lupus erythematosus. Systemic lupus erythematosus is an autoimmune disease affecting connective tissue. Many organs are involved, including the kidneys, spleen, and endocardium. The renal involvement in lupus varies from asymptomatic albuminuria to severe renal failure. The condition is treated with large doses of corticosteroids (60–80 mg prednisone/day) plus cytotoxic drugs—azathioprine (Imuran) or cyclophosphamide (Cytoxan). This treatment sometimes causes remission, but it is usually unsuccessful after severe proteinuria and azotemia appear.

Scleroderma. Scleroderma, an autoimmune disease characterized by sclerosis of the connective tissue of the skin and other organs, affects the kidneys in a majority of patients. Renal failure is the cause of death in about one third of patients with the disease. Symptoms vary from mild to severe uremia. There is no effective treatment for scleroderma.

Polyarteritis nodosa (hypersensitivity angiitis). Polyarteritis nodosa is characterized by inflammatory damage to the arteries, especially the small and medium-sized ones; this results in altered function of the involved organs. Most patients with the disease have renal involvement, which varies from mild to severe. Treatment with large doses of steroids is sometimes successful.

Goodpasture's syndrome. Goodpasture's syndrome is a form of acute glomerulonephritis accompanied by extensive capillary hemorrhage in the lungs. The disease seems to be caused by a circulating antibody against the capillary basement membranes of the kidneys and lungs, which are immunologically similar. Symptoms are hemoptysis, pulmonary hemorrhage, and acute glomerulonephritis with hematuria. The patient usually dies from either renal failure or pulmonary hemorrhage. Occasionally, patients have been successfully treated with corticosteroids.

THE NEPHROTIC SYNDROME

The nephrotic syndrome is a complex of symptoms caused by increased permeability of the glomerulus to plasma proteins. The disease occurs in both children and adults. Among children, most cases of the syndrome are due to unknown causes and are termed idiopathic; some cases occur following streptococcal infections. In adults, also, the majority of cases are idiopathic, but some are due to specific conditions such as systemic lupus erythematosus, amyloidosis, and toxic nephropathy, or follow streptococcal infections.

The patient with the nephrotic syndrome typically exhibits proteinuria, hypoalbuminemia, hyperlipemia, and generalized edema. The patient's urine is reduced in volume and contains large amounts of protein. In the active phase of the disease, the patient may excrete 5–10 gm protein/day (normal urinary loss is 0.01–0.15 gm/day). Most of the excreted protein is albumin. The blood level of albumin is low, usually about 2.5 gm/100 ml (normal blood level is 3.5–5.5 gm/100 ml). The total globulin level is normal, but the usual concentration of globulin fractions is altered. The blood level of all lipids is high; patients with the lowest albumin levels tend to have the highest lipid levels. The patient has edema that may vary from slight puffiness to incapacitating fluid retention. The blood pressure is usually normal. Renal function is normal or reduced, depending on the severity and type of underlying disease. The severity of these symptoms varies a great deal; some patients are debilitated, while others feel well enough to pursue their usual activities.

The nephrotic syndrome is treated with large doses of adrenal corticosteroids – 2 mg prednisone/kg/day for children and 60–100 mg prednisone/day for adults. Antibiotics are given for any accompanying infection.

Most children with the nephrotic syndrome recover. Some adults, however, go on to develop renal insufficiency.

HYPERTENSIVE NEPHROPATHY

Some damage to renal vessels occurs in most patients with hypertensive disease. Most of these patients do not develop clinical renal disease, but about 10 per cent of those who eventually die from hypertension do develop significant renal insufficiency.

With hypertensive nephropathy, the renal arteries, especially the small and medium-sized ones, show thickening of the intima and consequent reduction of lumen size, hyalinization, and other changes.

Symptoms of nephrosclerosis range from mild to severe proteinuria, hematuria, and renal failure. The disease sometimes enters a malignant phase characterized by extremely high blood pressure, retinal hemorrhage, papilledema, heart failure, hypertensive encephalopathy, and progressive renal failure. This malignant hypertension is usually fatal.

There is no specific treatment for nephrosclerosis itself. The accompanying hypertension is treated with medication and diet as described in Chapter 5.

Toxemias of pregnancy

Toxemias of pregnancy are diseases that occur during or shortly after gestation. Pre-eclampsia is characterized by hypertension, edema, and proteinuria. Eclampsia, a more severe form of the disease, is characterized by the additional symptoms of convulsions and coma.

The disease is usually self-limited and disappears following delivery. However, it can lead to permanent renal damage. The likelihood of permanent damage increases with the duration of the toxemia.

To prevent the development of severe toxemia, pregnant women should be checked regularly for edema, excessive weight gain, hypertension, and proteinuria. If these symptoms develop, the patient is treated promptly with antihypertensive agents, diuretics, sodium restriction, sedation, and bed rest.

Obstructive nephropathy

Obstructive nephropathy is renal damage caused by obstruction anywhere along the genitourinary tract, from the kidney to the urethra. Obstruction is a very significant cause of renal failure. Lytton and Epstein state that two thirds of the deaths from uremia are wholly or partially due to obstruction.[8]

Obstruction is due to several causes: inadequacy of the lumen, as in bladder neck contracture and ureteral stricture; intrinsic obstruction, as with calculi and clots; extrinsic compression, as with aberrant vessels and prostatic hyperplasia; anomalies of form such as angulation and diverticula; disease of the wall such as ureteritis and periureteral fibrosis; and functional inadequacy such as atonic or neurogenic bladder.

Obstruction can cause renal damage, and, unfortunately, the obstruction is often not detected until extensive destruction has occurred. Symptoms of obstruction include: infection, especially recurrent infection; abnormal urinary sediment; micturition abnormalities such as slow onset of voiding, frequency, and infrequency; and gastrointestinal complaints such as nausea, vomiting, and failure to thrive. Regarding the significance of infection, Schreiner says, "Infection is the calling card of obstruction." Infection "... should be an invitation to investigate."[10]

Numerous diagnostic procedures can be used to determine whether obstruction is present: direct visualization of the genitourinary tract, various x-ray studies such as the intravenous pyelogram, and blood and urine studies.

Treatment of the patient with obstruction includes immediate relief of the obstruction, treatment of any associated infection, and the attainment of adequate fluid and electrolyte balance, by dialysis if necessary. The obstruction is then definitively corrected, if possible. Various surgical techniques for such correction are described in standard nursing or medical textbooks of urology. Patients with irreversible renal damage are treated for chronic renal failure.

TUMORS

Malignant and benign tumors occur at many points along the genitourinary tract. These tumors can cause urinary obstruction, and produce renal insufficiency. Benign tumors of the kidney are usually small and asymptomatic. The malignant tumors can cause death from primary invasion and metastases.

Nephroblastoma, or Wilms' tumor, is the most common malignant renal tumor of childhood. It is treated by a combination of surgery, chemotherapy, and radiation therapy. Carcinoma of the kidney is the most common malignant renal tumor in adults. It is treated by surgery and, in some cases, radiation therapy.

Carcinoma of the bladder occurs in two main forms – papillary and solid. It is usually treated by partial or total cystectomy, sometimes in combination with radiation therapy.

Benign prostatic hypertrophy is quite common. About 50 per cent of males over 50 develop the clinical symptoms of difficulty "starting the stream" and urinary retention. However, only about 10 per cent require surgery to relieve the obstruction.

Adenocarcinoma of the prostate accounts for about 10 per cent of deaths from cancer among males. It occurs commonly in about the fifth decade of life. Many cases (80–90 per cent) are asymptomatic and are diagnosed only by tissue examination at autopsy. When the disease is diagnosed during life, the treatment of choice for nonmetastatic tumors is radical prostatectomy. Unfortunately, only about 5 per cent of cases are diagnosed before metastases occur, because most of the tumors develop in the posterior lobe of the prostate and, therefore, do not cause early urinary symptoms.

Renal calculi

Renal calculi are kidney stones or nephroliths. They vary in size and in the severity of symptoms produced, some causing no symptoms, while others cause excruciating pain. Some stones cause obstruction and, if not removed, can cause renal failure.

Kidney stones are caused by several mechanisms, among them increased urinary excretion of calcium, as in hyperparathyroidism or when intake of milk, alkali, and vitamin D is excessive; increased urinary excretion of uric acid, as in gout; increased urinary excretion of cystine, arginine, ornithine, and lysine, called cystinuria; and renal infection with formation of stones containing blood and pus.

A typical attack of ureteral colic (misnamed renal colic) is caused by a stone in the ureter. It is characterized by excruciating pain radiating down the course of the ureter, sometimes to the tip of the urethra and midthigh. The patient may experience concomitant nausea, vomiting, sweating, syncope, and shock. The pain is intermittent and spastic during an attack. An attack may last for a few minutes or several hours.

Attempts are usually made to pass the stone without surgery. The patient is hydrated and given analgesics, and the urine is carefully examined. If the stone is not passed, it is removed by instrumentation or surgery. To prevent further stone formation, the patient is kept well hydrated, and the underlying metabolic defect is treated. The patient with calcium stones is treated with diet and medications to reduce hypercalcinuria and with parathyroidectomy if hyperparathyroidism is present. The patient with cystine or uric acid stones is treated with diet and medication to keep the urine alkaline.

Congenital and hereditary disorders

Polycystic disease. Polycystic disease is a hereditary condition in which the kidneys contain multiple cysts. These cysts occur in grapelike clusters and are filled with clear or bloody fluid. Normal renal tissue is interspersed between them. The disease occurs with greatest frequency during infancy and, in adulthood, during the fourth to sixth decades. The patient with polycystic disease often has palpable kidneys. He may complain of pain and aching in the kidney area. The disease often causes renal failure and the uremic syndrome. The infantile form is usually rapidly fatal, while the adult form usually progresses more slowly and is sometimes compatible with a normal life span.

Congenital anomalies. Numerous congenital anomalies of the kidneys, ureters, and bladder occur. Some of these, such as stricture at the ureterovesical junction, predispose to obstruction, hydronephrosis, and infection, and can lead to irreversible renal damage. A variety of surgical procedures is available to correct some of the symptom-producing anomalies. It is important that these anomalies be corrected before permanent kidney damage occurs.

Toxic Nephropathy

Toxic nephropathy is functional or structural damage to the kidney caused by chemical or biological agents. Toxic nephropathy accounts for a significant portion of cases of acute renal failure; in a study at Georgetown University Hospital, it accounted for 20 per cent of such cases.[11]

A classification and a partial list of nephrotoxins are shown in Appendix C. The most frequently encountered nephrotoxins in the Georgetown series were carbon tetrachloride, mercury, sulfonamide drugs, radiographic contrast media, analgesics (phenacetin), ethylene glycol, and antimicrobials.

The treatment of toxic nephropathy varies with the poison, but it follows some general principles. The patient is removed from the toxic environment, and any undissolved toxin is removed by gastric lavage and, in some cases, the induction of diarrhea. The renal failure is managed medically, with balancing of fluid and electrolytes, restriction of protein intake, and other measures described in Chapter 5. Peritoneal or hemodialysis is used as indicated to remove dialyzable poisons and to substitute for the malfunctioning kidneys. With specific types of toxins, specific therapeutic agents are used. For example, dimercaprol (BAL) is used in the treatment of mercury poisoning.

Other Diseases Affecting the Kidney

Diabetes mellitus. About 25 per cent of patients with diabetes mellitus develop vascular changes of the kidney, called diabetic nephropathy or Kimmelstiel-Wilson disease. Important histological changes characteristic of the disease are the presence of nodular hyaline masses at the periphery of the glomerular tufts and hyalinization of afferent and efferent arterioles.

The patient with diabetic nephropathy usually has had diabetes for several years. He then develops proteinuria, renal function declines, and BUN increases. He is prone to develop urinary tract infections, which can increase the severity of the disease. He develops retinopathy and visual impairment. He may develop congestive heart failure or suffer myocardial infarction or cerebrovascular accident due to generalized vascular disease.

The diabetes mellitus and diabetic nephropathy are treated symptomatically by medical measures. There is no evidence that strict control of blood sugar decreases the development of diabetic nephropathy.

The patient with diabetic nephropathy can die from renal failure, but more often death is caused by cardiac disease or cerebrovascular accident.

Amyloidosis. Amyloidosis is a condition in which amyloid, a protein, is deposited in various tissues including the kidney. Secondary amyloidosis, which is the more common form of the disease, occurs in association with chronic suppurative diseases such as tuberculosis, osteomyelitis, and Hodgkin's disease. Typically the kidneys, liver, and spleen, and occasionally the adrenal cortex are affected. Primary amyloidosis occurs less often and is not associated with other diseases; typically the heart, gastrointestinal tract, nerves, and joints are affected.

There is no specific treatment for amyloidosis. Eradication of the primary suppurative disease by antibiotic therapy or surgery sometimes reverses or stops amyloid deposition, but this is rare. The patient usually dies from the suppurative disease, from renal failure or heart disease due to amyloid deposits, or from infection.

Gout. Gout, a disease characterized by high serum levels of uric acid and reduced urinary excretion of the substance, may affect the kidneys as well as the joints and other tissues. Uric acid may collect in the kidney, form urate stones and interstitial deposits, and cause renal failure. The renal disease is treated by maintenance of high fluid intake, administration of uricosuric agents, administration of allopurinol (Zyloprim), which blocks uric acid formation, and maintenance of alkaline urine. It is especially important to maintain a high fluid intake when uricosuric agents are given, to avoid further precipitation of uric acid stones.

Sickle cell nephropathy. Patients with sickle cell anemia often develop renal damage due to multiple small hemorrhagic and ischemic infarcts. Some adult patients eventually develop renal insufficiency.

Multiple myeloma. Many patients with multiple myeloma have impaired renal function characterized by azotemia, anemia, and proteinuria. Hypertension, retinitis, and edema are usually absent. The proteinuria consists of albumin, certain globulins, and Bence Jones protein—a characteristic mixture of proteins found in the urine of patients with multiple myeloma. Patients with multiple myeloma have a marked tendency to form kidney stones, so care must be taken to avoid dehydration when preparing them for procedures such as an intravenous pyelogram.

Radiation nephritis. Renal damage occurs when large doses of radiation (for example, 2300 rads in five weeks) are administered for malignant disease of the abdomen. Following a latent period of about six months, symptoms of renal failure appear. The patient develops azotemia, slight proteinuria, hypertension, retinopathy, congestive heart failure, and anemia. The kidneys are fibrotic with atrophic tubules. The uremia is often progressive, but some patients begin to show improvement about six months after the onset of symptoms.

References

1. Beeson, P. B., and McDermott, W. (Eds.): *Cecil-Loeb Textbook of Medicine.* Twelfth and thirteenth editions. Philadelphia, W. B. Saunders Co., 1967 and 1971.
2. Black, D. A. K. (Ed.): *Renal Disease.* Second edition. Philadelphia, F. A. Davis Co., 1967.
3. Brest, A. N., and Moyer, J. H. (Eds.): *Renal Failure.* Philadelphia, J. B. Lippincott Co., 1968.
4. De Wardener, H. E.: *The Kidney. An Outline of Normal and Abnormal Structure and Function.* Third edition. Baltimore, Williams & Wilkins Co., 1968.
5. Douglas, A., and Kerr, D. N. S.: *A Short Textbook of Kidney Disease.* Philadelphia, J. B. Lippincott Co., 1968.
6. Hamburger, J., Richet, G., Crosnier, J., Funck-Brentano, J. L., Antoine, B., Ducrot, H., Mery, J. P., and De Montera, H.: *Nephrology.* Philadelphia, W. B. Saunders Co., 1968.
7. Harrison, T. H., and Mason, M. F.: The pathogenesis of the uremic syndrome. *Medicine, 16:*39, 1937.
8. Lytton, B., and Epstein, F. H.: Obstructive uropathy. In Wintrobe, M., Thorn, G., Adams, R., Bennett, I. L., Jr., Braunwald, E., Isselbacher, K. J., and Petersdorf, R. G. (Eds.): *Harrison's Principles of Internal Medicine.* Sixth edition. New York, McGraw-Hill Book Co., 1970.
9. Schreiner, G. E.: Acute renal failure. In Beeson, P. B., and McDermott, W. (Eds.): *Cecil-Loeb Textbook of Medicine.* Twelfth edition. Philadelphia, W. B. Saunders Co., 1967.
10. Schreiner, G. E.: Obstructive nephropathy. In Beeson, P. B., and McDermott, W. (Eds.): *Cecil-Loeb Textbook of Medicine.* Thirteenth edition. Philadelphia, W. B. Saunders Co., 1971.
11. Schreiner, G. E.: Toxic nephropathy. In Beeson, P. B., and McDermott, W. (Eds.): *Cecil-Loeb Textbook of Medicine.* Thirteenth edition. Philadelphia, W. B. Saunders Co., 1971.
12. Tests of Renal Function. *Nurs. Clin. N. Amer., 2:4:*800–803, 1967.
13. Wintrobe, M. M., Thorn, G. W., Adams, R. D., Bennett, I. L., Jr., Braunwald, E., Isselbacher, K. J., and Petersdorf, R. G. (Eds.): *Harrison's Principles of Internal Medicine.* Sixth edition. New York, McGraw-Hill Book Co., 1970.

CHAPTER 5

Conservative Treatment of Renal Failure

Conservative treatment, and the accompanying nursing care, of the patient in renal failure involves diet, medication, and symptomatic management of uremic manifestations. It excludes peritoneal dialysis, hemodialysis, and transplantation.

Conservative treatment is appropriate for patients with mild renal failure whose symptoms can be relieved or lessened by these measures. Patients suitable for conservative treatment include those with diminished renal reserve, renal insufficiency, and some with acute renal failure. Patients with severe chronic renal failure and many with acute renal failure require more aggressive treatment—dialysis and transplantation. Unfortunately, aggressive treatment cannot be offered to all these patients at present, because of insufficient facilities and funds. Many of them are, therefore, also treated by conservative measures, although these are inadequate for their needs.

Conservative treatment includes dietary treatment, treatment of infection, treatment of alterations in body biochemistry, treatment of alterations in organ systems, and teaching the patient to live within the limitations imposed by his disease.

Dietary Treatment

Dietary regulation is extremely important in renal failure. Because the kidney cannot adequately balance the concentrations of certain substances, the ingestion of these substances must be regulated.

In the usual diet for patients with renal failure, protein, potassium, sodium, and water are regulated.

Protein intake is usually restricted in patients with renal failure, because the products of protein metabolism are excreted at a decreased rate. Sufficient protein to meet the needs for maintenance and repair of body tissue is given. The minimum requirement for this is 10–20 gm/day for an adult. (The normal diet contains 1 gm protein/kg body weight/day, or 60–80 gm/day.) The protein content can be increased if the patient can tolerate it. Most of the dietary protein should be complete protein—milk, eggs, meat, fish, and poultry. These foods provide essential amino acids that the body cannot manufacture. Adequate calories are given to prevent breakdown of body protein for energy; this is about 2000 calories/day for an adult.

In certain types of renal conditions, such as the nephrotic syndrome, urinary loss of protein is great. Patients with these conditions are often given a high-protein diet.

Potassium is usually restricted in uremia, because of decreased renal excretion of this substance. Potassium is found in most plant and animal tissue, and it is, therefore, difficult to restrict to less than 1.5 gm/day. In the diuretic phase of acute renal failure and in other conditions characterized by polyuria, however, much potassium is lost in the urine, and in these circumstances the dietary intake of potassium must be increased.

Sodium is usually restricted in uremia, because of decreased renal excretion of the substance. It may be severely restricted when hypertension and congestive heart failure are also present. When polyuria is present, as in the diuretic phase of acute renal failure, increased dietary sodium is given to replace urinary sodium loss.

Water intake is balanced with water loss, as the ability of the kidneys to maintain this balance is impaired in renal failure. Water balance involves both *sensible loss*—water lost in urine, stool, emesis, and drainage—and *insensible loss*—water lost in respiration and perspiration. Water losses are replaced with water intake to maintain a state of balanced hydration. Sensible loss from urine, stool, emesis, and drainage is measurable and is replaced with equal amounts of fluid. Insensible loss is replaced, on the average, by 4.8 ml/kg/24 hr; for the average male, this would be 300–700 ml/day. The figures for replacement of sensible loss and insensible loss are added together to give the day's fluid allowance. Ten per cent is added to the basic figure for each degree centigrade elevation of the patient's temperature.

For example, a 70 kg male in acute renal failure excreted 200 ml urine in 24 hours; he had one 50 ml diarrheal stool; he had no emesis or drainage; he was afebrile. His fluid allowance for that day was approximately 600 ml—250 ml to replace sensible loss and 336 ml to replace insensible loss.

Fluid is restricted in most types of renal failure, because of decreased renal excretion of water. Particularly in acute renal failure, when the patient is oliguric, the water restriction may be quite severe, as in the foregoing example. In conditions characterized by polyuria, such as the diuretic phase of acute renal failure, fluid intake is greatly increased to replace urinary losses.

Dietary regulation varies with the severity of the uremia and with the type of treatment the patient is receiving. If the uremia is severe, the restriction of protein, sodium, potassium, and water will be severe. If the renal failure is less advanced, the diet will be more liberal. If the patient is receiving intermittent dialysis, the diet may be liberal even if his disease is severe.

The following are typical diets for given clinical conditions. A patient with severe uremia who is not receiving dialysis may be on a 20–40 gm protein diet. One such diet was developed by Giovanetti and Maggiore; it contains 22 gm protein, 600–900 mg sodium, 1400–2000 mg potassium, and 2000–3000 calories.[10] A patient with renal insufficiency or a patient receiving long-term dialysis may be on a 40–60 gm protein diet. The diet for patients in the chronic dialysis program at Downstate Medical Center, Brooklyn, New York, is 40 gm protein, 325 mg sodium, and 1700 mg potassium.[8] Occasionally, patients receiving maintenance dialysis are on a 60–80 gm protein diet, which is essentially normal. The diet for some patients in the dialysis program at The New York Hospital-Cornell Medical Center is 60–80 gm protein, 500–1000 mg sodium, and 2000 mg potassium.[18] This liberal diet is possible only when adequate staff and facilities are available to dialyze the patient an optimal amount of time each week.

A fairly typical diet for the uremic patient is one used at Peter Bent Brigham Hospital in Boston. It consists of 40 gm protein, 500 mg sodium, and 1500 mg potassium and is constructed with exchange lists that allow for patient choice.[19] The diet, exchange lists, and a sample menu are shown in Appendix D.

Nursing care. The nurse is responsible for helping the patient to maintain adequate nutrition in the hospital and to follow the prescribed diet at home. In the hospital the nurse checks the patient's tray to be certain he is receiving the proper diet. She makes certain the food is served at the proper temperature in order to make it more palatable. For example, dietary supplements consisting of liquids with high carbohydrate and fat content are more tolerable when served ice cold.

The nurse allows the patient a choice in his diet whenever possible. It is preferable for the patient to select his food by using exchange lists or similar devices, rather than be given a fixed menu.

The nurse also gives the patient choice in the distribution of his fluid allowance. For example, if the patient is restricted to 1000 ml/day, the nurse lets him decide how this fluid will be distributed over the three shifts.

When the fluid restriction is severe, the nurse helps "stretch" the allowed fluid. She can give the patient a wet cloth to suck on to keep his mouth from becoming dry. She can give him ice chips as part of his fluid. One unit of ice chips is equal to approximately half that unit of fluid. The nurse helps evaluate the patient's fluid balance by keeping an accurate record of his intake and output, and by weighing him daily on the same scale.

If the patient is not eating most of his diet, the nurse reports this to the physician, as other methods of maintaining nutrition may be necessary. Nutrients can be given via nasogastric tube in the form of high-carbohydrate, high-fat mixtures. Nutrients can also be given by intravenous infusion of 50 per cent dextrose and fat emulsions. The hypertonic intravenous solutions are infused in larger, more central veins, as they tend to sclerose smaller veins. When administering solutions with high glucose content, the nurse changes the IV tubing with each bottle, as the sugar makes an excellent medium for bacterial growth.

If the patient will have to remain on a special diet after discharge from the hospital, the nurse helps teach him about the diet. (In many hospitals the dietitian is responsible for teaching, but in most settings this is at least partially within the domain of the nurse.) Teaching must be started early and be done gradually. It is folly to hand the patient a diet sheet and give him a 20-minute talk on the day of discharge and think that he will follow the diet. Teaching can be started by discussing with the patient the types and portions of food that he receives on his hospital tray. Lists with food analysis and the prescribed diet are given to the patient. The nurse should make an effort to spend some time teaching the patient each day, even if only a few minutes.

In order to help the patient realize the importance of diet, the nurse can show him the relationship between his diet and blood chemistry. If he goes on a binge and his BUN increases, she can show him the blood chemistry results.

The nurse teaches the patient to read labels of processed foods to determine whether they contain protein, sodium, and potassium. Most processed foods, including bread, pastries, and cereals, do contain these substances and should be avoided unless the exact amounts of these constituents are known and are within the dietary limitations.

The nurse cautions the patient about using salt substitutes. Most salt substitutes are low in sodium, but high in potassium, and are, therefore, unacceptable.

The nurse teaches the patient about special products and recipes that are low in protein, sodium, and potassium. Low-protein baking mixtures, which can be used instead of wheat, are commercially available.* The companies furnish recipes for the use of their products. Some of these companies make additional products useful to the uremic patient. For example, Chicago Dietary Supply, Inc., also makes low-protein potato starch. Further information can be obtained by writing to the companies. The nurse may discover other products and companies by visiting the local health food or diet food store.

Some recipes that are low in protein, sodium, and potassium are given in Appendix D. It is helpful for the nurse working with renal failure patients to begin a recipe collection of her own.

Patients and their families can often help each other by exchanging recipe and diet ideas. The nurse can help arrange informal get togethers for this purpose.

Dieting is usually difficult, and the nurse gives the patient continuing support and motivation for staying within his restriction. She gives him opportunity to vent his feelings about dieting. She shows him the results of dietary indiscretions; she praises him for a job well done.

Treatment of Infection

Treatment of infection is very important in the management of patients with renal failure. Now that better methods are available for treating the renal failure itself, infection is becoming an important cause of death among uremic patients. In two series of patients with renal failure, infection was the leading cause of death.[21, 22]

Infection is to be avoided if at all possible. Unnecessary surgery and instrumentation are avoided, as this increases the chance of infection. When instrumentation is necessary, good aseptic technique is used. The patient is protected from exposure to hospital personnel or other patients with infectious diseases.

If infection does occur, it is treated promptly with antibiotics. Many antibiotics are given in reduced dosage because excretion of the drugs is reduced in uremia. Appendix B contains information about dosages of antimicrobials in renal failure.

Nursing care. The nurse plays an important part in preventing infection. She is meticulous about sterile technique when performing sterile procedures such as venipuncture, nasotrachael suctioning, tracheotomy care, shunt care, and bladder catheterization.

---

*Cellu Wheat Starch (Cellu-Featherweight Products, Chicago Dietary Supply, Inc., 405 East Shawnaut Avenue, La Grange, Illinois 60525); Paygel Wheat Starch Flour (Prescription Ltd., 1151 Madison Ave., New York, N. Y. 10028); Resource Baking Mix (The Doyle Pharmaceutical Company, Highway 100 at West 23 Street, Minneapolis, Minn. 55416).

When a patient with renal failure is admitted to the hospital, the nurse preferably places him in a single room. If he cannot have a single room she puts him in a room with patients who do not have infections. The charge nurse does not assign persons with colds or other infections to care for patients with renal failure.

The nurse recognizes and reports any signs of infection to the physician. The patient with uremia may have a low body temperature, even with an infection. Also, he may have an elevated white blood cell count without having an infection. The nurse is, therefore, also alert for other less specific symptoms of infection—malaise, listlessness, rapid heart rate, and rapid respiration. Symptoms of local infection do occur in uremia; these are pain, swelling, redness, and warmth of the infected area.

When infection does occur, the nurse administers the ordered antibiotics and continues to protect the patient from other sources of infection.

Treatment of Alterations in Body Biochemistry

SUBSTANCES DERIVED FROM PROTEIN METABOLISM

The build-up of substances derived from protein metabolism, such as urea, creatinine, and uric acid, is treated in several ways: by limitation of dietary intake of protein and avoidance of infection as just described, and by avoidance of unnecessary surgery and manipulation, by exercise, and by anabolic hormones. Unnecessary surgery and unnecessary instrumentation such as the insertion of an indwelling catheter are avoided; these procedures, in addition to increasing chances of infection, lead to breakdown of traumatized tissue. The patient is encouraged to exercise, rather than remain at absolute bed rest, as muscle disuse leads to muscle atrophy and breakdown. Occasionally, anabolic hormones are given; these are male hormones that cause tissue build-up and can reverse tissue breakdown.

Nursing care. The nurse helps and encourages the patient to ambulate. He should walk, not just once, but several times a day. When the patient is too ill to be out of bed, the nurse helps him exercise in bed.

POTASSIUM IMBALANCE

Hyperkalemia is a constant danger to many uremic patients. Symptoms of hyperkalemia include EKG changes. Decreased amplitude of the P wave, widened QRS complex, and peaked or "tent-shaped" T waves occur when the potassium level is 6.5–8 mEq/L (see Fig. 13). Cardiac arrhythmias and standstill are likely when the potassium increases to 9–10 mEq/L. Other symptoms of hyperkalemia are flaccid paralysis, slow respirations, anxiety, convulsions, and anesthesia. These clinical symptoms usually occur after early EKG changes.

Hyperkalemia is treated in several ways. Dietary intake of potassium is limited as explained in the preceding section. Drugs containing potassium, such as potassium penicillin, and diuretics that "spare" potassium, such as spironolactone, are not given.

Ion exchange resins are given on an emergency basis, or on a regular basis to allow more freedom for dietary intake of potassium. Kayexalate is the most commonly used exchange resin. It contains sodium in a compound that is not absorbed from the gastrointestinal tract. While in the gut, the sodium "exchanges" places with serum potassium, and the potassium becomes part of the nonabsorbable compound. The bound potassium is then excreted in the feces. Kayexalate is often mixed with sorbitol, a liquid that promotes osmotic diarrhea and thus insures adequate gastrointestinal loss. Kayexalate is given orally or as a retention enema. The usual dose is 15 gm once to four times/day. Fifteen grams four times daily usually reduces the serum potassium by 1–2 mEq/L over 24 hours.

Intravenous calcium gluconate or calcium chloride is given as an emergency measure when the potassium level is dangerously high and cardiac arrhythmias are imminent. Calcium protects the heart from the effects of hyperkalemia, but does not actually reduce serum potassium.

Intravenous sodium bicarbonate is another emergency treatment for hyperkalemia. When the patient is acidotic, intracellular proteins help buffer the hydrogen ion, and intracellular potassium is released. Sodium bicarbonate causes the potassium to go back inside the cell, and thus lowers the serum potassium level.

The administration of insulin and glucose is a fourth emergency measure for the treatment of hyperkalemia. Insulin causes glucose to go into the cell. As glucose moves inside the cell, it takes potassium with it and reduces the serum potassium.

A deficiency of serum potassium occasionally occurs in renal failure. Symptoms of hypokalemia are muscle weakness and paralysis with loss of reflexes. Cardiac arrhythmias—ventricular premature contractions and ventricular tachycardia—can occur. Digitalis intoxication can develop, as described later in this chapter. Electrocardiographic changes characteristic of hypokalemia are sagging ST segment, depressed T wave, and elevated U wave. The presence of the U wave indicates hypokalemia (see Fig. 12). Hypokalemia is treated with oral or parenteral potassium supplements.

Nursing care. The nurse is familiar with the EKG signs of hyperkalemia and reports their development to the physician immediately. These early EKG manifestations occur before clinical symptoms such as flaccid paralysis. The nurse, therefore, relies more on the cardiac monitor or rhythm strip to detect hyperkalemia than on clinical symptoms.

When administering Kayexalate, the nurse explains to the patient that mild diarrhea is expected and desired. She teaches the patient who will be taking Kayexalate at home to administer it himself. When administering insulin and glucose, the nurse observes the patient for signs of hypoglycemia – weakness, nervousness, shaking, diaphoresis, and loss of consciousness. She checks the urine for glucosuria.

The nurse observes the patient for hypokalemia. She administers intravenous and oral potassium supplements as ordered. Oral potassium supplements can be made more palatable by mixing them with orange, tomato, or other juices.

SODIUM IMBALANCE

Hypernatremia usually occurs when the patient is oliguric. Signs of hypernatremia are fluid retention, weight gain, systemic edema, congestive heart failure, pulmonary edema, and hypertension. Hypernatremia is treated by limiting sodium intake and administering diuretics, digitalis, and antihypertensive agents.

Hyponatremia occurs occasionally and is characterized by dehydration – dry mouth, loss of skin turgor, and decreased blood pressure. Other symptoms are listlessness, fatigue, confusion, anorexia, and nausea. As hyponatremia increases, muscle cramps, generalized muscle twitching, convulsions, and coma develop. Hyponatremia is treated by increasing dietary intake of sodium or by giving sodium supplements – sodium bicarbonate and sodium citrate. Intravenous replacement with hypertonic sodium solution is rare, owing to the danger of causing hypernatremia.

Nursing care. The nurse observes the patient for signs of hypernatremia or hyponatremia. If the patient is hypernatremic, she helps him restrict sodium intake; if he is hyponatremic, she administers ordered sodium supplements.

CALCIUM, PHOSPHORUS, AND BONE DISEASE

Calcium and phosphorus derangements and bone disease are interrelated. In most uremic patients, the serum calcium level is low. (The EKG change characteristic of hypocalcemia is a prolonged QT interval while the T wave remains of normal shape and duration.) The hypocalcemia is associated with a high level of serum phosphate and bone disease that is characterized by loss of calcium from osteoid tissue. The parathyroid gland may hypertrophy in an attempt to compensate for the deficiency of serum calcium.

Many practitioners feel that these conditions should not be treated unless clinical bone disease or other symptoms are present; the treatment can be hazardous, and the results are often unsatisfactory. Other practitioners treat these conditions more readily. To increase calcium absorption from the gut, vitamin D can be given in larger doses than are required by the usual patient, as uremic patients are somewhat resistant to it. The usual dose of vitamin D is 400 units/day; the dose for uremic patients may be 50,000–200,000 units/day. Vitamin D intoxication can occur with such large doses; symptoms are lassitude, anorexia, nausea, an increase in serum calcium to more than 10 mg/100 ml, and an increase in BUN due to no other known cause. Vitamin D is withdrawn immediately if these side effects occur, as the effects persist for about two weeks after the drug is discontinued.

Calcium supplements—calcium lactate and calcium citrate—can be given in doses of 10–20 gm/day orally to raise serum calcium. Aluminum hydroxide gels can be given to retard the absorption of phosphate from the gut; this reduces serum phosphate and increases serum calcium. Acidosis can be corrected by the use of alkalies. Correction of acidosis combined with the use of vitamin D helps heal some bone lesions. Occasionally, partial or complete parathyroidectomy is performed when the patient has severe hyperparathyroidism, as described in Chapter 4.

Nursing care. The nurse is responsible for giving the ordered medication and observing for any side effects.

She gives the aluminum hydroxide gels with meals, to reduce absorption of the phosphorus in the ingested food. Commonly used gels are Amphogel and Basalgel. Gels that contain magnesium in addition to aluminum are usually not used because of the danger of magnesium intoxication. Gelusil M, Maalox, Mylanta, and milk of magnesia contain magnesium.

ACIDOSIS

Most uremic patients are somewhat acidotic. Symptoms of moderately severe acidosis include fatigue, malaise, anorexia, and nausea. Rapid, deep respirations occur and represent respiratory compensation—excess carbon dioxide is being exhaled by the lungs. These respirations become more pronounced in severe acidosis and are called Kussmaul's respirations.

Acidosis is generally not treated until the patient is bothered by these symptoms. The uremic patient often has a serum bicarbonate level of 16–18 mEq/L and is quite comfortable (normal is 25 mEq/L). When treatment becomes necessary, sodium bicarbonate or sodium lactate is given orally or intravenously. The serum bicarbonate is usually not brought back to normal levels, as this is difficult to achieve and may precipitate tetany in patients with insufficient serum calcium. Sometimes calcium lactate or gluconate is given along with the alkalyzing agent to prevent tetany. When the patient is retaining sodium, as in congestive heart failure and hypertension, the administration of alkalies is deferred as long as possible because of their high sodium content. When sodium bicarbonate or sodium citrate must be given, the dietary intake of sodium is sharply reduced.

Nursing care. The nurse observes the patient for signs of developing or increasing acidosis and reports significant changes to the doctor. She administers ordered medications and watches for the development of any side effects. Both sodium bicarbonate and sodium citrate can cause nausea and vomiting when given orally, but sodium bicarbonate does so more often. She observes for symptoms of sodium retention, which can be caused by these drugs, and is alert for the development of hypocalcemic tetany and convulsions. She has appropriate medication and equipment at hand should this occur—IV calcium, IV diazepam (Valium), padded tongue blade, suction, and oxygen.

Treatment of Alterations in Organ Systems

CARDIOVASCULAR SYSTEM

Hypertension

Hypertension of varying severity develops in more than 80 per cent of patients with chronic renal failure. Hypertension is a very important determinant of survival. It can set up a vicious circle of further parenchymal kidney damage, further sodium retention, and further hypertension. Treatment is sometimes aimed at returning blood pressure to normal. In other cases, however, elevated blood pressure is not treated; lowering the blood pressure can cause a drop in glomerular filtration rate, decreased renal perfusion, and further renal damage.

Many drugs are used to treat hypertension in renal failure. Some of the commonly used ones, their dosage ranges, and important side effects are given in Table 2.

TABLE 2. Drugs Commonly Used To Treat Hypertension in Uremic Patients

DRUG	DOSE	SIDE EFFECTS
Antihypertensive agents Methyldopa (Aldomet)	500–2000 mg/day	Sedation, dizziness, extrapyramidal signs, depression, allergic-type reactions – positive direct Coombs test, hemolytic anemia
Rauwolfia Alkaloid Reserpine (Serpasil and other names)	0.1–0.2 mg/day	GI symptoms – increased GI tone and motility with abdominal cramps and diarrhea; increased appetite and weight gain. CNS symptoms – sedation, nightmares, depression
Ganglionic blacking agent Guanethidine (Ismelin)	begin with 10 mg/day and increase as needed	Orthostatic and exercise hypotension, decreased myocardial competence secondary to decreased adrenergic nerve effects, diarrhea, inhibition of ejaculation
Propranolol (Inderal)	30–320 mg/day	Bradycardia, heart failure, increased airway resistance and asthma, hypoglycemia due to augmentation of hypoglycemic effect of insulin
Diuretics Thiazide diuretic Chlorothiazide (Diuril)	500–2000 mg/day	Hypokalemia, hyperuricemia, exacerbation of renal and hepatic insufficiency, hyperglycemia and aggravation of existing diabetes mellitus. Effective with GFR greater than 15 ml/min
Ethacrynic acid (Edecrin)	25–200 mg/day	Hypokalemia, hyperuricemia, and deafness. Effective with GFR greater than 5 ml/min
Furosemide (Lasix)	40–2000 mg/day	Hypokalemia. Effective with GFR greater than 5 ml/min

Fluid and sodium intake are often restricted to treat hypertension.

Nursing care. The nurse measures the blood pressure accurately; it should fall gradually in response to therapy. She reports any sudden or severe drops in blood pressure to the physician immediately. Sudden hypotension can cause decreased renal blood flow and further renal damage.

If the patient is receiving ganglionic blocking agents, the nurse measures the blood pressure when the patient is lying down, standing up, and after he has exercised, as these drugs cause exercise and postural hypotension. The nurse teaches the patient taking these drugs to stand up slowly in order to avoid dizziness and fainting. She checks that the patient is having normal bowel movements, as these drugs tend to cause diarrhea.

The nurse checks the patient's pulse each time before giving propranolol. She withholds the drug and checks with the doctor if the pulse is below 50.

She also observes for the other side effects of drugs used to treat hypertension.

Congestive Heart Failure and Pulmonary Edema

Congestive heart failure and pulmonary edema are treated with sodium and water restriction, diuretics, and digitalis glycosides. Peritoneal dialysis and hemodialysis are sometimes used to remove excess fluid from the body.

Digoxin seems to be the best digitalis glycoside for uremic patients, according to Reidenberg.[20] The dose of digoxin is reduced in proportion to reduction in renal function. Jelliffe suggests the following schedule for maintenance doses of digoxin.[13]

Creatinine clearance (ml/min)	*Percentage of usual dose*
0	42
25	63
50	75
75	90

The use of digitalis can be hazardous in renal failure, because of the patient's abnormal potassium level. A patient with excess serum potassium requires more digitalis for the same therapeutic effect than a patient with normal serum potassium. If the patient's serum potassium is reduced quickly, as in dialysis, digitalis intoxication may occur. The peritoneal dialysis clearance for potassium is about 21 ml/min; it is about 10 ml/min for digoxin.[2, 20]

Nursing care. The nurse observes the patient for symptoms of congestive heart failure and pulmonary edema and notifies the physician should they develop. Important symptoms include orthopnea, rales, distention of neck veins, pallor, cool skin, and diaphoresis. The nurse can detect early signs of pulmonary edema by listening to the patient's lungs with a stethoscope at regular intervals.

The nurse is alert for the toxic effects of digitalis, which can result in prolongation of the PR interval, ventricular premature contractions, bigeminy, and almost any other arrhythmia. The nurse counts the patient's apical pulse before giving digitalis, and withholds the drug and checks with the doctor if the pulse is below 60. She withholds the drug and checks if any new arrhythmias are present. Other signs of digitalis intoxication are nausea, vomiting, and disturbances of color vision.

Systemic Edema

Systemic edema caused by heart failure and sodium and fluid retention is treated with digitalis, diuretics, and sodium and fluid restriction. Occasionally, as in the nephrotic syndrome, the edema is caused by hypoproteinemia; lack of serum protein results in low oncotic pressure in the blood and movement of fluid out of the capillaries and into body tissue. Edema in the nephrotic syndrome is treated primarily with sodium restriction and diuretics. A high-protein diet and, occasionally, intravenous infusions of salt-poor human albumin may be prescribed. However, this extra protein is quickly lost in the urine.

Nursing care. The nurse gives the patient with systemic edema special skin care, as his skin is likely to break down. She turns the patient at least every two hours and gives him backrubs with lotion, talcum, or other nondrying agents.

Pericarditis

The development of pericarditis, or inflammation of the pericardial sac, often means that the patient is in poor chemical control. Symptoms of pericarditis are pain and a friction rub. Pericarditis is treated symptomatically—analgesics are given to relieve the pain.

The pericarditis sometimes causes pericardial effusion and cardiac tamponade—a condition in which the pericardial sac fills with fluid and exerts pressure on the heart, thus making cardiac contractions ineffective. Symptoms of cardiac tamponade are lowered blood pressure, paradoxical blood pressure, lowered pulse pressure, increasingly distant heart sounds, cold and poorly-perfused extremities, and distended neck veins. Cardiac tamponade is treated by removing the effusion. A cardiac needle is inserted into the pericardium, and the fluid is withdrawn. Occasionally, after one or several attacks of pericarditis, the pericardium becomes thickened and adheres to the heart, causing constrictive pericarditis. In such cases, the pericardium is surgically removed.

Nursing care. The nurse is alert for signs of pericarditis. The patient may complain of left-sided or central chest pain, which can mimic a myocardial infarction. Sometimes the pericarditis is painless.

The nurse can detect the friction rub by listening with a stethoscope over the heart; the rub is an unusual heart sound, often loud. When pain is present, the nurse administers ordered analgesics.

The nurse watches carefully for the aforementioned signs of developing effusion and tamponade. She takes the blood pressure carefully to detect a paradoxical blood pressure; this is one in which the blood pressure falls more than 10 mm Hg on inspiration and then returns to the previous level on expiration. (The blood pressure normally falls only a few millimeters of mercury on inspiration.) The nurse listens to the heart at regular intervals so that she will be able to tell if the heart sounds are becoming increasingly distant, i.e., softer sounding or diminished in volume.

Cardiac tamponade often requires immediate treatment. The nurse has a paracentesis tray, with cardiac length needles, available for emergency pericardiocentesis.

HEMATOPOIETIC SYSTEM

Anemia

The anemia that occurs in chronic renal failure is apparently caused by lack of erythropoietin and consequent bone marrow depression and by shortened life span of red blood cells. Anemia does not usually cause symptoms unless the hemoglobin is less than 7 gm/100 ml. Below this level, anemia can cause extreme fatigue, dyspnea, increase in cardiac output and venous pressure, and angina.

Asymptomatic anemia is usually left untreated. When treatment is required, androgens can be given. These drugs act directly on the bone marrow and increase renal secretion of erythropoietin. Testosterone propionate 150 mg IM/week can be given to men; it may incidentally help to restore libido. A steroid of low androgenicity, such as nandrolone decanoate 25 mg IM every three weeks can be given to women. Side effects from androgen administration in females include hair growth, skin thickening, deepening of the voice, and other masculinizing effects.

Blood transfusions are sometimes given, but only when necessary. A transfusion decreases erythropoietin output and bone marrow production because of negative feedback. The transfused red blood cells, like the patient's own red blood cells, have a shortened life span. The patient's hemoglobin, therefore, quickly returns to the previous level, or even lower, and transfusions must be continued on a regular basis. Transfusion can give the patient serum hepatitis and can cause the development of antibodies that can endanger renal transplants. When a transfusion is necessary, buffy coat–poor cells or other preparations of low antigenicity are given. Packed cells may be given to avoid overhydration with unneeded plasma.

Nursing care. The nurse provides adequate rest for the anemic patient, as he tires easily. She provides him with an adequate night's sleep plus morning and afternoon rest periods, as needed.

The nurse reports the development of masculinizing effects from androgens to the physician and teaches the patient to do the same. The drug should be reduced or withdrawn if these effects appear. If the drug is not reduced or withdrawn, some of the effects can become permanent.

When a transfusion is being given, the nurse observes the patient for signs of a blood reaction—fever, chills, rash, pruritus, and hematuria. She stops the blood and calls the doctor if any of these signs develop.

Bleeding Tendency

The bleeding tendency common in uremia can be manifested by epistaxis, gastrointestinal bleeding, easy bruising, and excessive bleeding following trauma. The bleeding tendency is usually treated symptomatically. Trauma is avoided, if possible. Local bleeding is treated by the application of pressure, Gelfoam, and dilute solutions of epinephrine. Aminocaproic acid (EACA), an inhibitor of fibrinolysis, is sometimes given in dire emergencies for cases of internal bleeding refractory to other measures.

Nursing care. The nurse avoids unnecessary trauma to the patient. For example, if she is drawing blood, she collects all necessary specimens at one time. When inserting a nasogastric tube or performing nasotracheal suctioning, she lubricates the tube well to avoid damaging fragile mucous membranes. The nurse teaches the patient that he, too, must be careful. For example, he should use a soft toothbrush, avoid vigorous noseblowing, avoid constipation, and avoid rough contact sports such as football or hockey.

Gastrointestinal System

Anorexia, nausea, and vomiting are common, troublesome symptoms in uremia. These symptoms usually respond to a low-protein diet. Antiemetic drugs are also used for nausea and vomiting. Commonly used antiemetics are prochlorperazine (Compazine), orally or intramuscularly, and trimethobenzamide hydrochloride (Tigan) 100–250 mg orally, intramuscularly, or rectally.

Often the uremic patient's mouth is ulcerated and uncomfortable, as salivary flow is decreased and infections are common, and he needs frequent oral hygiene. If the mouth is infected with *Candida albicans*, as it frequently is, this can be treated with nystatin suspension 500 mg four times daily, amphotericin lozenges 10 mg, 10–20/day, or applications of 1 per cent gentian violet solution three times daily.

Nursing care. The nurse gives oral hygiene to the patient several times a day, using a soft toothbrush, Q-tips, or padded tongue blade. The unpleasant breath and taste that the patient experiences can often be relieved with chewing gum, sour balls, and other hard candy.

Skin

Dry, flaking, itching skin often occurs in uremia. This can be caused by disturbances in calcium and phosphorus balance, in which case it is treated with aluminum hydroxide gels or parathyroidectomy or both. The skin condition may be caused by a superficial *Candida albicans* infection, which is treated with nystatin, amphotericin, or gentian violet. The dermatitis is often due to no known cause and is, therefore, treated symptomatically with bland soaps, oils, and creams. Topical steroid creams can be used for rashes, and diphenhydramine hydrochloride (Benadryl) can be used for pruritus.

Nursing care. The nurse gives the patient frequent skin care. When the dermatitis is nonspecific and is being treated symptomatically, the nurse can suggest or try a variety of regimens. She should use a bland soap that does not contain perfume; baby soaps and Ivory soap are good. If the skin is very dry, she can use sodium bicarbonate in the bath, use plain tap water, or skip the bath every other day. Bland, unperfumed oils that may help include baby lotion, lanolin creams, Nivea Lotion, and Alpha-Keri lotion.

In terminal uremia, urea crystals precipitate out on the skin, forming "uremic frost." The nurse bathes the patient frequently to remove the crystals. These crystals are soluble in water, and therefore, it is not necessary to use soap on skin that is probably already dry.

Psychological manifestations and neuromuscular system

Most of the psychological and neuromuscular manifestations of uremia can be treated successfully only with dialysis and transplantation. When these forms of therapy are not available, these manifestations are treated symptomatically, usually with only limited success.

Confusion and agitation are treated with paraldehyde and chloral hydrate. Barbiturates are also used and should be given in minimal effective doses until patient sensitivity to the drug is established.

Peripheral neuropathy is sometimes caused by nitrofurantoin (Furadantin), a urinary antiseptic. This drug should not be given to uremic patients.

Muscle twitching and the "restless foot syndrome" can be treated symptomatically with diazepam (Valium) 5–10 mg orally, intramuscularly, or intravenously three to four times a day.

The seizures that occur in uremia are often secondary to hypertension, and are treated by reducing the blood pressure. Hypertensive convulsions and those due to other causes are treated initially with intravenous diazepam or phenobarbital. If the seizures recur, heavy sedation, tracheal intubation, and use of a respirator may be necessary. Some patients must continue to use maintenance doses of phenobarbital and diphenylhydantoin (Dilantin).

Nursing care. The uremic patient may experience periods of personality and intellectual deterioration, interspersed with periods of lucidity. This is, understandably, quite distressing to the patient and his family. The nurse should explain to both patient and family that this is an expected consequence of the disease and is not the patient's "fault" or own doing.

The confusion patients experience is sometimes precipitated or intensified by darkness. The nurse can try leaving a light on at night in the room of a confused patient.

The nurse teaches the patient with peripheral neuropathy to guard against foot and leg trauma. Sensation is dulled in the affected limbs, and the patient may be unaware of injury to these areas.

During an acute seizure, the nurse helps maintain the patient's respirations by inserting an airway, performing nasotracheal suctioning, and administering oxygen as necessary. She prepares emergency medication as needed.

Metabolism of drugs

Drugs that are metabolized and excreted by the kidneys must usually be given in decreased doses in uremia because these patients have poor renal function. Drugs that are metabolized to inactive substances by the liver and other means usually need not be given in decreased doses. Lists of appropriate dosage ranges of selected drugs in renal failure are given in Appendix B.

Nursing care. Drug toxicity is a common hazard to uremic patients. The nurse observes the patient carefully for the development of toxic effects from all drugs he is receiving.

Patient Teaching

Many patients are managed by conservative treatment for several years. They may come into the hospital for diagnosis and during exacerbations of their illness, but they spend much of their time outside the hospital, pursuing a fairly normal life. These patients should, therefore, be taught to care for themselves as much as possible. The patient with uremia is similar, in some respects, to the patient with diabetes mellitus; both are taught about their diseases and are relied upon to accept responsibility for certain aspects of their therapeutic management.

As indicated throughout this chapter, the nurse has very important responsibilities for teaching the patient. Indeed, she is usually the primary teacher. She begins the teaching early in the patient's hospitalization and continues it on a regular basis. Her teaching plan will vary, depending on the severity of the illness and the patient's prescribed therapy. The following topics, however, should be covered for almost all patients.

- Nature of the disease
- Diet
- Medications
  - Name
  - Action
  - Dose
  - Significant side effects
- Symptoms that should be reported to the doctor
  - Changes in urinary pattern such as increased output, decreased output, nocturia
  - Increased feeling of fatigue, malaise
  - Nausea, vomiting, and diarrhea, which can result in dehydration and electrolyte imbalance
  - Symptoms of infection
  - Symptoms of fluid retention
    - Edema
    - Sudden weight gain
    - Difficulty breathing
  - Symptoms of hypertension
    - Headaches
    - Dizziness
    - Blurred vision

Delivery of Treatment

Many patients with acute and chronic renal failure cannot be maintained by conservative measures alone. These patients will die if not treated with dialysis or transplantation. At present, these more aggressive forms of therapy cannot be offered to all patients requiring them, because of lack of funds and facilities.

It is an unfortunate state of affairs that a person who could live a fairly normal life should die while knowledge is available for keeping him alive and only funds and facilities are lacking. Lack of funds is a serious problem, but several things can be done to ameliorate the situation. Emphasis should be placed on prevention and early detection of renal disease, before extensive renal damage has occurred (see Chapter 9). Emphasis should also be placed on home dialysis and transplantation rather than on the more expensive long-term in-hospital dialysis, which makes treatment of large numbers of persons difficult. Governmental help and regional planning for efficient use of resources are essential.

In Australia a program based on these guidelines has made it possible to offer appropriate treatment to all renal failure patients—including dialysis and transplantation for all those who require it.[15] It is to be hoped that this will become more widespread in the near future.

CASE STUDIES

I

A 68 year old retired male elevator operator was seen in the CPMC clinic 10/71 with an acute attack of gout. His uric acid level at that time was 15.9 mg/100 ml. Further evaluation revealed that he had uremia, anemia, and chronic liver disease. Over the next four months, the patient's uremia progressed, his BUN increasing from 31 mg/100 ml in October to 156 mg/100 ml in February. He was admitted to CPMC 2/3/72, for evaluation of progressive renal failure.

On admission to the hospital, the following data were obtained. Na 136, K 5.3, CO_2 23, Cl 90, and Ca 10.5 mg/100 ml; BUN 156, serum creatinine 11.1, and uric acid 10.1 mEq/L; hbg. 12.6 gm/100 ml; and hct 36 per cent. The patient had had nocturia two times per night for several years.

On the night of admission, the patient was catheterized for residual urine, although he denied symptoms of retention. Residual urine amounting to 1900 ml was obtained. The diagnosis of bladder outlet obstruction was established.

An indwelling catheter was left in place for several days. With catheter drainage alone, the patient's BUN decreased from 156 to 87 mg/100 ml. The BUN did not return to normal, as the patient had some element of chronic underlying renal disease.

On 2/22, cystoscopy was performed. The patient was found to have bilobar benign prostatic hypertrophy. On 3/3, a retropubic prostatectomy and bilateral vas ligation were performed. The prostate gland weighed 30 gm (normal weight about 20 gm).

The patient did well postoperatively. He was discharged 3/13/72 in good condition with BUN of 51 and uric acid of 8.17 mg/100 ml, hbg of 11.2 gm/100 ml, and hct of 32.5 per cent.

II

A 23 year old female drug addict was admitted to CPMC 11/29/70, with the chief complaint of weight gain of about 30–35 lb over a period of one week. One year prior to this admission, the patient first noticed swelling of her ankles.

The following data were obtained on admission: weight 160.5 lb (usual 125–130 lb); 4+ pitting edema of feet and legs and milder edema of abdomen and periorbital region; BP 140/100; temperature 100°F; Na 136, K 4.0, CO_2 25, and Cl 109 mEq/L; BUN 24, serum creatinine 1.8 mg/100 ml; creatinine clearance 30.4 ml/min; urine specific gravity 1.015, pH 5, albumin 3+, glucose and acetone negative, many WBC's, bacteria 2+, culture more than 10,000 *E. coli*/ml; urinary protein loss/24 hr 8 gm.

An intravenous pyelogram showed mild hydronephrosis of the right kidney. An open renal biopsy demonstrated acute and chronic interstitial pyelonephritis, focal proliferative glomerulonephritis, and focal necrotizing glomerulonephritis.

The patient was restricted to bed rest and a high-protein diet, 2 gm Na, and 1500 ml fluid/day. She was given kanamycin and then ampicillin for the pyelonephritis. She was treated with methadone and then gradually withdrawn from this drug. The patient did well on this regimen; diuresis set in, and her creatinine clearance increased.

A decision was made not to treat the patient with azathioprine and steroids, as is often done in cases of glomerulonephritis, because of the pyelonephritis and because of the possibility of additional infection should she resume heroin use. These agents may be used in the future, however, if she does not continue to do well.

On 1/8/71, the patient was discharged. Her weight was 123 lb, creatinine clearance 53 ml/min, serum creatinine 1.0 mg/100 ml, urine culture negative, and 24-hour urinary protein loss 6.75 gm. Her discharge medications were folic acid 5 mg orally daily, diazepam 5 mg orally every six hours, and ampicillin 500 mg orally every six hours.

References

1. Beeson, P. B., and McDermott, W. (Eds.): *Cecil-Loeb Textbook of Medicine.* Twelfth and thirteenth editions. Philadelphia, W. B. Saunders Co., 1967 and 1971.
2. Boen, S. T.: *Peritoneal Dialysis in Clinical Medicine.* Springfield, Ill., Charles C Thomas, 1964.
3. Brest, A. N., and Moyer, J. H. (Eds.): *Renal Failure.* Philadelphia, J. B. Lippincott Co., 1968.
4. Bricker, N., discussant: Renal osteodystrophy. *J.A.M.A., 211*:97–101, 1970.
5. Chicago Dietary Supply, Inc. (Makers of Cellu Wheat Starch, Cellu-Featherweight Products), 405 East Shawnaut Avenue, La Grange, Ill. 60525.
6. Douglas, A., and Kerr, D. N. S.: *A Short Textbook of Kidney Disease.* Philadelphia, J. B. Lippincott Co., 1968.
7. Downing, S. R.: Nursing support in early renal failure. *Amer. J. Nurs., 69*:1212–1216, 1969.
8. Downstate Medical Center, Chronic Dialysis Program, Brooklyn, N.Y.
9. Doyle Pharmaceutical Company (Makers of Resource Baking Mix), Highway 100 at West 23 Street, Minneapolis, Minn. 55416.
10. Giovanetti, S., and Maggiore, Q.: A low-nitrogen diet with proteins of high biological value for severe chronic uremia. *Lancet, 1*:1000–1003, 1964.

11. Goodman, L. S., and Gilman, A.: *The Pharmacological Basis of Therapeutics.* Fourth edition. New York, Macmillan Co., 1970.
12. Hampers, C., Katz, A. I., Wilson, R. E., and Merrill, J. P.: Disappearance of uremic itching after subtotal parathyroidectomy. *New Eng. J. Med., 179*:695–697, 1969.
13. Jelliffe, R. W.: An improved method of digoxin therapy. *Ann. Intern. Med., 69*:703–717, 1968.
14. Kerr, D. N. S.: Chronic renal failure. In Beeson, P. B., and McDermott, W. (Eds.): *Cecil-Loeb Textbook of Medicine.* Thirteenth edition. Philadelphia, W. B. Saunders Co., 1971.
15. Kincaid-Smith, P.: Treatment of irreversible renal failure by dialysis and transplantation. In Beeson, P. B., and McDermott, W. (Eds.): *Cecil-Loeb Textbook of Medicine.* Thirteenth edition. Philadelphia, W. B. Saunders Co., 1971.
16. Mitchell, H. S., Rynbergen, H. J., Anderson, L., and Dibble, M. V. (Eds.): *Cooper's Nutrition in Health and Disease.* Fifteenth edition. Philadelphia, J. B. Lippincott Co., 1968.
17. Mitchell, M. C., and Smith, E. J.: Dietary care of the patient with chronic oliguria. *Amer. J. Clin. Nutr., 19*:163–169, 1966.
18. New York Hospital–Cornell Medical Center, Department of Nutrition, New York, N. Y.
19. Peter Bent Brigham Hospital, Department of Dietetics, Boston, Massachusetts, and Handbook Number 8, Composition of Foods, U. S. Department of Agriculture, 1963. Mitchell, H. S., Rynbergen, H. J., Anderson, L., and Dibble, M. (Eds.): *Cooper's Nutrition in Health and Disease.* Fifteenth edition. J. B. Lippincott Co., 1968.
20. Reidenberg, M. M.: *Renal Function and Drug Action.* Philadelphia, W. B. Saunders Co., 1971.
21. Schreiner, G. E.: Acute renal failure. In Beeson, P. B., and McDermott, W. (Eds.): *Cecil-Loeb Textbook of Medicine.* Twelfth edition. W. B. Saunders Co., Philadelphia, 1967.
22. Schreiner, G. E., and Maher, J. F.: *Uremia: Biochemistry, Pathogenesis and Treatment.* Springfield, Ill., Charles C Thomas, 1961.
23. Williams, S. R.: Nutrition and Diet Therapy. Saint Louis, C. V. Mosby Co., 1970.
24. Wintrobe, M. M., Thorn, A. W., Adams, R. D., Bennett, I. L., Jr., Braunwald, E., Isselbacher, K. J., and Petersdorf, R. G. (Eds.): *Harrison's Principles of Internal Medicine.* Sixth edition. New York, McGraw-Hill Book Co., 1970.

CHAPTER 6

Peritoneal Dialysis

Peritoneal dialysis dates back to 1877 when Wegner conducted experiments on the effects of peritoneal temperature on body temperature. He instilled cold saline solution (14–16°C) into the peritoneal cavity of rabbits and noted that this caused a drop in their body temperature. He also noted that when he instilled a hypertonic glucose solution, more fluid was withdrawn from the peritoneal cavity than was originally introduced.[4] Study of the peritoneum was continued by other investigators.[4]

In 1923 Ganter performed the first dialyses on uremic subjects—rabbits and guinea pigs with anuria due to ligation of the ureters. He introduced 50 ml normal saline solution into the peritoneal cavity and removed the fluid two to four hours later. The cycle was repeated again and again. The saline solution withdrawn from the peritoneal cavity contained the same concentration of nitrogenous wastes as the blood, and the experimental animals showed clinical improvement following the dialysis.[4]

Ganter attempted the first peritoneal dialysis in humans in 1923. He instilled 1.5 L normal saline into the peritoneal cavity of a patient with ureteral obstruction due to uterine carcinoma. The patient showed slight clinical improvement.[4]

Other early investigators of human peritoneal dialysis include: Heusser and Werder, Balázs and Rosenak, and Rhoads. In 1938 Wear et al. dialyzed five patients for periods of two to eight hours. Each patient demonstrated a reduction of serum nonprotein nitrogen (NPN) and creatinine concentrations. One patient was so much improved by the dialysis that he could be operated on for bladder stones.[4]

Since 1946, much investigation has been carried out and many publications have appeared on peritoneal dialysis in man.

Basic Concepts of Peritoneal Dialysis

Peritoneal dialysis involves the use of the peritoneal membrane as a dialyzing membrane to remove nitrogenous waste products from the body and to normalize body fluid and electrolytes.

The peritoneum, the serous membrane that lines the abdominal cavity and covers the visceral organs within, is composed of two sections—the parietal peritoneum and the visceral peritoneum. The parietal peritoneum lines the inside of the abdominal wall; the visceral peritoneum covers the abdominal organs, making many folds. The two sections are continuous; thus, the peritoneum forms a sac, and the space between its parietal and visceral layers is the peritoneal cavity. The filtering surface of the peritoneum is about 22,000 sq. cm.[18] The area is this large because of the many folds and reflections of the visceral peritoneum (Fig. 16).

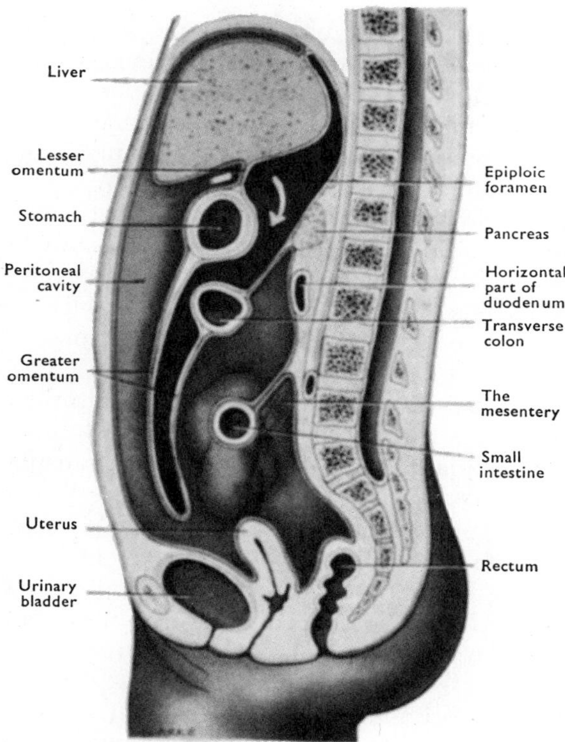

Figure 16. A diagrammatic median section of the abdomen and pelvis to show the arrangement of the peritoneum. Normally the abdominal viscera completely fill the abdominal cavity and the peritoneal cavity is reduced to a slit. In the diagram the cavity has been distended to make it obvious. The arrow traverses the epiploic foramen. (From Romanes, G. J. (Ed.): *Cunningham's Manual of Practical Anatomy.* Thirteenth edition. New York, Oxford University Press, 1968.)

The peritoneum acts as an inert, semipermeable membrane. Permeable to substances of low molecular weight such as urea, electrolytes, and glucose, it is impermeable to substances of high molecular weight such as large proteins. Osmosis, diffusion, and filtration occur across the peritoneum, between fluid in the peritoneal cavity and the rich blood supply of the abdominal organs.

In peritoneal dialysis, fluid is introduced into the peritoneal cavity. Osmosis, diffusion, and filtration take place across the peritoneal membrane, between the dialysis solution (dialysate) and the blood. After this equilibration period, the dialysate is drained from the peritoneal cavity. A new cycle is then begun with the introduction of more dialysate.

Indications for Peritoneal Dialysis

Peritoneal dialysis is used to treat patients with a variety of conditions, including some that are not primarily renal disorders.

Acute renal failure. Peritoneal dialysis is used to treat patients with acute renal failure. The kidney damage can be from many causes, such as acute glomerulonephritis, extensive burns, and carbon tetrachloride poisoning.

Accentuated chronic renal insufficiency. Patients with chronic renal insufficiency are treated with peritoneal dialysis when they have temporary exacerbations. These patients manage well most of the time without dialysis, but events such as trauma, infection, vomiting, diarrhea, or excessive protein intake temporarily worsen their clinical condition.

Chronic renal failure. Peritoneal dialysis is used as a temporary maintenance measure for patients with end-stage chronic renal failure who are awaiting places in hemodialysis and transplantation programs.

Occasionally peritoneal dialysis is used as a permanent measure to maintain the life of a patient with end-stage chronic renal failure. However, the feasibility and value of the long-term use of peritoneal dialysis is not established, and it is not routinely used for this purpose. Hemodialysis and renal transplantation are the treatments of choice in this situation.

Intoxication. Peritoneal dialysis is used to treat patients who are intoxicated with dialyzable poisons, when hemodialysis is unavailable or contraindicated. Common dialyzable intoxicants include: salicylates, barbiturates, methyl alcohol, amphetamines, and meprobamate (Miltown) (see Appendix E for a complete list).

Fluid retention. In patients with severe fluid retention, as in congestive heart failure and pulmonary edema, peritoneal dialysis is used to remove water when other measures are ineffective.

Electrolyte imbalance. Sometimes, peritoneal dialysis is used to correct electrolyte imbalance, such as hyponatremia, hyperkalemia, hyperuricemia, and acidosis, when other measures are dangerous or ineffective.

Peritonitis. Peritoneal dialysis is sometimes used as an adjunct to the treatment of generalized peritonitis. Antibiotics are added to the dialysis solution.

Contraindications to Peritoneal Dialysis

Contraindications to peritoneal dialysis are associated with unsuitable conditions of the peritoneal membrane and cavity. They include extensive abdominal adhesions, localized infection of the peritoneum (peritoneal dialysis may spread a localized infection), and a gangrenous or perforated bowel.

Kinetics of Peritoneal Dialysis

Substances diffuse across the peritoneal membrane at varying rates. Urea diffuses rapidly. The amount of urea that diffuses across the peritoneal membrane per minute, called the peritoneal urea clearance, is 26 ml/min at a dialyzing rate of 2.5 L/hr.[4] The peritoneal clearance of other substances, expressed as milliliters per minute, at a dialyzing rate of 2.5 L/hr is: potassium 21, inorganic phosphate 16, creatinine 15, uric acid 14, magnesium 11, calcium 9.5, and indican 8.5.[4] Clinically this means, for example, that BUN will be reduced at a faster rate than creatinine.

Comparing the efficiency of peritoneal dialysis to other methods, the urea clearance by peritoneal dialysis is 26 ml/min; the urea clearance by hemodialysis (twin-coil) is between 70 and 170 ml/min. The urea clearance by normal human kidney is 40–65 ml/min.

Peritoneal clearance is influenced by other factors in addition to the nature of the peritoneal membrane and the substances diffusing across it. The dialyzing rate, or the rate of flow of the dialysate, influences peritoneal clearance. For example, if the dialyzing rate is high, the gradient between urea in the blood and in the dialysate will always be high, and the peritoneal urea clearance will be rapid. If the dialysate flow rate is slower, the urea concentration in the dialysate will increase, the urea gradient between the blood and dialysate will decrease, and peritoneal urea clearance will decrease.

The optimal dialysate flow rate, according to Boen, is 2.5 L/hr. The peritoneal clearance increases when the flow rate is greater, but the gain in clearance is small, and more dialysis solution is required, which increases cost. So, considering both peritoneal clearance and financial aspects, the usual optimal dialysate flow rate is 2.5 L/hr.[4]

To achieve this dialyzing rate of 2.5 L/hr, one dialysis cycle lasts about 48 minutes. The inflow period, when dialysate flows into the peritoneal cavity, is 5–10 minutes; the equilibration or dwell period, when the dialysate remains in the peritoneal cavity, is about 20 minutes; and the outflow or drainage period, when the dialysate drains out of the peritoneal cavity, is about 20 minutes.

The temperature of the dialysate affects peritoneal clearance. Warming the dialysate from 20° C (room temperature) to 37° C (body temperature) increases urea clearance by 35 per cent.[17] (Warming the dialysate to body temperature also avoids discomfort for and heat loss from the patient.)

Increasing the glucose concentration in the dialysate increases peritoneal urea clearance. This increased urea clearance occurs primarily because of solvent drag associated with ultrafiltration. It is also partially due to increased peritoneal permeability.[17]

Other substances added to the dialysate increase peritoneal clearance of specific solutes. Albumin increases the clearance of substances that bind to protein—calcium, bilirubin, salicylates, and barbiturates. Oil increases the clearance of lipid-soluble substances such as glutethimide (Doriden).[17]

Composition of the Dialysis Solution

The dialysis solution is composed so that it accomplishes removal of the metabolic wastes, correction of fluid balance, and correction of electrolyte balance. Commercially prepared dialysate is generally used and is made by several companies in the United States.*

Removal of metabolic wastes such as urea, creatinine, and uric acid is accomplished by using a dialysate that is devoid of these substances. These waste products readily diffuse from the patient's blood into the dialysate, moving from the area of higher concentration to the one of lower concentration.

Fluid balance is attained by using dialysates of varying tonicity. Dialysate usually contains 1.5 per cent dextrose (15 gm/L) or 4.25 per cent dextrose (42.5 gm/L).†

---

*Abbott Laboratories (Inpersol), North Chicago, Illinois 60064; Cutter Laboratories (Peridial), Berkeley, California 94710; McGraw Laboratories, Glendale, California 91201; Travenol Laboratories, Inc. (Dianeal), Morton Grove, Illinois 60053.

†Dialysate containing 7 per cent dextrose (70 gm/L) was available formerly, but has been withdrawn from the market, as it is too hypertonic.

If the patient is in adequate fluid balance, 1.5 per cent dialysate is used. This usually maintains the fluid balance status quo. However, 1.5 per cent dialysate is slightly hypertonic; it contains approximately 365 mOsm/L, as compared with blood, which contains 285–295 mOsm/L, and can, therefore, sometimes cause fluid loss, especially if the dialyzing rate is rapid.[8, 17]

If the patient is retaining fluid, 4.25 per cent dialysate (approximately 504 mOsm/L) is used. This more hypertonic solution results in more rapid water removal.

Some companies also make dialysate with sorbitol instead of dextrose to give the solution the desired tonicity.* Sorbitol does not cause hyperglycemia, as dextrose sometimes does.

Electrolyte balance is attained by using a dialysate with an electrolyte composition similar to blood. The dialysate and blood equilibrate, and the patient's electrolyte abnormalities are corrected. The concentration of electrolytes in commercial dialysate is approximately:

Na	140–141 mEq/L
Ca	3.5–4.0 mEq/L
Mg	1.5 mEq/L
K	4 mEq/L in some solutions
	0 mEq/L in some solutions
Cl	101–102 mEq/L
Lactate or acetate	43–45 mEq/L per cent
Dextrose	15 gm/L (1.5 per cent)
	42.5 gm/L (4.25 per cent)
Osmolality	365 mOsm/L (1.5 per cent)
	504 mOsm/L (4.25 per cent)

Dialysate is available with or without potassium.† If the patient's potassium level is high, dialysate without potassium is used in order to remove potassium more quickly; after the potassium level has become normal, dialysate with potassium is used to avoid body depletion of this electrolyte. Potassium is added to the solution manually if the commercial dialysate containing it is not available.

Lactate or acetate is used as the base element instead of bicarbonate for technical reasons—dextrose and bicarbonate cannot be sterilized together because caramelization will occur. Lactate and acetate are converted to bicarbonate after absorption.

Commercial dialysate is available in 1 and 2 L bottles.‡

---

*McGraw Laboratories; Travenol Laboratories, Inc.

†Abbott Laboratories and Travenol Laboratories, Inc., make dialysate with potassium.

‡Abbott Laboratories, McGraw Laboratories, and Travenol Laboratories, Inc., prepare dialysate in 1 and 2 L bottles; Cutter Laboratories prepares dialysate in 1 L bottles.

To summarize, dialysate usually contains no metabolic waste products, a dextrose concentration of 1.5 per cent or 4.25 per cent, and a physiological concentration of electrolytes, with or without potassium.

Equipment for Peritoneal Dialysis

The equipment needed for peritoneal dialysis is as follows:

Dialysis solution. Dialysis solutions are discussed in the preceding section.

Peritoneal catheter. The catheter is inserted into the peritoneal cavity. Its intra-abdominal portion is perforated with numerous holes to facilitate rapid flow of fluid. Commercial plastic catheters are made by several companies; if these are not available, a large rubber stomach tube with holes punched along the tip can be used.

Trocar or stylet. A trocar or stylet is used to insert the peritoneal catheter. The trocar fits around the outside of the catheter; the stylet fits inside it. A stylet is preferable because it makes a smaller wound and thus minimizes pain and leakage around the catheter (Fig. 17).

Administration tubing. Tubing similar to IV tubing, but of larger diameter, is used to infuse and drain the dialysate. The first section of tubing connects the bottle or bottles of dialysate to the peritoneal catheter; the second section connects the peritoneal catheter to the drainage receptacle on the floor (Fig. 18).

Equipment for catheter insertion. Surgical equipment needed to insert the peritoneal catheter includes: skin preparation material,

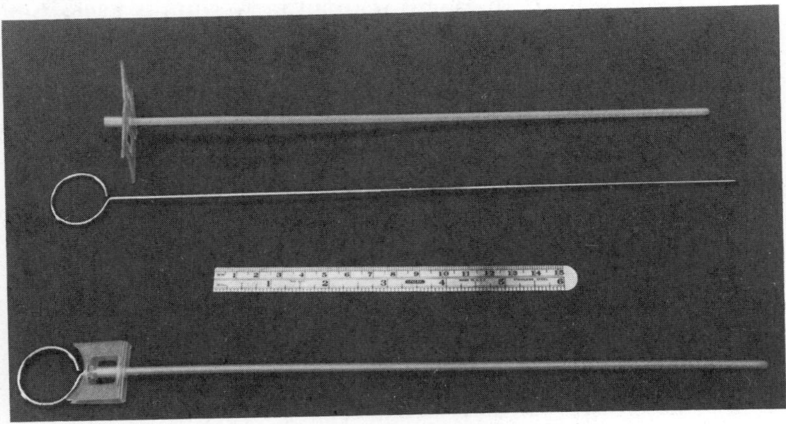

Figure 17. Peritoneal catheter and stylet.

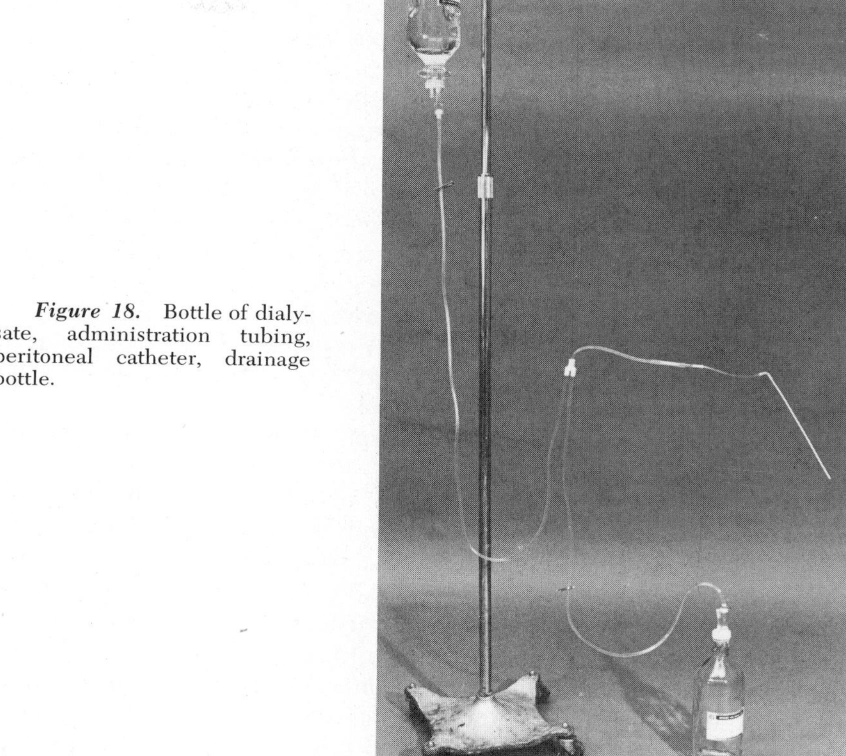

Figure 18. Bottle of dialysate, administration tubing, peritoneal catheter, drainage bottle.

needle, syringe, local anesthetic, scalpel, suturing material, scissors, and sterile dressing material.

The Dialysis Procedure

Before the peritoneal catheter is inserted to begin the dialysis, the patient is asked to void in order to prevent accidental perforation of the bladder. If he cannot void, and the bladder is distended, the patient is catheterized.

The skin is then prepared. Most parts of the abdominal wall can be used for catheter insertion. The preferred section is midway between the umbilicus and the pubic bone, at or near the midline. The skin is shaved, scrubbed with antiseptic solution, and covered with sterile drapes.

A local anesthetic such as procaine is administered. One to two liters of dialysate are infused into the peritoneal cavity through a needle. This expands the peritoneal space and lessens the danger of perforating the intestines during catheter insertion.

A small incision is made through the skin, subcutaneous tissue, muscle, and fascia, leaving the peritoneum exposed. Capillary bleeding is controlled by pressure or topical application of dilute epinephrine. The stylet is inserted through the incision, and the peritoneum is penetrated by a short thrust. The peritoneum itself is sometimes incised with the scalpel, especially when adhesions are present. The stylet is removed, and the peritoneal catheter is pushed further into the abdominal cavity, downward, toward the anterior portion of the pelvis. The tip of the catheter is placed in the lowest part of the abdominal cavity to insure good outflow of fluid. The edges of the skin incision are sutured snugly around the catheter, and the surrounding skin is cleaned with an antiseptic solution and covered with a sterile dressing.

The catheter is connected to the administration tubing, and a dialysis cycle is begun. The inflow clamp is opened, the dialysate infuses rapidly into the peritoneal cavity, and the inflow clamp is then closed. To achieve a dialyzing rate of 2.5 L/hr, the inflow period is 5–10 minutes. Two liters of dialysate are usually used for each cycle in an adult. Less solution is used for a child.

The dialysate remains in the peritoneal cavity for an equilibration or dwell period, during which osmosis, diffusion, and filtration take place. To achieve a dialyzing rate of 2.5 L/hr, the equilibration period is about 20 minutes. The equilibration period is increased or decreased as required by the patient's condition. If, for example, rapid removal of potassium is critical to life, the equilibration period is shortened. Often there is no equilibration period for the first cycle of a dialysis; the dialysate is drained immediately after infusion to determine if the catheter is functioning properly and to prevent clot formation.

At the end of the equilibration period, the outflow clamp is opened, and the dialysate drains from the peritoneal cavity. To achieve a dialyzing rate of 2.5 L/hr, the outflow period is about 20 minutes. At the completion of the outflow period, the outflow clamp is closed (Fig. 19).

This cycle of inflow, equilibration, and outflow is repeated until the dialysis is completed. The duration of dialysis varies and depends on factors such as the severity of the uremia and the size and weight of the patient. The usual dialysis lasts for 24–72 hours.

Blood samples are drawn at intervals during the dialysis to determine the patient's electrolyte status. Samples of outflow dialysate are

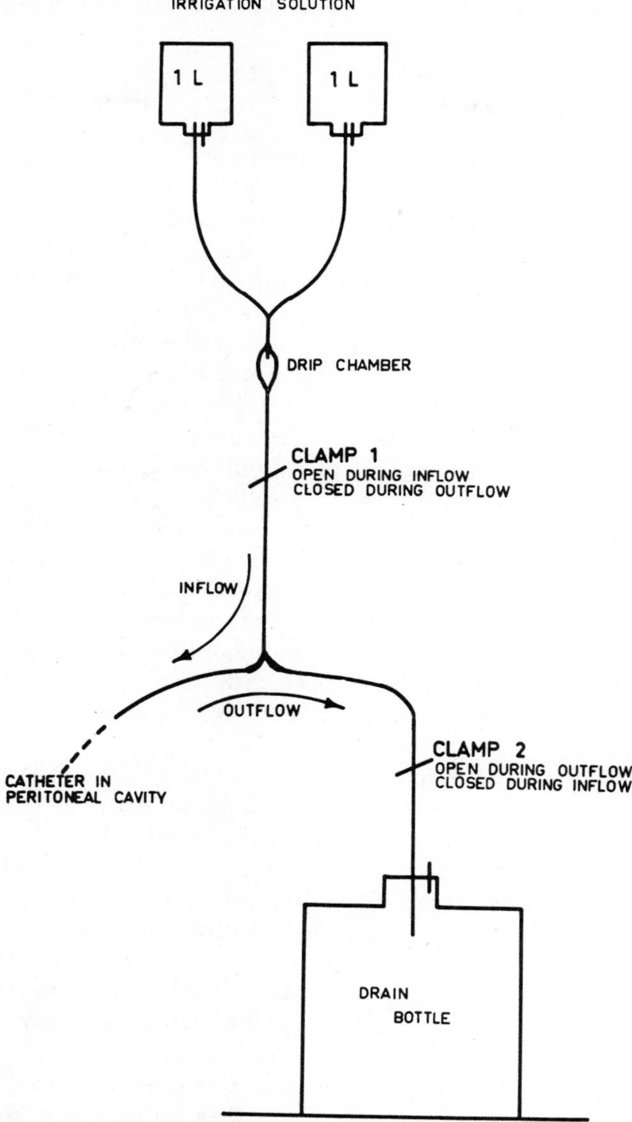

Figure 19. Schematic drawing of the intermittent method of peritoneal dialysis. (From Boen, S. T.: *Peritoneal Dialysis in Clinical Medicine.* Springfield, Ill. Charles C Thomas, 1964.)

also collected at intervals to be examined for bacteria. The patient is weighed before dialysis and at intervals during the procedure to help determine his state of hydration; his vital signs are monitored during the procedure.

When the dialysis is completed, the catheter is removed. The abdominal wound is sutured closed, cleaned with antiseptic solution, and covered with a sterile dressing.

Complications of Peritoneal Dialysis

Several complications can result from peritoneal dialysis:

Peritonitis. Peritonitis, or inflammation of the peritoneum, is the most common complication. It occurs in 5–50 per cent of patients receiving peritoneal dialysis.[17] Peritonitis occurs when there is leakage around the abdominal wound, or when dialysate, administration tubing, or peritoneal catheter is contaminated because of faulty sterile technique. The symptoms are: diffuse abdominal pain, tenderness on palpation, rigidity of the abdominal wall, and cloudiness of the outflow dialysate. Peritonitis is treated with systemic antibiotics and with antibiotics added to the dialysis solution.

Protein loss. Serum protein diffuses from the blood into the dialysate. About 0.5 gm protein is lost in each liter of drained dialysate; occasionally as much as 1 gm/L is lost.[4] Protein loss from one or two dialyses does not usually affect the patient seriously, but repeated dialysis can result in protein depletion, malnutrition, ascites, and impairment of his immune defenses. The protein loss is treated by increasing the oral intake of complete proteins such as eggs, meat, and fish.

Hyperglycemia and hyperosmolar coma. Glucose is absorbed from the dialysate into the blood. When 2 per cent glucose dialysate is used, 5–12 gm of glucose is absorbed after 30 minutes. At a dialyzing rate of 2.5 L/hr, this implies an absorption of 300–720 gm glucose/24 hr.[4] Glucose absorption can cause hyperglycemia and hyperosmolar coma. It is especially likely to cause difficulties in the diabetic patient. The complication of glucose overload is treated by monitoring the patient's blood and urinary glucose and by administering insulin as needed. Sorbitol dialysate may be used to avoid hyperglycemia, but it, too, can cause hyperosmolar coma.

Pulmonary edema. Acute pulmonary edema occasionally develops during dialysis, especially at the beginning of the procedure. The pulmonary edema occurs because the volume of dialysate is too large and compresses the thoracic organs. Decreased cardiac output and decreased perfusion of lung bases occurs, and the patient develops symptoms of pulmonary edema—dyspnea, orthopnea, tachypnea, rales, and tachycardia. The pulmonary edema is treated by promptly draining out the dialysis solution. Dialysis can then be tried with a smaller volume of fluid.

Perforation. Perforation of the intestines can occur when the peritoneal catheter is inserted. Symptoms of this complication are pain and the presence of intestinal contents in the outflow fluid. If this occurs, the dialysis is stopped and the perforation is surgically repaired.

Nursing Care During Peritoneal Dialysis

The nurse has many responsibilities during peritoneal dialysis. Before the dialysis is started, the nurse, or the doctor, explains the dialysis procedure to the patient. The explanation includes information regarding the purpose of the dialysis, insertion of the catheter, cycling of fluid, permitted activity during the dialysis, and expected length of the procedure. The nurse allows the patient ample opportunity for questioning and discussion.

The nurse gathers the necessary equipment for inserting the peritoneal catheter:

- Sterile dialysis solution
- Sterile administration tubing
- Sterile peritoneal catheter
- Skin preparation material
  - Razor and blade
  - Antiseptic solution
- Sterile surgical equipment
  - Syringe and needle
  - Lidocaine (1 or 2 per cent)
  - Gloves
  - Scalpel and blade
  - Suturing material and needle
  - Needle holder
  - Hemostat
  - Scissors
- Dressing material
  - Sterile gauze pads
  - Antibiotic ointment
  - Tape

She then assists the doctor with the insertion procedure.

The nurse is responsible for cycling the dialysis fluid. She connects the bottle or bottles of dialysate to the administration tubing, allows the dialysate to infuse rapidly, waits for equilibration to occur, allows the fluid to drain, and then closes the outflow clamp and begins a new cycle. A time schedule for the cycles is ordered by the physician.

Sterile technique must be used during the dialysis; infection is the most frequent complication of this procedure. The nurse is very careful to maintain sterility when she changes dialysate bottles. If possible, she uses 2 L instead of 1 L bottles. This reduces the number of bottle changes and consequent chances for contamination by half. If 1 L bottles must be used, all the medications for one cycle are added to one bottle only. They will mix together in the abdomen, and there will be less chance of contamination, as only one bottle will have been opened. For example, if the doctor orders 4 mEq/L of potassium chloride, the nurse adds 8 mEq to one bottle and then uses this bottle together with one that has no medication added. She changes the administration tubing and drainage bottle every 24 hours.

The nurse warms the dialysis solution to body temperature (37°C) before infusion. This warming helps increase peritoneal clearance, helps the patient maintain a constant body temperature, and usually seems more comfortable to the patient than room temperature fluid. The fluid is warmed by placing bottles of dialysate in a bedside warmer equipped with a thermometer; one must be careful not to overheat the dialysate, as hot fluid can damage the abdominal organs.

The nurse is careful to keep air out of the administration tubing and to remove any that enters accidentally. Air that gets into the tubing and, consequently, into the peritoneal cavity can cause abdominal discomfort and drainage difficulties.

The nurse observes the color of the outflow fluid—usually a clear, pale yellow. It is sometimes blood-tinged for the first few cycles owing to the trauma of inserting the catheter. Blood-tinged dialysate, after the first few cycles, indicates abdominal bleeding. Fecal-colored dialysate indicates bowel perforation. Cloudy dialysate usually indicates peritonitis.

Accurate records of each dialysis cycle are kept on a dialysis "flow-sheet" (Fig. 20). The nurse records the type of dialysate and any added medication, the amount of dialysate introduced and drained from the peritoneal cavity, the timing of the inflow and outflow periods, and the character of the drained dialysate. She also records the net fluid balance for that cycle and the cumulative net fluid balance.

The net fluid balance for a cycle indicates how much fluid the patient retains or loses during that cycle. For example, if, during one cycle, 2000 ml were infused and 2400 ml drained out, the net fluid balance for that cycle would be 400 ml lost by the patient. If during the subsequent cycle, 2000 ml were infused and 1700 ml drained out, the net fluid balance for that cycle would be 300 ml retained by the patient. The cumulative net fluid balance for these two cycles would be 100 ml lost.

The nurse informs the doctor about the fluid balance at intervals, at least every eight hours. And she notifies him if there are any sig-

PERITONEAL DIALYSIS RECORD

DETACH FOR INDIVIDUAL USE

PATIENT__________ ROOM ______

ATTENDING PHYSICIAN __________

HOSPITAL NUMBER______ AGE____ SEX ____

DIAGNOSIS__________

WEIGHT PRIOR______ WEIGHT ON COMPLETION______

DATE	SOLUTION TYPE				MEDICATION ADDED TO SOLUTION	OTHER MEDICATION OR REMARKS	SOLUTION IN			SOLUTION OUT			DIFFERENCE PLUS OR MINUS	CUMULATIVE DIFFERENCE
	1.5%	1.5%K	4.25%	7%			STARTING TIME	FINISH TIME	VOLUME	STARTING TIME	FINISH TIME	VOLUME		
	✓				8 mEq. KCL		$8\frac{00}{A}$	$8\frac{10}{A}$	2,000	$8\frac{30}{A}$	$8\frac{50}{A}$	2,400	−400	−400
	✓				8 mEq. KCL		$8\frac{50}{A}$	$9\frac{00}{A}$	2,000	$9\frac{20}{A}$	$9\frac{40}{A}$	1,700	+300	−100

Figure 20. Dialysis flow sheet. (Courtesy of Abbott Laboratories, Chicago, Ill.)

nificant changes in the balance—if the patient is retaining or losing large amounts of fluid. If the patient loses fluid too rapidly, for example, 1 L per cycle for a few cycles, there is danger that he will develop hypovolemic shock. If the patient retains large amounts of fluid, he is in danger of fluid overload.

It should be noted that the terms "retain" and "lose," "plus" and "minus," and "ahead" and "behind" are used interchangeably at different hospitals. The nurse should understand clearly what the terms mean in her particular institution.

In addition to keeping a record of the dialysis, the nurse keeps a record of the patient's other intake and output. Intake includes oral and parenteral fluid. Output includes urine, stool, emesis, and drainage.

The nurse weighs the patient as another indication of fluid balance. She weighs him before the dialysis begins and at intervals during the procedure, usually daily. She weighs the patient at the same point in the dialysis cycle each time—either with the fluid in the peritoneal cavity or with the fluid drained out. Two liters of dialysate weighs approximately 4.4 lb.

The nurse collects ordered specimens for analysis. She may be responsible for drawing blood for electrolyte determinations, which are taken every 12 hours or more often. She collects samples of drained dialysate in sterile containers for bacteriological examination. This is usually done daily and at the conclusion of the dialysis. She tests the patient's urine, usually every six hours, for glucose. The

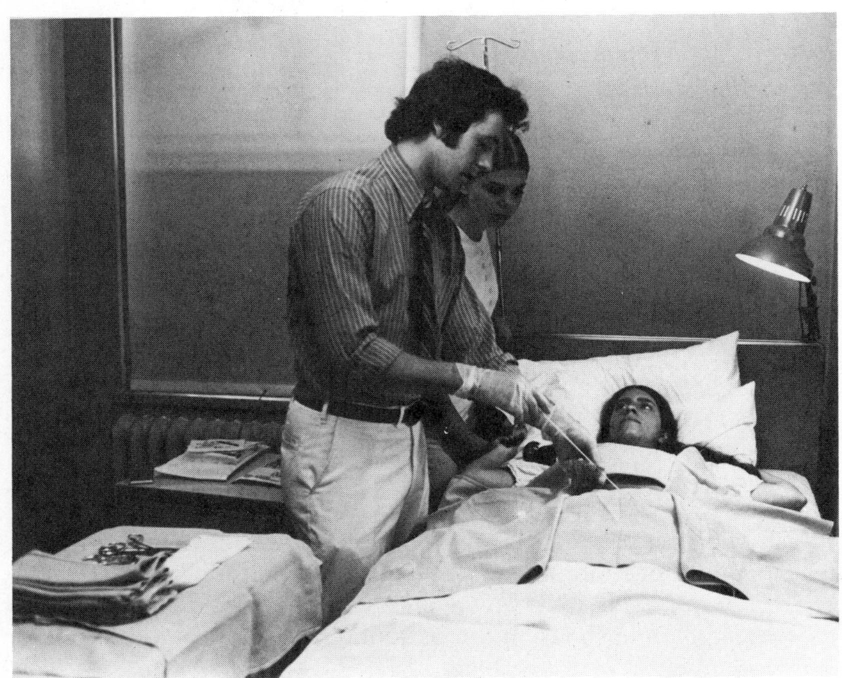

Figure 21. Insertion of the peritoneal catheter.

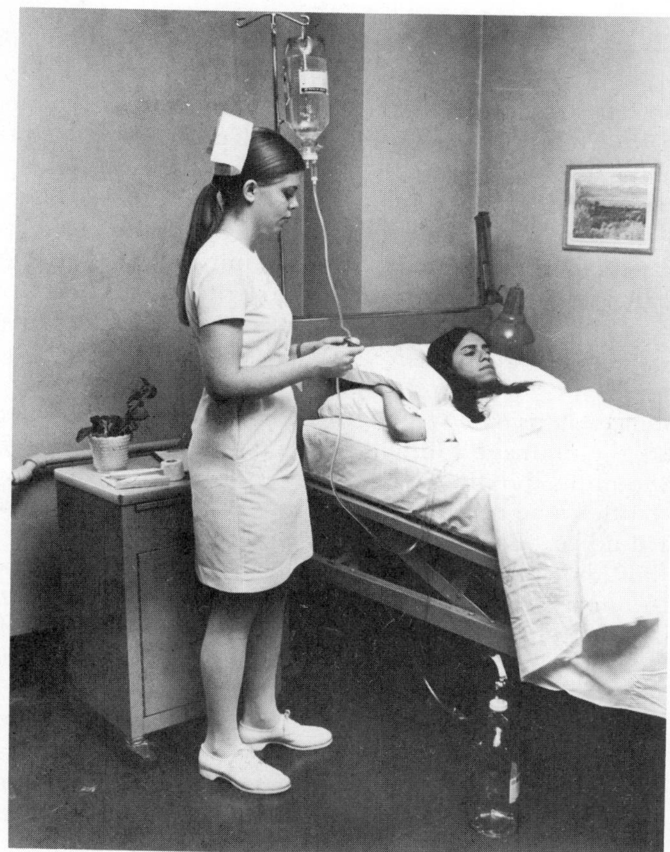

Figure 22. Nurse cycling dialysis solution.

urine should be tested for every patient; even a nondiabetic patient can absorb large quantities of glucose from the dialysate and become hyperglycemic.

The patient's vital signs—temperature, pulse, respirations, blood pressure, and central venous pressure—are taken at intervals during the dialysis, usually every two hours. Any significant changes such as a fall in blood pressure or a temperature elevation are reported.

The nurse gives the patient hygienic care during the dialysis. The best time for baths, backrubs, and other hygienic procedures is during the equilibration and outflow periods. During the inflow period, movement is often uncomfortable. Sometimes, moving about during the outflow period interferes with drainage, and the bath will have to be stopped. The patient helps with his care, if he is able. Backrubs are important, as the patient must spend most of his time in bed, lying on his back or side.

Occasionally a patient will be permitted to get out of bed for a few minutes to relax and change his position. The nurse disconnects the administration tubing from the peritoneal catheter and covers the catheter with sterile material.

The nurse will often encounter difficulties with dialysate drainage. To help prevent drainage difficulties, she adds ordered heparin to the dialysate. The usual dose is 50 – 100 units heparin/L. She keeps air out of the administration tubing and peritoneal cavity, as the air can form pockets and impair drainage. At the end of the inflow period, she closes the inflow clamp before air gets into the administration tubing.

If drainage stops or slows, there are several things the nurse tries. She checks the drainage tubing to be certain it is not clamped off or kinked. She milks the drainage tubing. She checks the airway in the drainage bottle to be certain it is patent, as air must escape from the bottle for fluid to enter it. She may need to loosen the cap on the drainage bottle or put a needle in the airway to establish airway patency. The nurse changes the patient's position, trying back and side positions. She often finds that a particular position promotes effective drainage in a particular patient. She irrigates the peritoneal catheter with heparinized saline or changes the position of the catheter slightly, as it may be blocked by omentum (a fold of the peritoneum) or a fibrin clot. She can sometimes leave a reservoir of 1–2 L of dialysate in the peritoneal cavity in order to maintain speed and ease of drainage. This reservoir keeps omentum from blocking the drainage holes and maintains a fluid level high enough so that the catheter is in constant contact with the dialysate. If the nurse cannot restore adequate drainage despite these measures, she notifies the physician. A new catheter may have to be inserted because the old one remains occluded or is poorly positioned.

The patient may complain of abdominal discomfort during the dialysis. The nurse puts an ordered local anesthetic, such as procaine 50 mg/L, into the dialysate. She gives ordered systemic analgesics, such as propoxyphene hydrochloride (Darvon) 65 mg orally, as needed. If the discomfort occurs during the inflow period, the nurse tries infusing the dialysate at a slower rate. Abdominal discomfort can be a sign of peritonitis, so the nurse looks carefully for any signs of this complication. The pain can be caused by air in the abdomen, so the nurse is careful to keep air out of the administration tubing and peritoneal cavity.

The nurse observes the patient carefully for signs and symptoms of any of the complications described earlier. If peritonitis develops, the patient has abdominal pain and tenderness and ri-

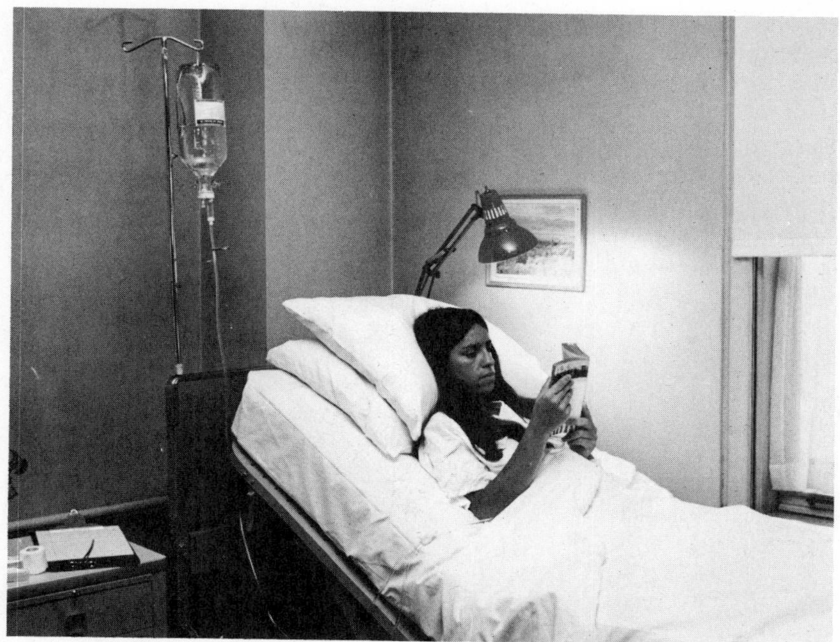

Figure 23. Patient resting comfortably during peritoneal dialysis.

gidity of the abdominal wall, and the drained dialysate is cloudy owing to the presence of bacteria. The nurse sends an aliquot of this dialysate for culture and notifies the physician. If the bowel is perforated, the patient experiences pain, and fecal matter is present in the dialysate. The nurse stops the dialysis and notifies the physician. If the symptoms of pulmonary edema—rapid respirations, rales, and tachycardia—develop, the nurse begins dialysate drainage immediately and notifies the doctor. If the drained dialysate is bloody after the first few exchanges, the nurse notifies the doctor, as this indicates abdominal bleeding. The nurse checks the patient's urine for glucose, to ascertain if he is developing hyperglycemia.

Automatic Dialysis Machines, Permanent Peritoneal Access Devices, and Long-Term Peritoneal Dialysis

Automatic cycling machines for peritoneal dialysis are available. The first machine of this type was developed by Boen, Mulinari, Dillard, and Scribner in 1962.[4] The operation of the machine is as follows. Sterile dialysate is pumped from a 20–40 L container into an elevated reservoir, where the cycle volume is preset, usually at 2 L. At the beginning of dialysis, an inflow valve opens, and the desired volume of fluid flows into the abdomen by gravity. The inflow valve then closes, and the reservoir refills. The dialysate remains in the peritoneal cavity during the equilibration period. At the start of the outflow period, an outflow valve opens, and dialysate then drains into a sterile calibrated bottle. This completes the cycle. An alarm sounds if too much dialysate remains in the patient because of drainage difficulties (Fig. 24).

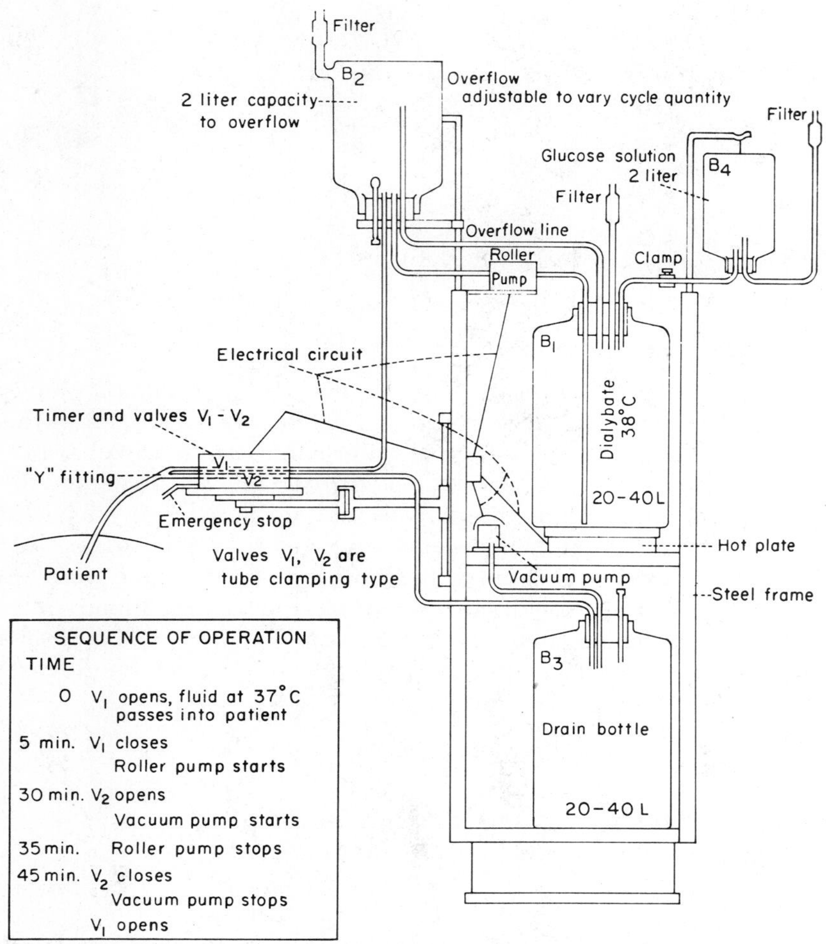

Figure 24. Schematic drawing of automatic cycling machine for peritoneal dialysis. (From Boen, S. T.: *Peritoneal Dialysis in Clinical Medicine.* Springfield, Ill. Charles C Thomas, 1964.)

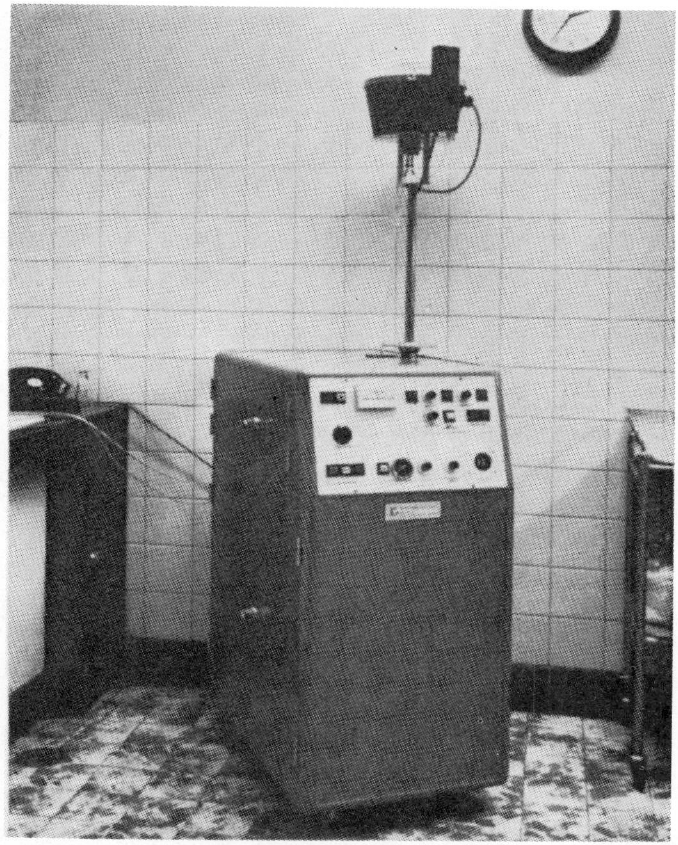

Figure 25. The "Sefton" automatic peritoneal dialysis machine. (From Peachey, J.: Automatic peritoneal dialysis. *Bio-med. Engin.*, *4*:461, 1969.)

Several other automatic peritoneal dialysis machines are available. These function in the same basic manner as the one designed by Boen et al. (Figs. 25 and 26).[2, 21]

Permanent peritoneal catheters are implanted in some patients who require long-term peritoneal dialysis. One such catheter, developed by Tenckhoff et al., is made of Silastic tubing and has Dacron felt cuffs. The catheter is 40 cm long and is divided into three sections: the intra-abdominal section is 20 cm long and has numerous perforations; the middle section is 10 cm; the section that is external to the body is 10 cm. A rubber cap fits over the end of the external section. Two felt cuffs are located on the catheter; one is just superficial to the peritoneum and the other is just beneath the epidermis. These felt cuffs help anchor the catheter securely and help prevent infection by

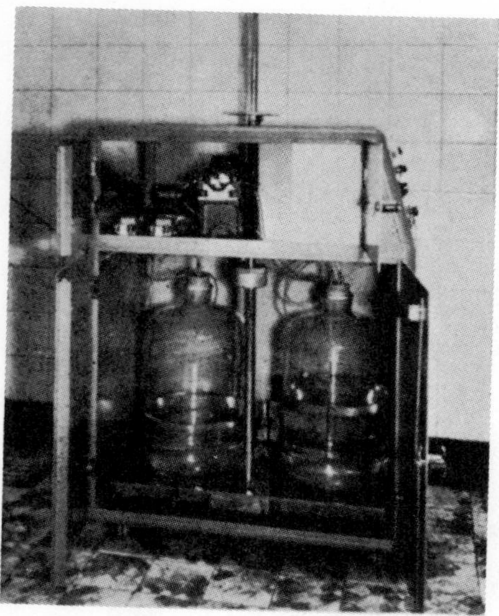

Figure 26. Side view of the "Sefton" machine with its doors open. (From Peachey, J.: Automatic Peritoneal Dialysis. *Bio-med. Engin., 4*:463, 1969.)

encouraging closure of the sinus tract around the catheter (Figs. 27 and 28).[26, 30]

Other permanent peritoneal access devices are being developed and are in use.[7, 12, 14, 35] But permanent peritoneal catheters are not widely used. They often eventually lead to peritoneal infection, and

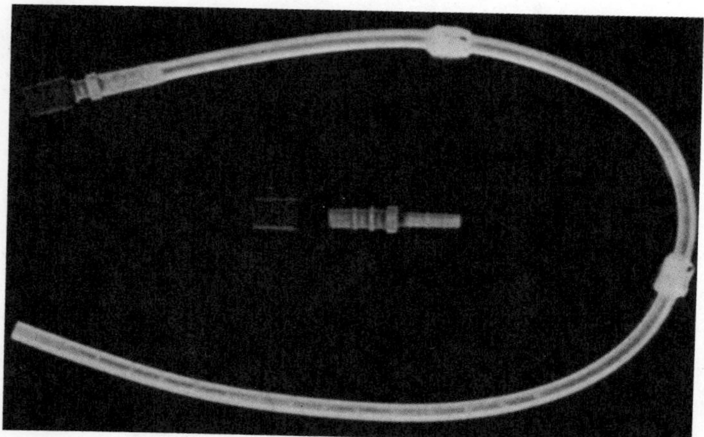

Figure 27. Straight Silastic catheter with Dacron felt cuffs, connector, and cap. (From Tenckhoff, H., and Schechter, H.: A bacteriologically safe peritoneal access device. *Trans. Amer. Soc. Artif. Inter. Organs, 14*:182, 1968. Reprinted with the specific permission of the editor, Dr. George E. Schreiner, Georgetown University, Washington, D.C.)

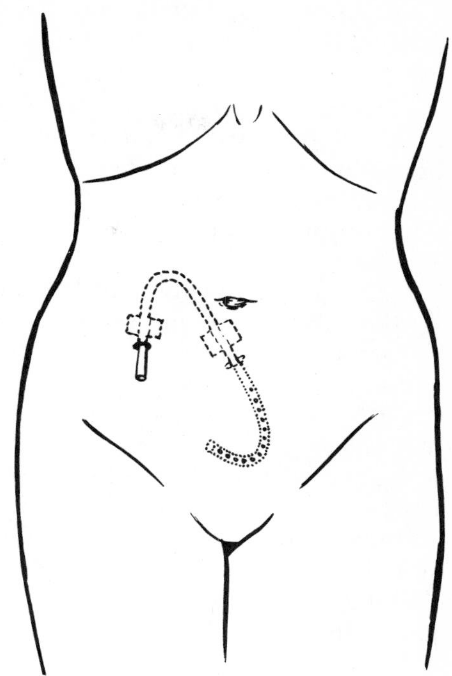

Figure 28. Cuffed Silastic catheter implanted, skin exit in right lower abdominal quadrant, short subcutaneous tunnel. (From Tenckhoff, H., and Schechter, H.: A bacteriologically safe peritoneal access device. *Trans. Amer. Soc. Artif. Intern. Organs, 14*:183, 1968. Reprinted with the specific permission of the editor. Dr. George E. Schreiner, Georgetown University, Washington, D.C.)

many practitioners, therefore, prefer to insert a new catheter each time dialysis is performed.

In some centers, peritoneal dialysis is used as a permanent measure for maintaining the lives of patients with chronic renal failure who are medically or financially unsuitable for hemodialysis. These patients usually have permanent peritoneal catheters, and automatic cycling machines are used. Some of these patients receive dialysis in the hospital. Others are taught to perform dialysis at home.[13, 20, 29, 31]

As an example of the effectiveness of long-term peritoneal dialysis, Tenckhoff and Curtis reported that they had, for periods up to four years, maintained 19 patients with long-term peritoneal dialysis. Sixteen of the patients performed self-dialysis at home; three were dialyzed in the hospital. They felt that, in general, the patients were well and rehabilitated.[29]

However, the feasibility of using long-term peritoneal dialysis as an alternative to hemodialysis or transplantation is not clearly established. Problems of peritoneal infection, economy of time, and preparation of sterile dialysate in the home remain. At present, peritoneal dialysis is generally considered desirable for short-term therapy only.

Comparison of Peritoneal Dialysis and Hemodialysis

The same chemical results can usually be achieved by either peritoneal dialysis or hemodialysis. But there are important differences between the two forms of therapy, and one is often more appropriate than the other for given circumstances.

The disadvantages of peritoneal dialysis compared to hemodialysis are:

1. Peritoneal dialysis is slower than hemodialysis. Urea clearance is about 26 ml/min with peritoneal dialysis; it is between 70 and 170 ml/min with hemodialysis. The same removal of wastes and normalization of fluid and electrolytes can be achieved with both types of dialysis, but it takes about four times as long with peritoneal dialysis. Hemodialysis is, therefore, preferable when rapid removal of wastes is critical to life. Hemodialysis is also preferable when long-term dialysis is necessary. A patient receiving hemodialysis spends about 12 hr/week on a Kiil dialyzer, while one receiving peritoneal dialysis spends 30–48 hr/week undergoing dialysis. The amount of time spent undergoing peritoneal dialysis can interfere with leading a normal, productive life.

2. A satisfactory permanent peritoneal catheter has not been developed. Several types are in use, but none has been developed that affords adequate safety from peritoneal infection. The shunts and fistulas used for hemodialysis are reasonably satisfactory.

3. Peritoneal dialysis causes protein loss. The patient loses about 20–30 gm of protein/day while undergoing peritoneal dialysis. This serum protein depletion does not occur with hemodialysis.

4. Peritoneal dialysis requires sterile irrigating fluid. This causes supply problems, especially for patients at home. Hemodialysis does not require sterile bath solution.

5. Peritoneal dialysis cannot be performed on patients with extensive abdominal adhesions, bowel perforation or localized peritonitis. Hemodialysis can be performed on such patients.

The advantages of peritoneal dialysis compared to hemodialysis are:

1. Peritoneal dialysis is a fairly simple procedure. The equipment needed is simple and the dialysis procedure itself is fairly simple and does not require extensive training for doctors or nurses. Thus, peritoneal dialysis can be performed in nearly every hospital. By contrast, hemodialysis requires elaborate equipment and training, and, therefore, is usually performed only in special centers.

2. Peritoneal dialysis can be instituted quickly. It can be started in one half to one hour, while more time is required to start hemodialysis—an artery and vein must be cannulated, and the machine must

be prepared. This aspect of time can be critical, as when the patient has a high serum potassium concentration. A few quick cycles of peritoneal dialysis can bring the patient out of danger, while he might die awaiting hemodialysis.

3. Peritoneal dialysis does not require heparinization. Hemodialysis does, however, require heparinization. Peritoneal dialysis is, therefore, preferable when the use of heparin would be dangerous. This drug is hazardous for patients who have recently undergone major surgery or who have gastrointestinal bleeding or bleeding defects.

4. Peritoneal dialysis is efficient and safe for infants and young children. It is more efficient in infants and young children than in adults, because the size of the peritoneum in the child is greater in relation to body size than in the adult. It is also a fairly safe procedure for infants and young children. Hemodialysis, however, is technically difficult to perform on these small people.

The cost of peritoneal dialysis and hemodialysis is approximately the same, although in some cases the former may be slightly less expensive. At the University of Washington, Seattle, according to Tenckhoff, in-hospital peritoneal dialysis costs about $185: $50 for catheter insertion and $135 for each 80 L dialysis, using an automatic peritoneal dialysis machine. (The cost would be greater if an automatic machine were not used, as more nursing care would be required.) Inhospital hemodialysis is about $300: $150 for cannulation and $150 for each dialysis.[32]

Costs of home peritoneal dialysis during the first year include $7500 for equipment, an average of $100 for home modification, $1500 for three weeks of home training, and approximately $23 per 80 L dialysis for supplies. The total cost during the first year for a patient requiring three dialyses per week would be approximately $12,688. During subsequent years, the cost of home peritoneal dialysis continues at about $23 per 80 L dialysis, or $3588 per year for a patient requiring three dialyses per week.[32]

Cost of home hemodialysis is approximately $10,000–$12,000 for the first year, including equipment and training. During subsequent years, home hemodialysis costs about $3000–$5000 per year.

CASE STUDIES

I

A 23 year old male waiter in a Chinese restaurant was admitted to CPMC 4/12/72, with the chief complaint of malaise and nausea. He had a blood pressure of 150/110, cardiomegaly, and pulmonary vascular congestion. The following laboratory data were obtained: Na 138, K 5.0, CO_2 18, Cl 95, and Ca 5.5 mEq/L; BUN 158, creatinine 18.9, and uric acid 10.67 mg/100 ml; hbg 5.4 gm/100 ml; and hct 16.9 per cent. The diagnosis was end-stage renal disease, probably secondary to chronic glomerulonephritis, although the patient gave no history of previous acute glomerulonephritis or streptococcal infection. Application was begun for a hemodialysis program.

The patient was initially treated conservatively with Amphojel, phenobarbital, and a diet of 20 gm protein, 2 gm sodium, no potassium, and 800 ml fluid/day. In spite of this treatment, his clinical condition deteriorated. He had several episodes of epistaxis, probably secondary to hypertension and impaired platelet function, and he complained of increasing malaise. On 4/17, his BUN was 216 ml/100 ml.

Peritoneal dialysis was begun on 4/17, and continued until 4/20, in order to prevent further clinical deterioration before a slot in a hemodialysis program became available. The following dialysis solutions were used:

Exchanges 1–11 – 4.25 per cent dialysate + 50 units heparin/L + 1.25–4 mEq potassium/L

Exchanges 12–49 – 1.5 per cent dialysate + 50 units heparin/L + 3 mEq potassium/L

The dialyzing rate was approximately 1.6 L/hr.

When the first 2 L of dialysate were infused into the peritoneal cavity, the nurse noted that the patient became acutely short of breath. His blood pressure rose to 190/130, pulse to 120, and respiration to 40. She summoned the physician. Pulmonary edema secondary to fluid overload was diagnosed. The patient was treated with oxygen, morphine, furosemide (Lasix), and hyperosmolar dialysis, with resolution of the pulmonary edema. A second episode of pulmonary edema occurred during the dialysis. It was treated successfully with oxygen, rotating tourniquets, morphine, aminophylline, digoxin, and continued dialysis. The peritoneal dialysis was otherwise uneventful and well-tolerated by the patient.

At the completion of the dialysis, the patient's BUN was 91, serum creatinine 11.4, and uric acid 8.58 mg/100 ml; potassium 3.8, CO_2 29, and calcium 6.79 mEq/L; hbg 6.4 gm/100 ml; and hct 21.0 per cent. He had a net fluid loss of 5675 ml. Malaise, nausea, and epistaxis had disappeared.

On 4/25/72, the patient was accepted into a hemodialysis program. He was discharged from CPMC on the following regimen: folic acid 5 mg orally/day, multivitamins one tablet orally once a day, and a diet consisting of 50 gm protein and 1 gm sodium. He is now receiving hemodialysis on an outpatient basis and is awaiting a kidney transplant.

II*

A 33 year old patient, pregnant for the fifth time, gave birth to a normal boy on 6/22/58. In the morning and evening of the following day, she had seizures, became comatose, and developed a temperature of 102.7° F. She was hospitalized and treated with phenobarbital, chlorpromazine, penicillin, streptomycin, estradiol (dimenformon), and ACTH. The patient regained con-

*Data from Boen, G. T.: *Peritoneal Dialysis in Clinical Medicine.* Springfield, Ill., Charles C Thomas, 1964.

sciousness, and her temperature returned to normal. On 6/24, the patient's urine output was 600 ml, decreasing to 60 ml by 6/26.

The patient was admitted to the hospital on 6/26 in a drowsy condition. Blood pressure was 175/100. The following laboratory data were obtained: Na 134.5, K 5.15, CO_2 12.2, CL 99, and Ca 3.6 mEq/L; BUN 282 and creatinine 11.6 mg/100 ml; and hbg 11.5 gm/100 ml.

The patient was placed on a butter and sugar diet with a fluid restriction of 750 ml/day. Despite the diet, her clinical condition continued to deteriorate because of the obligatory protein breakdown following birth due to involution of the uterus and breasts. On June 28, the patient's CO_2 was 9.4 mEq/L, blood pH 7.25, K 6.9 mEq/L, and BUN 470 mg/100 ml.

Peritoneal dialysis was instituted 6/28, and continued for 39 hours. The peritoneal catheter was inserted carefully, behind the uterus, to avoid perforation of this organ. Dialysate of 1.5–2.5 per cent glucose with 2 mg heparin/L and no potassium was used.

Following dialysis, the patient's CO_2 was 21.4 mEq/L, blood pH 7.47, K 4.0 mEq/L, and BUN 216 mg/100 ml. The patient had a net fluid loss of 800 ml. She showed mental improvement.

During the next week, the BUN again increased rapidly, as involution of the uterus was not completed. On 7/4, the diuretic phase set in. During the early part of the diruretic phase, the patient was given sodium and potassium supplements to replace urinary losses of these substances. Kidney function and blood chemistry gradually returned to normal. On 8/11, the creatinine clearance was 83 ml/min, and the plasma creatinine was 0.8 mg/100 ml. The patient was discharged in excellent condition with normal blood pressure and no dietary restrictions.

References

1. Abbott Laboratories, North Chicago, Ill. 60064.
2. Automated peritoneal dialysis. *Biomed. Engin.*, *5*:312, 1970.
3. Beeson, P. B., and McDermott, W. (Eds.): *Cecil-Loeb Textbook of Medicine,* Thirteenth edition. Philadelphia, W. B. Saunders Co., 1971.
4. Boen, S. T.: *Peritoneal Dialysis in Clinical Medicine.* Springfield, Ill. Charles C Thomas, 1964.
5. Cutter Laboratories, Berkeley, Calif. 94710.
6. Dunea, G.: Peritoneal dialysis and hemodialysis. *Med. Clin. N. Amer.*, *55*:155–175, 1971.
7. Ersek, R. A.: Peritoneal access device for dialysis. J.A.M.A., *215*:1326, 1971.
8. Gault, H. M., Ferguson, E. L., and Cobin, R. P.: Fluid and electrolyte complications of peritoneal dialysis, choice of dialysis solutions. *Ann. Intern. Med.*, *75*:253–262, 1971.
9. Jones, H. J.: Peritoneal dialysis. *Brit. Med. Bull.*, *27*:165–169, 1971.
10. Kintzel, K. C. (Ed.): *Advanced Concepts in Clinical Nursing.* Philadelphia, J. B. Lippincott Co., 1971.
11. Lasker, N.: Chronic peritoneal dialysis. *Pa. Med.*, *74*:67–69, 1971.
12. Lewkonia, R. M.: Simple indwelling cannula for repeated peritoneal dialysis. *Lancet*, *2*:123–135, 1970.
13. McDonald, H. P., Jr : An automatic peritoneal dialysis machine for hospital or home peritoneal dialysis: preliminary report. *Trans. Amer. Soc. Artif. Intern. Organs*, *15*:108–111, 1969.
14. McDonald, H. P., Jr., Gerber, N., Mishra, D., Wolin, L., Peng, B., and Waterhouse, K.: Subcutaneous Dacron and Teflon cloth adjuncts for Silastic arteriovenous shunts and peritoneal dialysis catheters. *Trans. Soc. Artif. Intern. Organs*, *14*:176–180, 1968.

15. McGraw Laboratories, Glendale, California 91201.
16 Meltzer, L. E., Abdallah, F. G., and Kitchell, J. R.: *Concepts and Practices of Intensive Care for Nurse Specialists.* Philadelphia, The Charles Press Publishers, Inc., 1969.
17. Miller, R. B., and Tassistro, C. R.: Peritoneal dialysis. *New Eng. J. Med., 287*:945–949, 1969.
18. Nienhuis, L. I.: Clinical peritoneal dialysis. *Arch. Surg., 93*:643–653, 1966.
19. O'Neill, M.: Peritoneal dialysis. *Nurs. Clin. N. Amer., 1*:2:309–322, 1966.
20. Palmer, R. A., Newell, J. E., Gray, J. E., and Quinton, W. E.: Treatment of chronic renal failure by prolonged peritoneal dialysis. *New Eng. J. Med., 274*:248–254, 1966.
21. Peachey, J.: Automatic peritoneal dialyzer. *Biomed. Engin., 4*:460–463, 1969.
22. Persky L., and Cumming, W. S.: Peritoneal dialysis. *Surg. Clin. N. Amer., 49*:3, 665–669, 1969.
23. Schreiner, G. E., and Teehan, B. P.: Dialysis of poisons and drugs—annual review. *Trans. Amer. Soc. Artif. Intern. Organs, 17*:513–544, 1971.
24. Schwartz, F. D., Kallmeyer, J., Dunea, G., and Kark, R. M.: Prevention of infection during peritoneal dialysis. *J.A.M.A., 199*:79–81, 1967.
25. Secor, J.: Peritoneal dialysis: a nursing challenge. *RN*, 67–72, 102, August, 1965.
26. Sticker, G. E., and Tenckhoff, H. A. M.: A transcutaneous prosthesis for prolonged access to the peritoneal cavity. *Surgery, 69*:70–74, 1971.
27. Swartz, C., Onesti, G., Maillous, L., Neff, M., Ramirez, O., Germon, P., Kazen, I., and Brady, L. W.: The acute hemodynamic and pulmonary perfusion effects of peritoneal dialysis. *Trans. Amer. Soc. Artif. Intern. Organs, 15*:367–372, 1969.
28. Tenckhoff, H.: Editorial notes, choice of peritoneal dialysis solutions. *Ann. Intern. Med., 75*:313–314, 1971.
29. Tenckhoff, H., and Curtis, F. K.: Experience with maintenance peritoneal dialysis in the home. *Trans. Soc. Artific. Intern. Organs, 16*:90–95, 1970.
30. Tenckhoff, H., and Schecter, H.: A bacteriologically safe peritoneal access device. *Trans. Amer. Soc. Artif. Intern. Organs, 14*:181–186, 1968.
31. Tenckhoff, H., Shilipetar, G., Van Paasschen, W. H., and Swanson, E.: A home peritoneal dialysate delivery system. *Trans. Amer. Soc. Artific. Intern. Organs, 15*:103–107, 1969.
32. Tenckhoff, Henry. Personal communication.
33. Teviso, M. R.: Peritoneal dialysis. *Amer. J. Nurs., 59*:1560–1563, 1959.
34. Travenol Laboratories, Inc., Morton Grove, Ill. 60053.
35. Vidt, D. G., Somerville, J., and Schulty R. W.: A safe peritoneal access device for repeated peritoneal dialysis. *J.A.M.A., 214*:2293–2296, 1970.
36. Wenzl, J. E., Mills, S. D., and McCall, T.: Methanol poisoning in an infant, successful treatment with peritoneal dialysis. *Amer. J. Dis. Child., 116*:445–447, 1968.
37. Weston, R. E., and Roberts, M.: Clinical use of stylet-catheter for peritoneal dialysis. *Arch. Intern. Med., 115*:659–662, 1965.
38. Wintrobe, M., Thorn, G. W., Adams, R. D., Bennett, I. L., Jr., Braunwald, E., Isselbacher, K. J., and Petersdorf, R. G. (Eds.): *Harrison's Principles of Internal Medicine.* Sixth edition. New York, McGraw-Hill Book Co., 1970.

CHAPTER 7

Hemodialysis

In 1943, Dr. Willem Kolff introduced the first practical artificial kidney to clinical medicine. With this machine he demonstrated that extracorporeal purification of the blood was feasible. At that time, however, the artificial kidney was used only in the treatment of potentially reversible acute renal failure. General acceptance of this radical treatment was very slow owing to the complexity of the procedure and the lack of convincing evidence that dialysis could reduce the mortality rates of uremic patients. Today the use of hemodialysis for the patient with severe renal failure is considered a standard form of therapy.

Dr. Kolff's rotating drum dialyzer was the forerunner of many dialyzers devised by other investigators. The early machines were expensive, cumbersome, and difficult to assemble and operate. These difficulties, combined with lack of enthusiasm for the treatment among practitioners, severely limited the widespread application of hemodialysis as a life-supporting procedure. The first disposable, presterilized, and reasonably priced unit was introduced by Dr. Kolff in 1956.[51] The development of this twin-coil artificial kidney greatly increased the number of hospitals equipped to perform hemodialysis. However, two things detracted from its use for patients needing long-term chronic dialysis; first, the machine required two units of blood for priming, and second, it required a pump to propel the blood.

In an attempt to overcome the disadvantages of the twin-coil dialyzer, Dr. Kiil, in 1960, developed a parallel-flow or layer dialyzer that is uncomplicated to construct and operate. Modifications of the Kiil dialyzer were adopted across the country in rapidly expanding long-term dialysis programs. Despite the large variety of machines developed, only two types are commercially available in this country at present, i.e., the disposable twin-coil kidney with its various models, and the two-layer, parallel-flow dialyzer.

Chronic dialysis programs grew slowly until 1961 when the development of cannula shunts by Quinton and Scribner made it possible to use the artificial kidney for repeated treatment of patients with irreversible renal disease. By 1964, hemodialysis as a therapeutic technique changed from an expensive research-type treatment to one that could be done by the patient himself in his own home. Developments such as these in the field of dialysis, together with improvements in renal homograft techniques, restore useful, productive lives to many of the 30,000 patients annually who otherwise would die of terminal kidney failure.

In light of these changes, the concepts of caring for patients with renal disease also had to be altered. Medical and paramedical professionals now view the management of chronic uremia as a continuum beginning with diagnosis of chronic renal failure and progressing to treatment with long-term hemodialysis and renal homotransplantation.

Principles of Hemodialysis

Diffusion

Dialysis, either peritoneal dialysis or hemodialysis, is based primarily on the physiological concept of diffusion. Essentials for any dialysis are two fluid compartments separated by a semipermeable membrane that contains microscopic pores. Small dissolved particles (ions and molecules) pass through the membrane pores and diffuse from an area of greater concentration to an area of lesser concentration until an equilibrium is reached. Thus waste materials such as urea, creatinine, and uric acid diffuse out of the blood into the dialysate. Large molecules such as protein and blood cells are unable to diffuse across the membrane. Figure 29 illustrates this principle. Dialysis specifically means the passage of particles in solution through a semipermeable membrane. Diffusion and filtration are the physiological processes that allow dialysis to occur. This is essentially the same mechanism as that used by the natural kidney to excrete waste products.

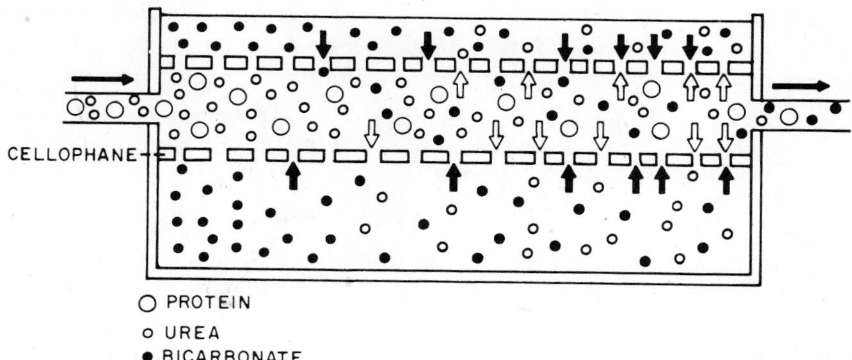

Figure 29. Schematic representation of diffusion and the function of the artificial kidney. (From Fellows, B. J.: The role of the nurse in a chronic dialysis unit. *Nurs. Clin. N. Amer., 1*:4:578, 1966.)

DIALYSIS

The primary function of the healthy kidney is the elimination of waste products and the maintenance of fluid and electrolyte balance in the body. The kidney accomplishes these goals by filtration in the glomeruli, and reabsorption and secretion in the tubules. The basic physiological principles involved in normal renal function are filtration, osmosis, and diffusion. The diseased kidney, however, is unable to perform one or more of these functions adequately. Hence, the artificial kidney was developed to accomplish them.

The primary purpose of the artificial kidney is identical to that of the normal kidney: to eliminate waste products and to maintain fluid and electrolyte balance. The artificial kidney accomplishes these goals by "duplicating" the functions of the natural kidney. For example, the artificial kidney mimics the function of the glomerulus by eliminating waste products from the blood by filtration and diffusion across a semipermeable membrane. The patient's blood flows within a cellophane or Cuprophane membrane and the dialyzing fluid flows on the outside of the membrane, continuously bathing the blood.

DIALYSATE

Dialysate is the solution used in the artificial kidney to bathe the blood. The chemical composition of dialysate is essentially that of normal serum (Table 3). It is not sterile, i.e., free of bacteria and other microorganisms, since bacteria are too large to pass through the membrane to the blood. In most dialysis units the water used to make up the

TABLE 3. Electrolyte Composition of Dialysate and Normal Serum (mEq/liter)

	DIALYSATE*	NORMAL SERUM†
Sodium	135	136–145
Chloride	100	96–106
Bicarbonate	35–40 (acetate)	24–30 (CO_2 content)
Potassium	0–1	3.5–5.0
Calcium	3	4.5–5.5
Magnesium	1	1.5–2.5
Glucose	200	60–100

*Data from Pendras, J. P., and Stinson, G. W.: *The Hemodialysis Manual.* Seattle, Wash., Edmark Corp., 1970.

†Data from Beeson, P. B., and McDermott, W. (Eds.): *Cecil-Loeb Textbook of Medicine.* Thirteenth edition. Philadelphia, W. B. Saunders Co., 1971.

dialysate solution is de-ionized tap water, i.e., tap water that has been treated to remove calcium, magnesium, sodium, and other electrolytes that would affect the dialysate concentration.

Like the glomerular membrane, the artificial membrane is impermeable to blood colloids and larger molecular complexes. Waste products of metabolism and water and electrolytes pass freely across the membrane until an equilibrium is reached.

CONCENTRATION GRADIENT

The direction of the movement of diffusable substances depends on the difference in concentration on both sides of the membrane, i.e., the concentration gradient. The specific electrolyte concentration of the dialyzing fluid, plus the length of the dialysis, determines the final composition of the patient's blood. Since the dialyzing fluid has the same composition as normal plasma, the more abnormal the patient's plasma, the greater will be the concentration gradient across the membrane and the more rapid the rate of clearance. Waste products such as urea, creatinine, and uric acid, and excess electrolytes such as sodium, potassium, and magnesium diffuse across the membrane from the patient's blood (the area of higher concentration) to the dialyzing fluid (the area of lower concentration). Conversely, electrolytes of greater concentration in the dialyzing fluid such as calcium and bicarbonate diffuse into the patient's blood and correct deficits (see Fig. 29). Deficiencies or excesses of sodium or potassium can be corrected within hours by the artificial kidney. For this reason hemodialysis may be employed in treating patients with lethally high potassium levels.

Pressure

In addition to the movement of electrolytes, water also moves across the membrane because of osmotic and hydrostatic pressures within the system. Osmotic pressure is the force necessary to propel water molecules through a semipermeable membrane separating unequal solutions containing nondiffusable particles. Hydrostatic pressure is the force exerted by a liquid against a membrane wall.

If the total pressure of the blood on one side of the membrane is greater than the pressure of the dialysate on the other side of the membrane, then filtration of water occurs from the blood to the dialyzing fluid. If the pressure of the blood within the membrane is significantly higher than that of the dialysate, then ultrafiltration of water from the blood occurs. ("Ultrafiltration" refers to the filtration of fluids and dissolved substances across a semipermeable membrane at a very rapid rate due to exceedingly high pressure within the system. For comparison, normal glomerular filtration pressure is 70 mm Hg while the ultrafiltration pressures within the dialyzer range between 150 and 400 mm Hg.)

Ultrafiltration is employed during hemodialysis in order to remove greater quantities of excess water from the patient more rapidly. The Kolff twin-coil system utilizes a blood pump to increase pressure in the blood compartment, thereby increasing the ultrafiltration pressure. The Kiil system accomplishes the same thing by reducing the pressure in the dialysate compartment through the use of a negative pressure pump. Osmosis may also be employed to draw off excess water during dialysis. In this situation glucose is added to the dialyzing solution, thus increasing the osmotic pressure of the dialysate and causing water to move from the blood into the dialysate. Glucose is used since its molecules are too large to diffuse easily across the membrane.

Flow rates

Blood. In general, the greater the blood flow rate through the dialyzer, the more efficient the dialysis. The blood flow rate is determined by the ability of the patient's artery to provide blood, and this is based on the type and condition of his shunt, his cardiac output, and his blood pressure. Blood pressure becomes a particularly important factor when a mechanical blood pump is not used. When a blood pump is used and the pumping rate exceeds the ability of the artery, negative pressure causes the artery to collapse. Most dialyzers function efficiently at blood flow rates of 100–300 ml/min.

Another factor affecting the blood flow in the dialyzer is viscosity.

The more viscous the blood the slower the rate of flow. Exposure to air increases the viscosity of the blood. Outside the body blood normally clots in 6–17 min, and even at high blood propulsion rates there is a danger of clotting in the system. Therefore, an anticoagulant, heparin, is used to prevent clotting and to allow the blood to flow rapidly through the system.

Dialysate. Efficient dialysis occurs when the dialysate flow rate is three to four times the blood flow rate. Therefore dialysate flow rates range from 300–1200 ml/min. At slower flow rates the concentration gradient in the system is insufficient to provide adequate dialysis. At greater flow rates there is no significant gain in dialysis efficiency.

Temperature

The efficiency of dialysis is directly proportional to the temperature of the dialysate. Warming the dialysate to body temperature promotes the most efficient dialysis and also eliminates the need to rewarm the blood before returning it to the patient.

Nursing implications of physiological principles

Awareness of the principles of dialysis is essential to providing safe patient care. Many physiological changes occur in uremic patients during dialysis, and astute observation by the nurse is required to monitor these changes. Knowledge and understanding of the physiological principles involved in dialysis enable the nurse to delineate her expectations for each patient realistically and plan the nursing care accordingly. The following examples show the application of physiological principles of dialysis to patient care.

1. *Principle:* Electrolytes diffuse from an area of greater concentration to an area of lesser concentration according to the concentration gradient.

   Application: Dialysate normally contains little or no potassium. If a patient's predialysis serum potassium level is 6.9 mEq/L, the nurse can expect that it will decrease during dialysis. She can also expect that the most rapid decrease will occur in the first two hours of dialysis when the concentration gradient is greatest.

   Nursing action: In addition to her awareness of the diffusion of potassium, the nurse's knowledge of the physiological effects of a rapidly changing serum potassium level alerts her to watch for the electrocardiographic changes described in chapters 3 and 5. Therefore, she will have an EKG machine available so that the patient can be monitored during dialysis.

2. *Principle:* A decrease in circulating blood volume causes a decrease in blood pressure and a compensatory increase in pulse.
   Application: When dialysis is initiated the patient's blood is pumped or flows by gravity into the dialyzing coil and is replaced by a sodium chloride solution. Several minutes is required for the system to reach an equilibrium. During this time a greater amount of the patient's blood may be in the dialyzer than is replaced by sodium chloride, resulting in a decrease in his fluid volume.
   Nursing action: Therefore, the patient's vital signs are monitored very closely while dialysis is being initiated. Vital signs may also change during dialysis since ultrafiltration causes loss of fluids, which would result in a decrease in circulating blood volume.
3. *Principle:* Urea diffuses from an area of greater concentration to an area of lesser concentration according to the concentration gradient.
   Application: Patients with excessive serum nitrogenous wastes as indicated by an elevated BUN level are frequently confused and lethargic. A reduction of the BUN results in improved functioning.
   Nursing action: The patient is monitored closely for improvement in intellectual function. This can be assessed by any number of techniques including having the patient count backward from 100 by 3's or by giving him a mathematical problem or riddle appropriate for his normal mental ability.

Indications for Hemodialysis

Severe uremia, whether reversible or irreversible, is the primary indication for dialysis.[68] Dialysis is also indicated in some cases of acute poisoning.

Acute Renal Failure

There has been a complete reversal in the attitude toward the use of hemodialysis in the treatment of acute renal failure over the past 25 years. In the 1940's and 1950's hemodialysis was considered a radical, unsafe treatment to be employed only when all other modes of treatment failed. It was not until 1959 that Teschan recommended "daily dialysis."[47] Although the practice of daily dialysis was not instituted by most centers, the concept of early rather than late dialysis gained support.

In acute renal failure the indications for dialysis as listed by Papper are: (1) the development of uremic symptoms, (2) uncontrolled hyperkalemia, and (3) uncontrolled symptomatic acidosis.[65]

In cases of acute renal failure in which very rapid dialysis is required or when frequent dialyses are expected, hemodialysis is preferred to peritoneal dialysis. Hemodialysis is also used for patients in acute renal failure whenever dialysis is necessary and indicated but peritoneal dialysis is contraindicated, as with patients who have had recent abdominal surgery. A complete list of contraindications is given in Chapter 6. In general early and frequent dialysis is the treatment of choice for severe acute renal failure regardless of the underlying cause.

POISONING

Poisoning is another major indication for hemodialysis. Statistics show that accidental, as well as intentional overdoses and exposure to industrial toxins are increasing at an alarming rate.[81] Schreiner divides acute poisoning for which hemodialysis can be used into two categories: dialyzable poisons whose rate of removal is critical to the patient's welfare and nephrotoxic poisons that damage the kidneys and are therefore similar to other causes of acute renal failure. Schreiner lists four basic criteria for the use of hemodialysis in acute poisoning:

1. The poison molecule diffuses through cellophane from plasma water and has a reasonable removal rate or dialysance.

2. The poison is sufficiently well distributed in accessible body fluid compartments. If substantial fractions of the absorbed poison dosage are bound to protein molecules, concentrated in important compartments (e.g., cerebrospinal fluid), or attain a significant intracellular concentration, then effective dialysis will be sharply limited. This restriction is diminished, however, if the "loculated" portion easily equilibrates with the plasma.

3. A relationship exists between the toxicity of the poison, the blood concentration, and the duration of the body's exposure to the circulating poison.

4. A sufficient amount of poison can be removed to enable the body's normal mechanisms for dealing with that particular poison to work effectively. These include metabolism, conjugation, and elimination of the substance by bowel and kidney.[77]

A review and list of dialyzable poisons is compiled annually by Schreiner et al., and appears in *Transactions of the American Society for Artificial Internal Organs*. The reviews include guidelines to enable the physician to determine when and when not to dialyze and this publication may be consulted for further detail on this subject. A list of dialyzable poisons appears in Appendix E.

Chronic renal failure

It is difficult to state concretely which patients should and which should not participate in a chronic dialysis program. This is partly because the criteria change rapidly. As the technical aspects of hemodialysis are perfected, the procedure is successfully applied to a greater number and variety of patients. The most important single criterion for initiating long-term hemodialysis is disabling irreversible uremia. Disabling means that the patient's symptoms are so severe that he is unable to carry out his usual activities. Specific criteria for accepting patients are established by the director-physician or the selection committee for each unit. In some cases the criteria for selection have been established by the state Department of Public Health. However, the criteria for all long-term hemodialysis programs share some common elements. In general the patients selected are between the ages of 18 and 60; are free of systemic disease and have been free of malignant disease for five years; and are free of cardiovascular, musculoskeletal, and neurological debilitation. It is essential to the success of the treatment that all patients selected be rehabilitable, be motivated to co-operate with the program, and be psychologically acceptable.

Dialyzers

Coil dialyzer

Several manufacturers make coil kidney machines and coils but they are all based on the original twin-coil machine developed by Kolff in 1956. The twin Ultra-Flo coil made by Travenol Laboratories is the most widely used coil at present (Fig. 30). The coils and necessary connecting tubings to complete the system are presterilized and ready for assembly. Most coils are standard and can be used with the Kolff artificial kidney or with the newer models of this canister machine made by various companies.

The coils consist of two parallel lengths of cellulose dialysis tubing, approximately 8.2 m long, wound spirally with a rigid plastic mesh for support. The dialyzing surface area of the Ultra-Flo 145 coil

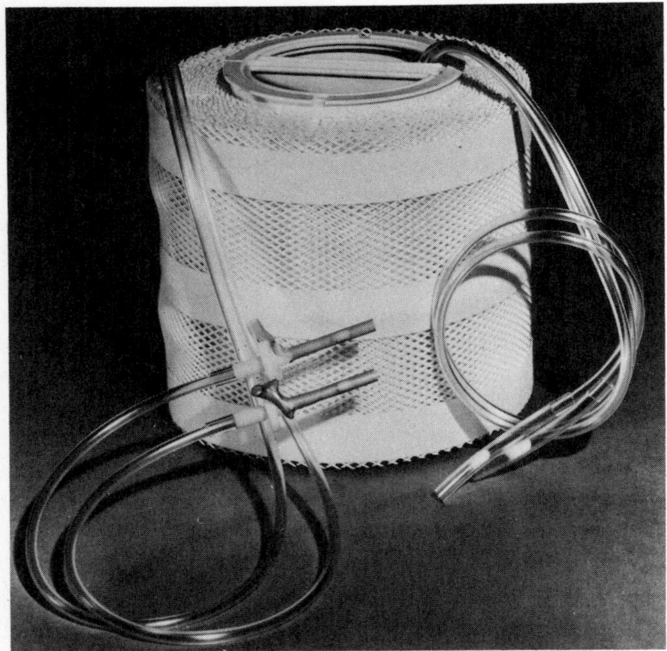

Figure 30. The coil dialyzing kidney. (Courtesy of Travenol Laboratories Incorporated, Morton Grove, Ill.)

is 14,500 sq cm. The original Kolff coil had a volume of 1200 ml and required blood to prime it. The coils used today have a volume of 200–500 ml and are primed with sterile isotonic saline.

As the patient's blood flows through the cellophane membrane, the dialysate fluid is forcefully pumped through and around the coil so that the blood in the tubing is constantly being bathed with dialysate. The fluid then spills over the top of the coil and back into the bath to be recirculated (Fig. 31). In the Kolff twin-coil dialyzer, the dialysate is continuously pumped and recirculated for two hours, at which time the blood and the bath are near equilibrium. The bath is then drained and a fresh dialysate solution is mixed. Thus every two hours there is a rapid shift in the concentration gradient as the fresh bath is circulated.

Several companies are producing coil dialyzers in which the bath is only slightly larger than the canister that holds the coil. These machines continuously deliver small amounts of fresh dialysate solution and allow continuous run-off of circulated dialysate (Fig. 32). The advantages with this system are that the bath does not require changing, thus less time and work are required maintaining the machine during dialysis; and that a continuous stable concentration gradient is maintained.

The coil dialyzers remove nitrogenous waste products and toxic substances efficiently; lethal amounts of potassium, urea, and certain drugs can be reduced in hours. Urea clearances achieved with the coil will vary in accordance with the initial level of the patient's blood urea, body weight, and blood volume and rate of flow through the

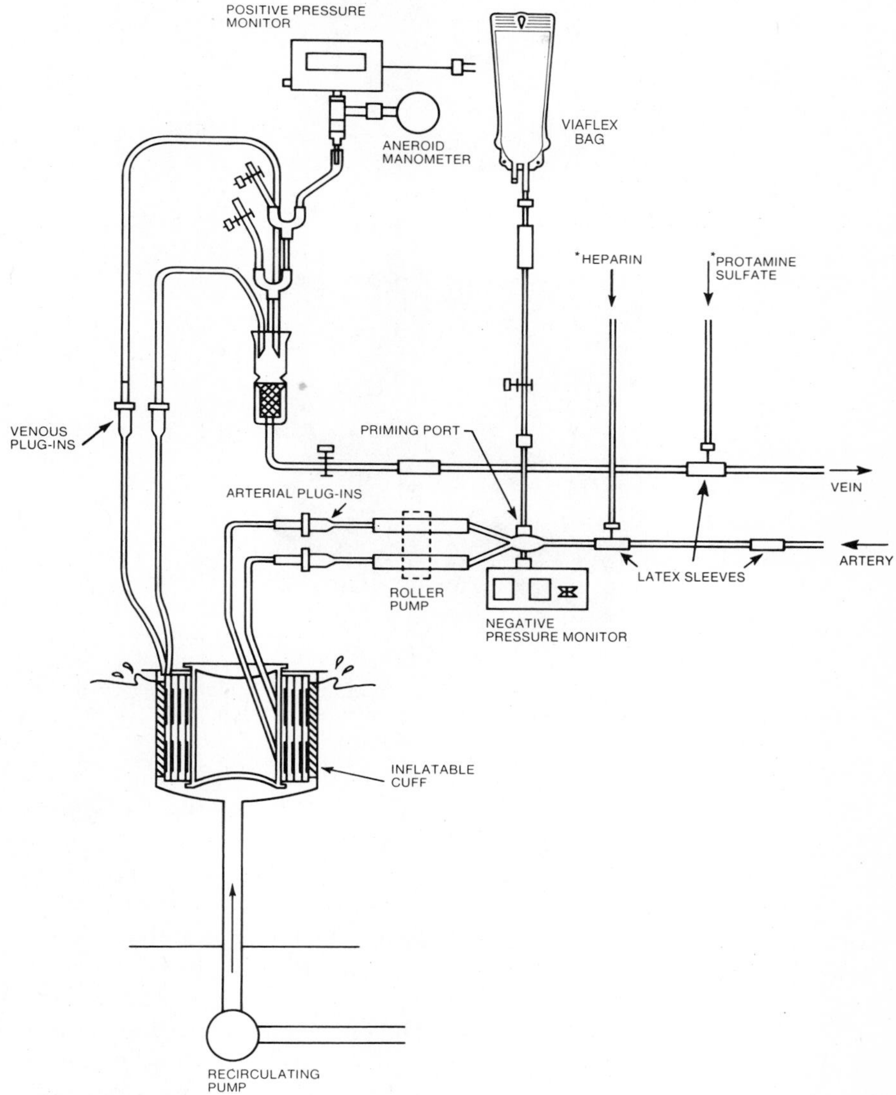

Figure 31. A drawing of the blood and dialysate circulation of the twin-coil artificial kidney system. (Courtesy of Travenol Laboratories Incorporated, Morton Grove, Ill.)

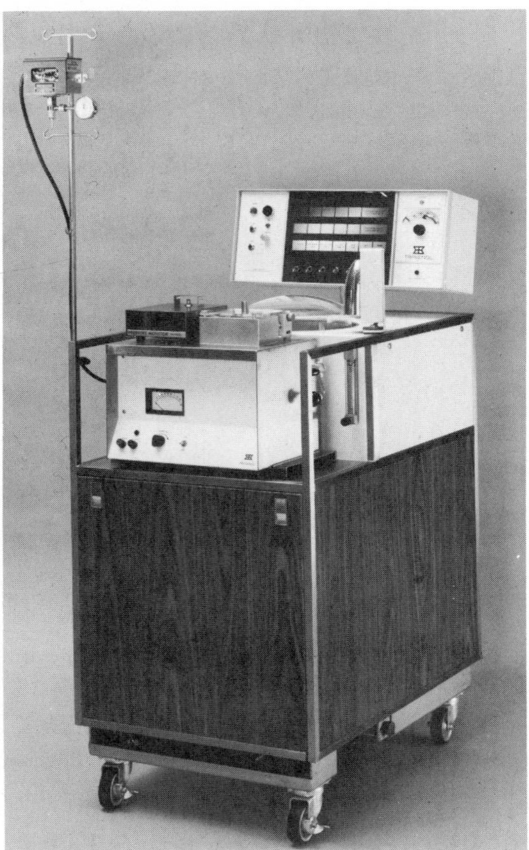

Figure 32. Recirculating single-pass (RSP) machine, a commonly used coil-type dialyzer. (Courtesy of Travenol Laboratories Incorporated, Morton Grove, Ill.)

dialyzing coil. At an average blood flow rate of 150–300 ml/min, urea clearance with Travenol's Ultra-Flo coil is in the range of 120–170 ml/min. These values are approximately 50 per cent and 70 per cent higher than those for the Kiil dialyzer.[94] Standard urea clearance in the natural kidney is 40–65 ml/min.[6] Creatinine clearance at these blood flow rates using the Ultra-Flo coil is approximately 80–120 ml/min. The normal creatinine clearance of a healthy male is 110–150 ml/min.

Due to the internal resistance of the coils, as much as 550 ml/hr of fluid can be ultrafiltered using only minimal (20 mm Hg) outflow resistance. Ultrafiltration can be increased by several milliliters per minute for every 100 mm Hg increment of pressure at the outflow. This is accomplished by placing a clamp on the venous return line and monitoring the pressure in the system. Weight loss due to ultrafiltration with the coil dialyzers has been reported up to 8.8 lb in a six-hour dialysis.[95]

The advantages of the coil dialyzers are that assembly of the coil is simple and can easily be managed by a woman within 20 minutes; coils are presterilized and ready for use; and coil machines are smaller and easier to clean. The greatest advantage to the patient is that dialysis for six hours on the coil accomplishes the same chemical results as 12 hours on the Kiil. Since the coil system utilizes a blood pump, hydrostatic pressure can be increased in the coil, causing greater ultrafiltration, which results in increased water loss by the patient.

There are also disadvantages to the coil dialyzer system. Coil dialyzers have high internal resistance and require a pump to propel the blood through them. A pump in the extracorporeal circuit increases the risk of hemorrhage if there is a leak in the system. A pump also makes it possible to introduce air emboli. However, this danger has been significantly reduced with the newer models of coil dialyzers that have pressure monitors that buzz when a negative pressure occurs in the line. The pump also causes trauma to blood cells, resulting in hemolysis. This is not a serious problem, however, since it has been shown that only 1 per cent of the total red blood cells are hemolyzed. If the pumping rates are increased beyond the capacity of the arterial cannula, the intima of the vessel may be traumatized. Rapid alterations of fluid and electrolytes occur more frequently with the coil-type dialyzer and may result in any number of disequilibrium symptoms including irritability, twitching, muscle cramps, nausea, headache, and vomiting. Another disadvantage of the coil dialyzer is that the coils are expensive. The cost of one coil with the tubings is approximately $35.00. This may be a great disadvantage to the patient whose income is average or limited. The patient on a high-flow coil dialyzer requires close supervision by a knowledgeable and well-trained person. This may present a problem for patients desiring home dialysis.

PARALLEL-FLOW DIALYZER

There are several models, including the Kiil artificial kidney, of layer or parallel-flow dialyzers. Since the most widely used of these is the Kiil model, this discussion is primarily limited to the Kiil.

It was in 1960 that Kiil first introduced this flat dialyzer, which at that time consisted of four parallel-flow cellophane blood chambers.[43] He quickly discovered that the large volume made it necessary to use a blood pump and to prime the machine with blood. Therefore his machine had no operating advantages over the coil kidney. A year later a new improved model was developed that is in wide use across the country today. This dialyzer consists of three longitudinally grooved polypropylene boards approximately 40 inches long by 15 inches wide by 6¾ inches high held together by a metal frame (Fig. 33). The patient's blood flows through two large flat cellophane membranes that are sandwiched between the boards. Since the volume of this model is only 300–400 ml there is no need to prime it with blood.

Unlike the coil dialyzers, the layer dialyzers have low internal resistance, which when combined with their small volume eliminates the need for a blood pump. The blood flow through the dialyzer is regulated by the patient's own blood pressure, the blood flow rate through the cannula, and the temperature of the dialysate. Blood flow rates average 100–200 ml/min but can be increased to as high as 300 ml/min by warming the dialysate to 37° C.[10] The dialysate solution flows in the opposite direction to the blood between the cellophane through the grooves in the boards (Fig. 34). The dialyzing surface area is approximately 1 sq m, which is just slightly less than that of the Ultra-Flo 145 coil dialyzer. For the parallel-flow systems, fresh dialysate continuously flows outside the cellophane from the inlet to the outlet and is discarded. In this system the concentration gradient remains high. The dialysate is either premixed or continuously mixed by a proportioning pump.

The advantages of the Kiil dialyzer are that: a blood pump is not

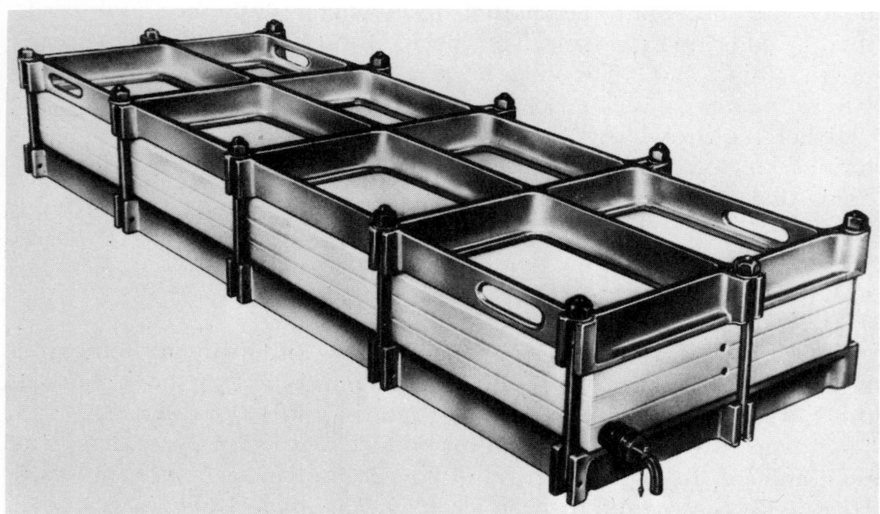

Figure 33. Full-size Kiil layer dialyzer with a blood volume of 300 to 400 ml. (Courtesy of Sweden Freezer Company, Seattle, Wash.)

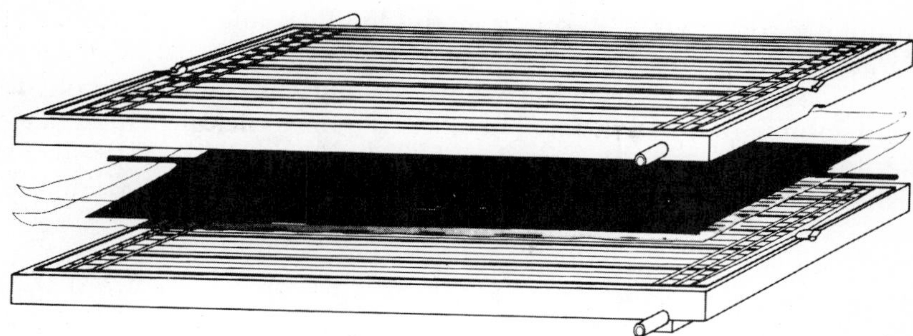

Figure 34. The layer or parallel-flow dialyzer. Schematic drawing of one of the two layers. The blood (dark portion) flows within the cellophane membrane and the dialysate fluid flows on either side of the membrane in the grooves of the epoxy resin boards. (From Fellows, B. J.: The role of the nurse in a chronic dialysis unit. *Nurs. Clin. N. Amer.*, *1*:4:580, 1966.)

always necessary and therefore the patient does not require as close supervision as does the patient using the coil kidney. Therefore, the Kiil is frequently used for home dialysis. It is easily adapted for home use and the cost of the membrane and tubings is about half the cost of a coil system. Once in operation the machine requires a minimum of attention; thus fewer personnel are needed in large dialysis units. The dialysate is automatically, continuously mixed by the machine, eliminating the element of human error. The dialyzer itself can be assembled in 45 minutes.

The disadvantages are that, in most models, the boards are heavy and must be assembled by a male technician. Sterilization and flushing of the unit are necessary prior to use. This takes approximately an hour in addition to the 45 minutes required to assemble the system, which makes it inconvenient for emergency dialysis. The boards must be inspected closely for foreign particles that may puncture the cellophane, causing leaks. Uneven blood flow through the dialyzer, due to unequal resistance, may cause a decrease in efficiency. The greatest disadvantage of the Kiil dialyzer, to the patient, is that it takes 12–16 hours of dialysis to accomplish the same blood chemistry changes as does six hours with the coil. Units that use the parallel-flow dialyzers employ full-time technicians who presterilize, assemble, and monitor the equipment, freeing the nurse to concentrate on caring for the patient.

Capillary dialyzer

The capillary dialyzer is a new design and is made up of many hollow capillary fibers in a parallel arrangement through which the patient's blood flows. It allows a small blood volume to be exposed to a large dialyzing surface area that has little internal resistance. An additional advantage is that the rigid structure maintains a constant blood volume in the dialyzer. The disadvantages include a high rate of clot formation and a relatively low ultrafiltration rate. However, further clinical testing is now in progress to correct these problems.

Ideal hemodialyzer

The criteria of an ideal hemodialysis system as outlined by Black are:

1. The cost of purchase and operation should be low.
2. The system must be safe, reliable, and simple to operate.
3. The volume in the system should be less than 500 ml to avoid priming with blood, and the blood remaining in the circuit after each dialysis should be minimal.
4. The blood circuit should be disposable.
5. The system should be efficient with a minimum urea clearance of 50 ml/min.
6. The hemodialysis system must be acceptable to the patient.[7]

Dialysate Delivery Systems

Since the development of long-term dialysis units where multiple dialyses are conducted simultaneously much research and experimentation has been devoted to improving the system of delivery of dialysate. At present, there are two basic systems for supplying dialysate during treatment: the batch system and the proportioning system, both of which can be used for an individual patient or for several patients simultaneously.

Batch system

The batch system consists of a reservoir that holds 100–400 L or more and a mechanism for mixing the chemicals with de-ionized tap water. The dialysate bath is mixed, tested for chemical accuracy, and in some cases warmed prior to circulation to the individual dialyzers. One example of the batch dialyzer is the Kolff tank model kidney (Fig. 35). With this system a fresh batch is mixed every two hours. The Travenol RSP also uses the batch system; however, in this machine the dialysate is mixed in a reservoir below the coil and is

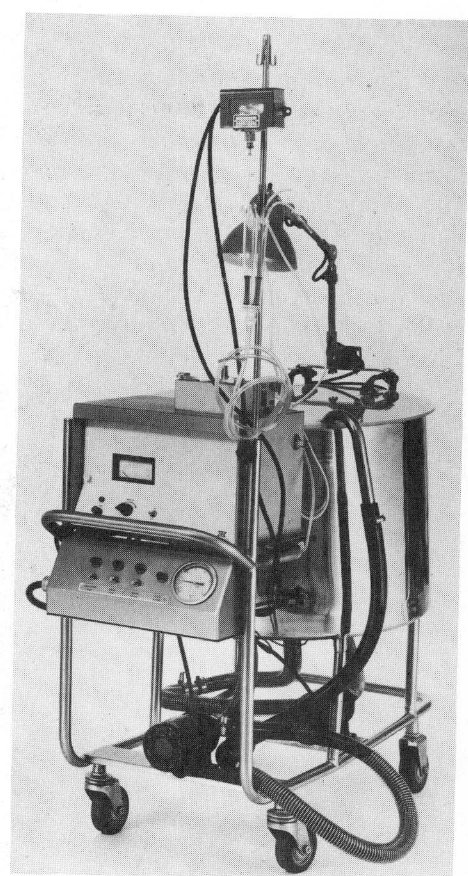

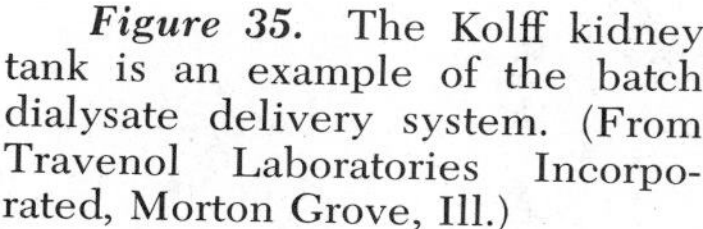

Figure 35. The Kolff kidney tank is an example of the batch dialysate delivery system. (From Travenol Laboratories Incorporated, Morton Grove, Ill.)

continuously circulated through the dialyzer at a rate of 300–500 ml/min until the supply is exhausted. The advantage of the batch design is that it is usually less expensive than the proportioning type; the disadvantage is that the volume of dialysate is fixed, thus limiting the flexibility of dialysis time. The bath concentrations for the small batch system are listed in Appendix F.

Another application of this system is used in large units where dialysate is centrally mixed in batches of 400 L or more and delivered to the individual dialyzers at varying flow rates. This central delivery system can be used with either the coil or parallel-flow dialyzer. Central batch mixing affords great flexibility in dialysate flow rate and length of dialysis; however, it requires expensive equipment for mixing and monitoring and a full-time chemical technician to operate it.

Proportioning System

The proportioning system requires two reservoirs, one with deionized tap water and one with concentrated dialysate, and pumping devices to proportion the desired amounts of each into a mixing line to form dialysate of the proper concentration. This is more expensive and complicated than the batch system. However, it has a great advantage in that it is very compact and offers complete flexibility in length of dialysis. Another advantage is that it practically eliminates the possibility of bacterial contamination of the bath that exists in the batch system. Figure 36 shows a Kiil board and a proportioning dialyzing system.

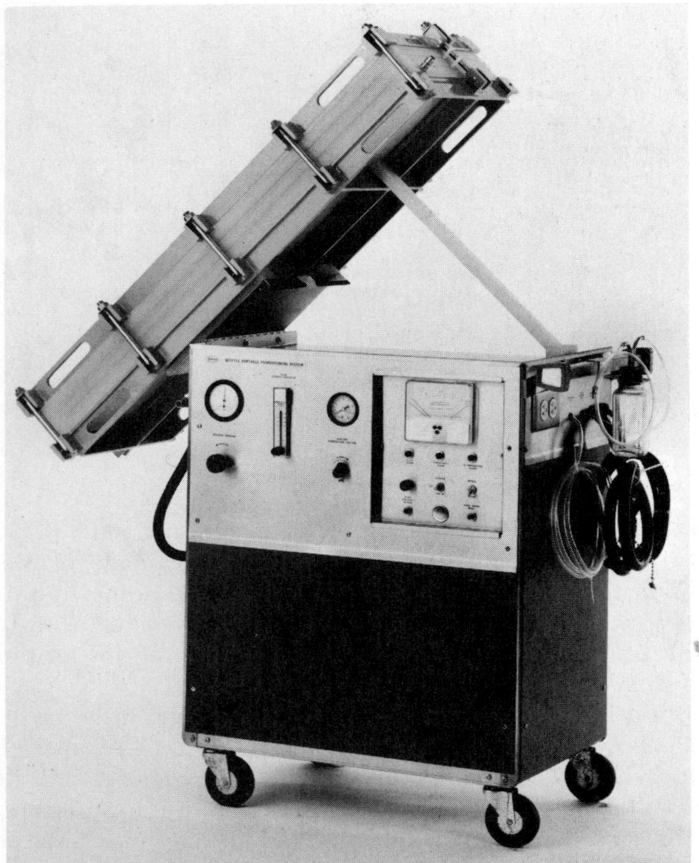

Figure 36. Kiil parallel-flow dialyzer and proportioning dialysate delivery system. (Courtesy of Sweden Freezer Company, Seattle, Wash.)

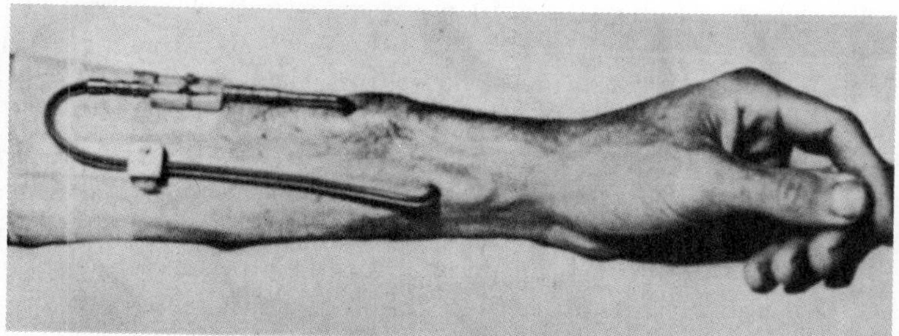

Figure 37. The cannula, the semipermanent appliance in the patient's arm. The Silastic material is shown coming out of the patient's skin; one side is inserted in an artery and the other side in a vein. The Silastic is connected to the Teflon joint, and the metal rings hold the Teflon inside the Silastic so that the cannula does not come apart. (From Fellows, B. J.: The role of the nurse in a chronic dialysis unit. *Nurs. Clin. N. Amer.*, *1*:4:579, 1966.)

Arteriovenous Shunts

An adequate access to the blood stream is essential for successful repeated hemodialysis. The ideal device should be easy to insert, easy for the patient or technician to manipulate, and should not limit the patient's activity. For long-term dialysis, the ideal shunt should allow repeated access to the blood stream for a period of two years or more. However, even in the treatment of acute renal failure, shunts are used to eliminate the need for repeated cut-downs. There are two types of shunts currently being used for repeated hemodialysis; the Teflon-Silastic cannula, and the subcutaneous arteriovenous fistula.

TEFLON-SILASTIC CANNULA

The Scribner shunt introduced in 1960 is the cannula most widely used in this country (Figs. 37 and 38). One tip of this cannula is

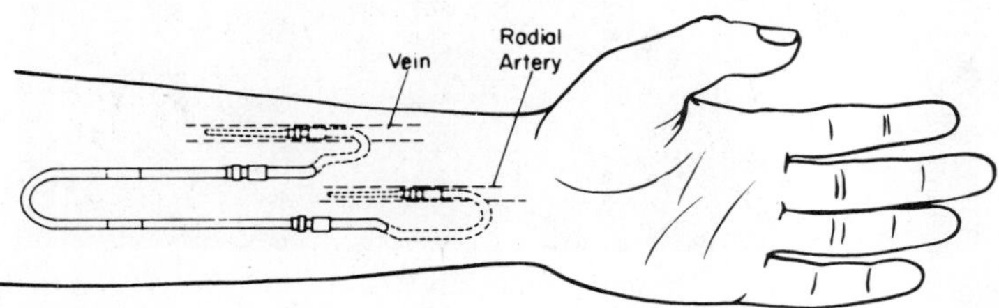

Figure 38. Schematic drawing showing a Silastic shunt with Teflon tips inserted into an artery and a vein. (From Fellows, B. J.: The role of the nurse in a chronic dialysis unit. *Nurs. Clin. N. Amer.*, *1*:4:259, 1966.)

surgically inserted and sutured in an artery, usually the radial artery in the arm or the posterior tibial artery in the leg; the other tip is sutured into a vein close to the artery. The ends are brought through the skin, and are connected by a Teflon joint; thus there is a continuous flow of blood through the cannula from the artery to the vein. The straight shunt and Shaldon catheters are Teflon-Silastic catheters also used in hemodialysis (Fig. 39).

The actual site of the cannula is determined for the individual patient. In general the cannula is placed in the nondominant limb so that the patient can favor the cannulated limb. If the patient's work involves use of both arms, the cannula is inserted in the nondominant leg. On the other hand, if the patient uses his legs extensively in his work, an arm site is preferred. A leg site is necessary for the patient who performs his own dialysis at home since both hands are needed to make the connections. The shunt area should ideally be allowed to heal for three to five days before the first dialysis. During this time the limb is kept immobilized to promote rapid healing. The cannulated arm should be kept in a sling and used as little as possible for a week to 10 days. In the case of a leg shunt, the patient is kept off his feet with his cannulated leg elevated for two to three days. He then

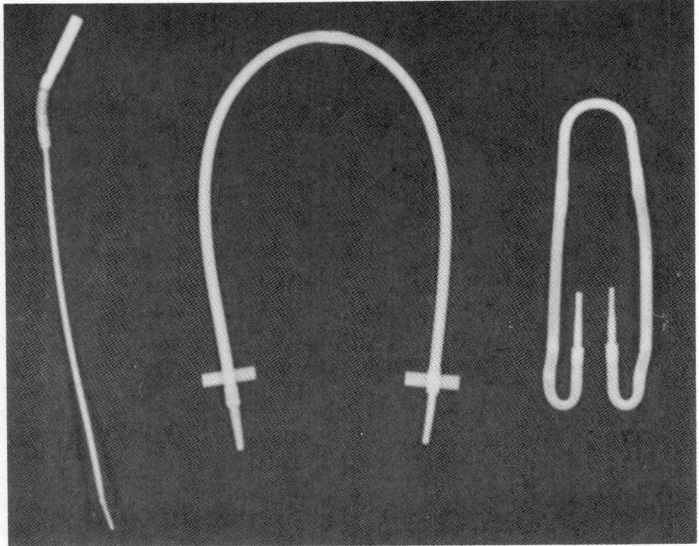

Figure 39. Catheters and shunts commonly used for hemodialysis: *left*, the Shaldon catheter; *center*, the straight shunt; *right*, the standard or U-shaped shunt. (From Kuruvila, K. C., and Beven, E. G.: Arteriovenous shunts and fistulas for hemodialysis. *Surg. Clin. N. Amer.*, *51*:5, 1221, 1971.)

progresses to a wheelchair with his leg elevated for a week, then to crutches with light weight bearing at 14 days, and finally normal weight bearing by three weeks after surgery.

At the time of dialysis the joint in the shunt is opened and the arterial cannula is attached to the blood tubing leading into the dialyzer while the venous cannula is attached to the tubing leading out of the dialyzer. Blood then flows from the patient's artery through the machine and then back to the patient via the venous cannula. During dialysis heparin is administered to prevent clotting of blood in the machine. However, when the cannulas are joined and the shunt is in operation, no heparin is needed; clotting does not ordinarily occur, because the circuit is short, the blood flow through it is rapid (150–300 ml/min), and the cannula is made of a material, Silastic, that does not cause clotting.

Theoretically, cannulas can be expected to last several years; however, the average "shunt life" is approximately six months.[56] The most frequent cause of shunt failure is thrombosis resulting in a decrease in the blood flow. If treated promptly, clots can be removed. Another complication of the cannula-type shunt is infection, usually caused by a staphylococcus organism and treated successfully with antibiotics.

The advantage of the cannula is that it offers painless, easy access to the patient's blood stream and can be used for repeated hemodialysis in patients with acute or chronic renal failure. The disadvantages are that it must be carefully cared for to prevent shunt failure and that the limb must be somewhat immobilized to prevent trauma to the cannula. The cannula requires daily washing and application of a sterile dressing that is kept on at all times. A procedure for shunt care appears in Appendix G.

Cannula complications

Infections. The most frequent cannula complication is infection. Approximately 90 per cent of cannula infections are caused by *Staphylococcus aureus* and 10 per cent are due to gram-negative organisms. Signs and symptoms of cannula infections are drainage (either bloody or serous), pain, redness, and swelling around the cannula sites. Small amounts of serous or bloody drainage at the cannula sites normally occur immediately after insertion or following excessive activity. However, continuous oozing at the openings arouses suspicion of infection. When infection is suspected, material from the area is taken for culture and antibiotic therapy is started promptly. The patient is instructed to limit the activity of the limb and to cleanse the cannula thoroughly daily. If the infection interferes with dialysis it may be necessary to remove the shunt and insert a new one at a different site.

Clotting. The next most common cannula complication is clotting, which may be caused by mechanical or physical abuse or by physiological factors in the blood vessels themselves. When clotting occurs the blood in the shunt turns very dark and may even separate into red cells and serum, giving a white frosted appearance to the cannula. The temperature of the shunt drops below body temperature so that it feels cool to touch. The shunt no longer pulsates nor can a bruit be heard through a stethoscope. The patient may complain of pain and tenderness. The treatment involves attempting to declot the cannula. If this is unsuccessful, a new shunt is inserted. Clotting is usually preceded by signs of cannula failure; if these are detected early, treatment can prevent the complication. Four signs of cannula failure and treatments to overcome them as described by Pendras and Stinson are:

1. A decreased blood flow (100 ml/min or less) during dialysis indicates difficulty in either the arterial or venous cannula. Irrigation of the partially occluded vessel may prevent a clot from occluding the cannula.

2. Venous spasm during dialysis can be caused by an obstruction or irritation in the vessel. Prompt treatment with warmth, massage, and anti-inflammatory or antispasmodic drugs may prevent cannula failure due to clotting.

3. Excessive fibrin formation in the shunt is treated with anticoagulants in order to prevent clotting.

4. Pain may be a warning sign of shunt failure due to clotting. Heat, heparin, and rest are used to prevent it.[68]

Erosion. Occasionally the subcutaneous loop of a cannula may erode through the skin because of excessive pulsation or the position of the loop over a pressure point. Erosion most frequently occurs at the arterial cannula site. The treatment consists of replacing the loop cannula with a straight one (see Fig. 39 *center*).

Phlebitis. Nonbacterial phlebitis frequently occurs because of irritation of the vein by attempts to declot the cannula. Treatment involves local heat, anti-inflammatory drugs, and heparin. Very rarely bacterial phlebitis may cause contamination of the venous cannula. Signs include spasm, redness, pain, fever, and chills. Treatment consists of removing the cannulas and administering antibiotics.

Accidents. Accidental separation has occurred and can result in dangerous or fatal blood loss. The cause of separation is not known, but frequent checks on the position of the shunt seem to minimize the problem. Each patient carries two clamps on his person at all times in case of a separation. Some patients use Silastic or Teflon bridges at cannula junctions to prevent separation.

Subcutaneous arteriovenous fistula

The subcutaneous arteriovenous (A-V) fistula is created surgically by an anastomosis of the cephalic vein and radial or brachial artery (Fig. 40). Leg arteries and veins have been used when no arm vessels are available. As a result of this fistula a large amount of blood is shunted into the venous circulation, producing venous engorgement with a high rate of blood flow. A bruit or thrill can be felt over the fistula because of turbulent blood flow. After creation of the fistula, a delay of 72 hours is recommended before the first dialysis.

At the time of dialysis a 12–16-gauge thin-wall needle is inserted into the distended vein in the distal forearm or leg and another large-bore needle is inserted into the proximal end of the same vein. Blood then flows from the distal needle through the dialyzer and back to the patient through the proximal needle (Fig. 41).

This fistula can provide blood flow rates of 100–350 ml/min and is used with both the Kiil and the Kolff dialyzers. However, inadequate blood flow is a frequent problem, particularly when no blood pump is used. There is also the possibility of fistula enlargement with increased shunt flow resulting in cardiac overloading, although no conclusive cases have been reported to date.

The advantage of the A-V fistula is that no prosthesis is necessary, allowing for greater freedom of activity for the patient between dialyses and eliminating the necessity of daily washing and bulky dressings. Infections are also eliminated since no external apparatus acts as a portal of entry for bacteria. There are no parts to become dislodged or cause bleeding or clotting.

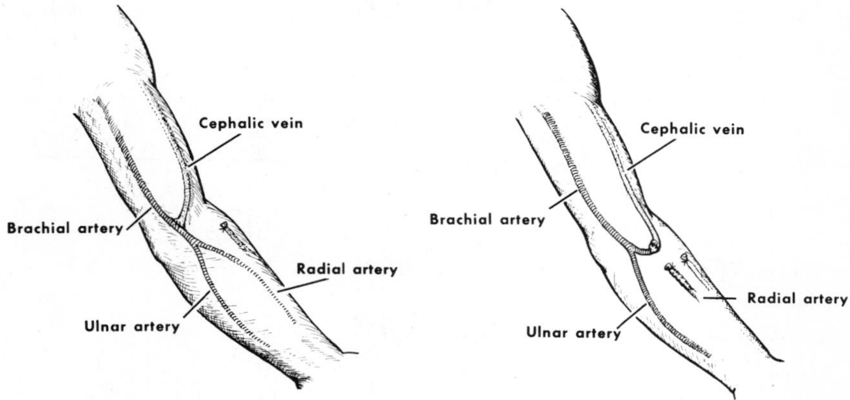

Figure 40. Construction of an arteriovenous fistula at the antecubital fossa: *left*, between the cephalic vein and brachial artery (end to side), and, *right*, between the cephalic vein and the radial artery (end to end). (From Kuruvila, K. C., and Beven, E. G.: Arteriovenous shunts and fistulas for hemodialysis. *Surg. Clin. N. Amer., 51*:5, 1229, 1971.

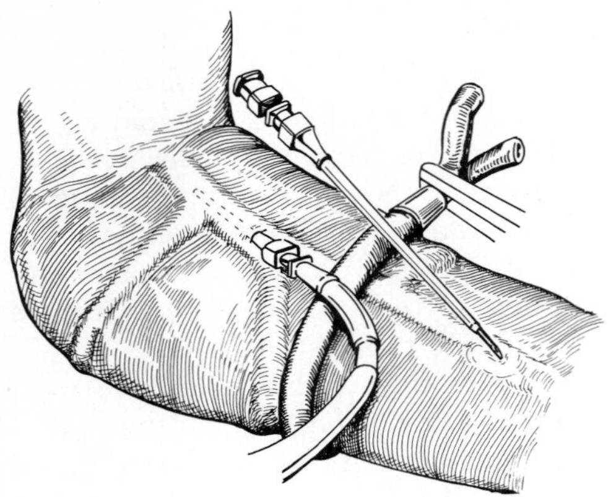

Figure 41. The arteriovenous fistula cannulated for dialysis. The blood is drawn out through the distal needle and returned through the proximal needle flowing in the direction of the patient's heart. A tourniquet may be used to increase the blood flow during dialysis. (From Nose, Y.: *Manual on Artificial Organs. I. The artificial kidney.* St. Louis, C. V. Mosby Co., 1969.)

The disadvantage of the fistula is the necessity of venipuncture for each dialysis and of strict immobilization of the limb during dialysis. A comparison of the advantages and disadvantages of the arteriovenous shunt and the fistula appears in Table 4.

Anticoagulation

The clotting of blood is an important defense mechanism of the body to protect it against excessive bleeding. It is only in abnormal states that the blood clots in the body vessels. However, outside the body, the blood clots very rapidly, particularly when it contacts rough and foreign surfaces. During hemodialysis the patient's blood comes

*TABLE 4. Comparison of Arteriovenous Shunts and Arteriovenous Fistulas**

Feature	Arteriovenous Shunt	Arteriovenous Fistula
Ease of use and training	Easier	More difficult
Limitations during dialysis	Can move limb	Movement restricted
Pain	Painless	Pain of needle puncture
Blood pump	Not required	Required
Activity	Restricted	Unrestricted
Thrombosis	Frequent	Infrequent
Infection	Frequent	Infrequent

*From Kuruvila, K. C., and Beven, E. G.: Arteriovenous shunts and fistulas. *Surg. Clin. N. Amer., 51*:5:1234, 1971.

in contact with the rough surfaces of the cannulas, the blood tubings, and the cellophane in the dialyzer. In order to prevent clotting, anticoagulation measures are used. Heparin, a short-acting anticoagulant, is used to prevent clotting during dialysis.

HEPARIN

Total heparinization is the technique most frequently used. Heparin is either administered periodically into one of the blood tubings with a needle and syringe or is injected continuously with a constant infusion pump. Since heparin inhibits the clotting of blood in vitro and in vivo, both the patient and the blood circuit are heparinized in this way.

Heparin is effective when administered parenterally. A single intravenous administration results in an immediate but transient effect reaching a peak in two hours and lasting four to six hours. The dose during hemodialysis is based on body weight and the clotting time, which is prolonged considerably over the normal Lee-White clotting time of 6–17 minutes. The usual heparin regimen is an initial dose of 1 mg/kg of body weight followed by intermittent clotting time determinations and additional heparin administration every two hours. Clotting time may be extended to more than an hour, and a clotting time of 30 minutes or less is the usual indication for additional heparin.

In circumstances in which a patient has a bleeding problem or an opened wound such as a new cannula site, care must be taken to avoid bleeding. In this case the blood circuit must be anticoagulated while the patient's coagulation system remains normal. The regional heparinization technique is utilized. This is accomplished by infusing heparin continuously into the arterial blood line leading from the patient to the machine and infusing protamine, a heparin antidote, into the venous line returning blood to the patient.

The greatest danger from heparin is hemorrhage. Bleeding may occur from unsuspected lesions such as peptic ulcers. Intramuscular injections are not given while the patient is receiving anticoagulants because of the danger of a hematoma at the puncture site.

COUMADIN

Some hemodialysis patients must be maintained with continuous anticoagulation therapy because of excessive fibrin formation, which causes sluggish cannula flow that leads to clot formation. Coumadin, an oral anticoagulant that has a slow onset and long duration of action (72 hours), is the drug of choice. The prothrombin test is used to determine the adequacy of anticoagulation which is ideally maintained at a prothrombin time of six to eight seconds longer than the normal control. The usual dose is 5–10 mg/day. Anticoagulation is discontinued or modified in cases of serious bleeding problems, excessive trauma or bruising, and prior to surgery.

Hemodialysis Technique

The majority of patients at present undergoing dialysis for renal failure are treated in the hospital in special units set up for hemodialysis. The nurse or the technician sets up the equipment before the patient arrives in the unit. Although the preparation time and procedure vary according to the type of dialyzer used, the system of dialysate delivery, and the individual patient, some things are essential for any dialysis and these include:

1. A dialysis machine set up with a sterile cellophane membrane and sterile inlet and outlet tubings, all of which are primed with sterile normal saline
2. Dialysate solution as prescribed by the physician and a system for dialysate delivery and disposal
3. A couch, chair, or bed for the patient to lie on
4. A preparation set containing antiseptic solution, 12–16-gauge metal or plastic needles for patients with fistulas, sterile clamps for patients with shunts, and a cut-down set for emergency patients
5. Masking tape or nonallergenic tape to secure needles or shunt during dialysis, and an arm board
6. Equipment for obtaining patient's weight, temperature, blood pressure, and blood samples
7. A chart for recording predialysis assessment data and specific dialysis information
8. A medical care plan including doctor's orders
9. A nursing care plan including nursing orders

The patient is admitted, weighed, interviewed, and attached to the artificial kidney. For the next 6 to 14 hours his blood circulates through the tubings and through the semipermeable membrane where the processes of diffusion, osmosis, and filtration remove waste products and replace serum electrolytes from the dialysate.

During the dialysis the nurse or technician monitors the machine for:

1. Rate of blood flow
2. Rate of dialysate flow
3. Temperature of dialysate

4. Negative pressure in the system
5. Air bubbles in the lines
6. Ultrafiltration pressure
7. Blood leaks
8. Bacterial contamination of dialysate
9. Dialysate concentration
10. Heparin delivery

In units where technicians are responsible for the assembly and operation of the dialyzers, the nurse is free to devote her time to monitoring, caring for, and teaching patients.

Complications of Hemodialysis

The complications of hemodialysis comprise technical failures of the procedure itself and its untoward effects on the patient at the time he is undergoing treatment as well as the ongoing medical problems inherent in the uremic state.

TECHNICAL COMPLICATIONS

Blood leaks. The most frequent technical complication is a blood leak caused by a tear or a hole in the dialysis membrane. The nurse or the technician or both constantly observe the outflowing dialysate for signs of blood. Small tears may allow only a small amount of blood to leak through the membrane, causing the outflow to turn pink. Large leaks occur early in dialysis and are easily observed since the outflow dialysate will dramatically turn red.

If the observer suspects a small leak he uses a dipstick (Hemastix) to test the dialysate outflow, and centrifuges a sample of the dialysate outflow. If both these tests are positive for red blood cells the dialysis is stopped and the membrane replaced. Some of the newer dialyzers are equipped with alarms that buzz when a membrane leak occurs. However, a human observer makes the final judgment. To avoid unnecessary blood loss, the blood in the circuit is returned to the patient. The nurse then reconnects the patient's shunt to maintain patency during the delay and prepares the equipment to resume dialysis.

Tubing separations. Another technical complication during dialysis is tubing separation. Most separations occur at the cannula–blood line connection and are easily detected by the patient or the nurse since blood will rapidly saturate the cannula dressing. The nurse immediately shuts off the blood pump and clamps both cannula and tubing. Contaminated lines are replaced and dialysis is resumed.

If clotting occurs in the tubings a new dialysis membrane and lines are used to complete the treatment.

Dialysate errors. Although errors in dialysate composition are rare they can occur and the nurse and technician must be alert to prevent them. In the batch system the danger lies in failure to add the concentrate to the bath water. Errors of this type are eliminated by conscientious chemical evaluation of each dialysate bath prior to initiation of the dialysis. In the proportioning dialysate system, dialysate pump failure is the cause for dialysate bath error. With this system the technician periodically analyzes the dialysate in the inflow and outflow lines for chemical composition during the dialysis.

Patient complications during the procedure

Dialysis disequilibrium syndrome. The dialysis disequilibrium syndrome is thought to be caused by removing urea nitrogen from the blood too rapidly in relation to its rate of removal from the brain. It is frequently seen in patients using coil dialysis because of the very rapid removal of urea. Two to four hours after the start of hemodialysis the concentration of urea in the blood is considerably lower than the concentration of urea in the brain, resulting in a reverse osmotic gradient that pulls water into the brain and causes cerebral edema. The symptoms include nausea, vomiting, mental confusion, hallucination, and convulsions. Convulsions most frequently occur in acutely ill patients with high BUN levels, in patients starting on maintenance hemodialysis, and in long-term hemodialysis patients who have a particularly high BUN value on the day of dialysis.

There are several solutions to the problem of disequilibrium syndrome. First, an acutely ill patient or one starting on a long-term hemodialysis program can be dialyzed more frequently than usual for shorter intervals using a smaller dialyzing surface area; i.e., he can be dialyzed every other day for four hours on a pediatric-size coil dialyzer or a one-layer parallel-flow dialyzer. Second, the flow rates of both blood and dialysate may be slowed to slow the rate of diffusion of urea. Last, the reverse osmotic gradient can be prevented by increasing the osmolality of the dialysate by adding 1–2 gm/100 ml of dextrose or by adding urea. This allows diffusion of water, electrolytes, and wastes of protein metabolism while maintaining a stable tissue fluid osmolality. Urea is added to the dialysate in amounts adequate to allow only a 20–30 per cent decrease in BUN with each dialysis.

Anticonvulsants are given prior to hemodialysis in patients with excessively high BUN levels due to acute renal failure, in patients undergoing initial hemodialysis treatments in a maintenance program, or in long-term dialysis patients when there is evidence of an increase in

BUN due to excessive ingestion of protein or a prolonged interval between dialyses. Diphenylhydantoin (Dilantin) is the drug of choice for controlling seizures. Patients on long-term hemodialysis are tested by means of EEG to determine whether there are any focal abnormalities; if there are, anticonvulsants are continued. Careful evaluation is essential, since uremia and dialysis lower the convulsive threshold and convulsions may be serious, particularly in a heparinized patient.

Acute hypertension. Acute hypertension during dialysis is usually caused by sodium and water excess. However, it also occurs with anxiety and disequilibrium syndromes. To determine the cause the nurse evaluates the patient's predialysis weight, emotional state, protein and fluid intake, and the interval since the last dialysis. Treatment is related to the cause and may include an increase in ultrafiltration for fluid overload, slow dialysis for the disequilibrium syndrome, sedatives for anxiety, and antihypertensive drugs.

Hypotension. The most frequent cause of hypotension is excessive ultrafiltration that occurs several hours after the dialysis is started. Hypotension is also common at the initiation of dialysis when blood moves rapidly from the patient into the dialyzer. Treatment, in either case, consists of maintaining the patient in supine position, decreasing the ultrafiltration pressure, and if necessary administering additional intravenous fluid. Persistent hypotension may be the result of excessive antihypertensive agents.

Nausea and vomiting. The most frequent causes of nausea and vomiting include the disequilibrium syndrome, hypertension, hypotension, anxiety, peptic ulcer, and a reaction to medication. Treatment consists of evaluating the patient carefully to determine the cause, and correcting or controlling the problem as indicated.

Headache. Headache occurs with anxiety, hypertension, and the disequilibrium syndrome and is treated by eliminating or controlling the cause. Analgesics and tranquilizers may be administered. Aspirin is not usually given concomitantly with anticoagulants.

Acute bleeding. Occasionally, in total heparinization, a patient may bleed from a peptic ulcer or a recent surgical wound. Minor bleeding around the cannula or body orifices is not uncommon. Treatment includes use of regional heparinization and if necessary discontinuance of the dialysis.

Fever. Fever occurs with infection, pyrogenic reactions to blood transfusions, and contamination of the blood or dialysate. A thorough investigation—including blood, dialysate and urine cultures as well as cultures of specimens taken from the cannula—is carried out to determine the cause, and the patient is treated accordingly. Appropriate antibiotics are used to control infections.

Blood reactions. Blood reactions occasionally occur owing to hypersensitivity to a blood transfusion. The transfusion is discontinued, the blood returned to the laboratory, and the patient treated with antihistamines.

Muscle cramps. Muscle cramps can be caused by rapid sodium and water removal, calcium shifts, or neuromuscular sensitivity. The usual treatment consists of reducing the ultrafiltration pressure or administering intravenous saline or both. Muscle relaxants or quinidine sulfate may be ordered. Heat and massage are temporary measures.

Cardiac arrhythmias. Arrhythmias are not infrequent during dialysis and may be due to hypotension, electrolyte disturbances, fluid overload, or anemia. However, regardless of the precipitating factor, since serious arrhythmias usually indicate cardiac disease, complete cardiac evaluation is indicated. Patients are often treated with quinidine, lidocaine, and diphenylhydantoin. Digitalis is used only when other medications fail, since the potassium fluctuations during dialysis increase the danger of digitalis intoxication.

Chest pain. Hypotension and cardiac arrhythmias frequently result in angina. An electrocardiogram is taken when there is any suspicion of cardiac malfunction. Treatment will depend on the cause as determined by the physician.

Shortness of breath. Causes of dyspnea include volume overload, congestive heart failure, and pulmonary embolism. The patient is examined by the physician, and a pulmonary evaluation may be ordered.

Restlessness. Restlessness during dialysis is frequently associated with anxiety. The nurse interviews the patient, makes pertinent behavioral observations and perhaps refers the patient to the psychiatrist, social worker, or physician. Sedatives may be necessary; however, patients often respond to the support and reassurance of the nurse, and further treatment is unnecessary.

Depression and hostility. Most patients display degrees of depression and hostility during the initial stages of the program and require tremendous understanding, support, and patience from everyone who relates to them. The nurse plays a major role in helping the patient to adjust to and accept dialysis and in helping the family understand this common reaction. A more detailed discussion of the psychological effects of hemodialysis on patients appears later in this chapter.

Medical complications

The medical complications associated with patients receiving maintenance hemodialysis include all the complications of uremia itself:

Electrolyte imbalance	Gastrointestinal upset
Acidosis	Bone disease
Fluid retention and edema	Bleeding tendency
Congestive heart failure	Pruritus
Hypertension	Peripheral neuropathy
Pulmonary edema	Infection
Pericarditis	Delayed wound healing
Anemia	Hypothermia

These complications and the required medical and nursing intervention are fully discussed in Chapters 4 and 5. In addition to the complications resulting from uremia itself there are a number of others that are seen in patients maintained by hemodialysis.

The shunt. Clotting, infection, and erosion—the most frequently seen cannula complications—have been discussed earlier in this chapter. Occasionally a cannula infection may result in bacteremia or septicemia that endangers the patient's health. Treatment consists of removing the infected shunt and vigorously treating the infection with appropriate antibiotics. A few cases of subacute bacterial endocarditis resulting from cannula infections have been reported. These cases were treated actively with massive doses of antibiotics. Loss of cannula sites due to frequent cannula complications has threatened continuity of treatment in some cases.

A possible complication of the *arteriovenous fistula* is the enlargement of the fistula with excess shunting of arterial blood to the venous system resulting in cardiac overload. Although no cases of this complication have been reported, it remains a real possibility. Treatment would consist of reconstruction or removal of the fistula and if necessary creation of a new fistula.

Hypertension. Hypertension is a frequent complication of uremia. The treatment of hypertension in uremic patients who are not receiving dialysis consists of restricting the salt and water intake and perhaps of administering antihypertensive drugs. Patients who are receiving intermittent hemodialysis are treated by limiting salt and fluid intake and also by removing excess salt and water during dialysis. Frequently, uremic patients remain normotensive with this therapy alone. In some cases however, antihypertensive drugs may be required. When both modes of treatment are utilized the nurse monitors the patient's blood pressure carefully during dialysis to avoid hypotension as a result of volume depletion.

Congestive heart failure and pulmonary edema. Removal of excess fluid during hemodialysis is an effective means of both preventing and treating congestive heart failure and pulmonary edema.

Peripheral neuropathy. Patients whose uremia is severe or mildly severe but long-standing prior to dialysis frequently develop peripheral neuropathy. In addition, patients who are maintained by hemodialysis for long periods may begin to have symptoms of neuropathy. Treatment consists of longer and more frequent dialysis until symptoms subside or are reversed. Neuropathy of long standing cannot be completely corrected; however, some improvement usually occurs with more frequent dialysis. Patients who have a tendency to develop neuropathy are usually treated effectively by frequent home dialysis.

Anemia. Anemia may be a complication of uremia or may be partially the result of dialysis when recovery of blood from the dialyzer is incomplete or when hemolysis of erythrocytes occurs. Heparinization, heparin rebound, and alteration of blood platelets can predispose to bleeding, thus complicating the already existing anemia. Iron may be given intramuscularly or orally and is particularly advisable in young women who are menstruating.

Hemosiderosis. Iron deposits in the tissue are seen in patients who have had multiple blood transfusions. The skin appears darker brown than the usual gray-tan color of uremia.

Hepatitis. Hepatitis is a serious complication of hemodialysis for the patient and the assistant. Hepatitis in the patient is felt to be the result of a contaminated blood transfusion. In general, patients develop a "subclinical" type of hepatitis in which fatigue and weakness are the main symptoms and jaundice is not evident.

Although hepatitis does not present severe symptoms in the patient, it can be a major threat to the dialysis nurse, technician, or assistant. Acute hepatitis transmitted from the infected patient to the dialysis assistant can be life threatening or even fatal. Hepatitis can be transferred to a staff member by a needle prick or contamination of an open wound or even by oral contamination with infected blood. Since patients may have undiagnosed hepatitis, staff members must maintain strict blood handling techniques. The staff member in a hemodialysis unit is constantly and unavoidably handling blood-filled equipment and containers. Careful handwashing, adequate protection of open wounds by wearing rubber gloves, and avoidance of contaminated needles are essential safety measures. In addition, one should never eat inside the dialysis area. Rubber gloves are worn whenever there is a possibility of direct contact with the patient's blood and while cleaning the kidney machines. Staff members exposed to patients discovered to have hepatitis are given prophylactic gamma globulin. In rare instances epidemics of hepatitis have broken out in hospital hemodialysis units.

Decreased sexual potency. One of the first signs of neuropathy in male patients is an inability to have an erection. Female patients have occasionally reported a decreased libido. This decreased sexual potency creates psychological as well as social problems that frequently require professional counseling.

Psychological Aspects of Hemodialysis

Since hemodialysis for chronic renal failure involves a tremendous amount of stress on the individual undergoing treatment, psychological factors are an important aspect of the total program.

Selection of Patients

After a careful medical examination and tentative acceptance, potential dialysis patients are seen and tested by a psychiatrist to determine their stability and maturity. The final selection of patients in most programs is ultimately dependent on the availability of space in the program and the final decision of a selection committee composed of medical and nonmedical members. In general, patients are selected on the basis of their motivation, emotional stability, and potential for rehabilitation. The individual's self-concept and ego strength greatly determine the success of his adjustment to the demands of long-term dialysis.

At one time it was believed that a high level of intelligence was essential to the process of adapting to dialysis. This has proved to be false; patients with normal or dull normal intelligence have adjusted well to hemodialysis programs. However, a favorable attitude toward health and health workers is essential, and this attitude can be related to IQ.

An increasing concentration of toxins in the patient's system adversely affects his behavior and response. The basic mechanisms of attention and concentration are among the first areas of function to be impaired. Consequently, the intellectual functions of abstraction and generalization are markedly decreased. Psychological data obtained in the predialysis period must therefore be interpreted with great caution. The family members are most helpful here in describing the patient's normal behavior prior to severe illness.

Stresses of Dialysis

The long-term hemodialysis patient is subject to frequent, recurring, stressful situations. In addition, he must tolerate the usual continuous stress of chronic illness. There is a constant uncertainty about his life expectancy as well as about immediate medical complications and emergencies. He and his family are forced to face great changes in their life style, not the least of which is a tremendous financial burden. Progressive kidney disease typically causes the patient to feel weak and lethargic and results in inability to perform normal functions. If he is the financial provider for the family, the time he will miss from work can cause deep concern and anxiety about financial status. Even the most generous employee's benefits rarely cover the amount of time lost during the initial treatment and maintenance in a dialysis program. The patient must spend anywhere from 12 to 36 hours every week in treatment and still maintain his role as family member and in many cases "bread winner." The cost of treatments have been a serious financial problem for the patient who did not have access to a funded program. The stress of treatment alone is severe, and in addition the patient must cope with the emotional and interpersonal conflicts involved in the family's adjustment. All this puts an extreme burden on his adaptive capacity.

In a study by Wright et al. of dialysis patients, psychological stress was evidenced by their concern over the following actual or threatened losses.

1. Parts of the body or body function: In the predialysis period most patients experience weakness, lack of energy and impaired concentration. They are concerned about the limitations involved in having a shunt or fistula in their arm. Other symptoms of uremia such as neuropathy, weight loss, and anemia also cause concern.

2. Loss of membership in groups: Patients with external shunts may have to withdraw from swimming, bowling, and other athletic groups. The patient may feel too poorly to continue active membership in social or charity groups.

3. Failure of plans or ventures: This may include anything from building or buying a new house to canceling vacation plans.

4. Changes in way of life and living: The unpredictability of feeling well leads to difficulties in planning social functions. This unpredictability despite regular dialysis represents a unique stress not shared by patients with other chronic diseases. In addition, the treatment process places the patient in a position of dependency. He is dependent on a machine to maintain his life. Patients see their shunts as life lines upon which their existence depends.

5. Loss of home, possessions, or financial status: Both patient and family show concern regarding their future financial obligations. Some patients fear the financial burden to the point of seeing it as a reason for discontinuing treatment.

6. Loss of job or occupation: Loss of job owing to physical restriction or reduction of job responsibilities is a frequent occurrence in dialysis patients. Some patients begin job retraining programs and in some cases the spouse assumes the financial burden.[97]

Dialysis patients frequently encounter other stresses, many of which vary with the individuals themselves. The decrease in sexual function adds its toll and creates marital problems that in some cases have led to divorce. Frustrations concerning dietary restrictions pose mild problems for most patients but more serious problems for "heavy eaters" and "meat eaters."

In addition to these stresses dialysis has a severe detrimental effect on the patient's self-image. The patient's psychological mechanism of role function is negatively altered. This presents more serious problems when the patient is a man and financial provider for the family. Suddenly, he is forced into a position of dependence that runs counter to his role as the head of the family in our culture. However, women patients also feel the strain of lack of the independence and self-determination that are so entrenched in our lives. Body image changes due to weight loss, presence of a cannula, skin color, leg braces, and bone and joint pain place additional demands on the adaptive mechanisms of the uremic patient, particularly of the woman, who is often more concerned about physical appearance and attractiveness. The stresses imposed on the patient's self-concept during long-term dialysis require some defense reaction that will permit him to "live with his illness." Depression, projection, and denial are the defense mechanisms most frequently observed.

Depression occurs in all patients at some time during treatment and is particularly frequent in the first three to six months in the program. Depression is so common that it has come to be expected and is considered a normal reaction. Absence of depression would be considered abnormal and a matter for investigation. No cases of depression are definitely known to have resulted in suicide, and psychiatrists agree that most patients need not be referred for a psychiatric evaluation for mild to moderate depression. Occasional cases of pathologically neurotic, psychotic, and psychopathic episodes have been reported in dialysis patients but these are rare.

Among defense mechanisms employed by dialysis patients, projection is a rather common and harmless one. It is characterized by the patient's belief that he is much better off than the other patients in the dialysis unit.

Denial, on the other hand, is a very dangerous coping mechanism. It is the most important and difficult psychological reaction the dialysis staff has to deal with. Psychiatric consultations are important for patients displaying this symptom. Simply defined, denial is a protective device used to reduce the anxiety caused by stressors and psychological reactions. Denial can be a temporary response in which the patient neglects to care for his shunt or cooperate with the staff. However, reports show that several patients' carelessness was so serious that it led to complications that eventually resulted in death. Some patients express denial by refusing to follow their diet in spite of repeated dietary instruction. Immature patients have used this "disobedience of rules" regarding diet to rebel against the staff. Some examples of denial from interviews with patients are:

"I didn't know I couldn't have salt." (After repeated instruction on the low-salt diet)

"You mean I shouldn't play golf." (Patient with repeated shunt infections)

"My home life is as simple and happy as it has always been."

"I really haven't given any thought to my future."

Another type of denial is withdrawal evidenced in patient behavior. This type of patient is pleasant and less anxious or depressed than others who are struggling with the realities of treatment. In spite of the fact that his intellectual capacities are unaffected he refuses to become involved in simple monitoring of instruments. He seems to be adapting well to the program in terms of morale, but closer observation will reveal trouble.

For a patient to adapt to the situation he needs an understanding of the basic functioning of the machine and his own kidneys. He must show signs of emotional acceptance of his physical status as explained to him by the physician. Signs of acceptance include social and vocational readjustment and awareness of his own feelings. Strong family support and backing is essential to the adaptation of a dialysis patient. The patient's flexibility and adaptiveness as displayed in other stressful situations in his life will predict the strength with which he can stand the stress of dialysis. Finally, it is the behavior of the dialysis staff—particularly the nurse—that will aid or hamper the patient's adaptation to dialysis.

Nursing care and stress of dialysis. The nurse is equipped with the same psychological mechanisms as the patients with whom she continuously interacts and to whom she responds. The nurse's role as a teacher is a very important one. Patients with uremia frequently function more slowly intellectually and need constant simple and concise information regarding their disease and treatment to reduce their anxiety. The nurse is the person in most constant contact with the patient. Therefore, other staff members depend on her for observations and evaluations of patient behavior. Her sensitive observation and skillful interviewing often offset serious problems of depression and denial. The effectiveness and appropriateness of the total program for the individual patient often depend on the nurse's ability to observe the patient's behavior accurately and consistently.

The nurse's ability to form a positive relationship with the patient has far-reaching effects on his eventual adaptation to dialysis. Trust, confidence, and warmth, in addition to technical skills, are the raw materials from which the ideal nurse-patient relationship is built. The nurse maintains her objectivity in order to help the patient face reality. If she allows herself to become too personally involved she may slip into the role of a "family member" and force the patient to rely completely on his own interpretation of the situation. Acceptance, respect, and honesty are antidotes for the patient's denial and low self-esteem.

Dialysis patients seem to be more aware of negative than positive information and therefore need a great deal of honest praise and reinforcement regardless of the length of time they have participated in the program. Praise helps the patient maintain the necessary motivation to follow the restrictions imposed on him. For example, praising a patient for keeping his weight down between treatments gives him recognition for following his diet. Weight charts at a "community scale" in the unit also provide recognition and motivation for patients. Group discussions with other patients have been effective in affording recognition by the group, thus elevating the patient's self-concept.

Another important nursing function is to provide information and support for the patient's family. The nurse again is the one who has the most continuous relationship with the family and can observe and evaluate their adjustment. She intervenes informally on a more social level—in the regular visits of the family to the unit. More formally, she gives emotional and intellectual support to families of newly accepted patients and those training for home dialysis. The family may be the nurse's only outside source of information regarding the patient between treatments, and frequent effective communication can help prevent complications before they can occur.

In addition, the dialysis nurse is mature, stable, sensitive, and interested in the individual patient. She has a thorough knowledge of herself and can accurately predict her personal reactions to various persons and situations. She also knows and admits her own weaknesses and limitations. It is no revelation that some personalities clash. In a close working situation such as a dialysis unit, it is essential that the staff discuss their problems and reach a comfortable working relationship. It is also necessary for the staff to understand and work through their problems with patients. Group therapy sessions conducted by the psychologist for all dialysis staff members have proved very effective in relieving tensions and improving morale.

The Roles of the Nurse in Long-Term Hemodialysis

Patients receiving long-term hemodialysis treatments in the United States are at present involved in one of three different types of program; hospital units, satellite units, and home dialysis. Large medical centers across the country house programs in which maximally supervised hemodialysis is performed on an outpatient basis. A rapidly expanding type of program is the satellite unit, which is used for patients who do not need maximal supervision but who do not qualify for home dialysis. The most desirable and economical program is home dialysis in which patients purchase the necessary equipment and conduct their own dialyses at their convenience.

The roles of the nurse will vary depending on the program the patient is involved in and on the individual patient. However, there are certain basic roles that the nurse assumes in any hemodialysis program—with variations for each of the three types.

THE NURSE IN THE HOSPITAL UNIT

The majority of patients at present receiving hemodialysis treatments for chronic renal failure are treated as outpatients in hemodialysis units of large hospitals or medical centers equipped to handle multiple dialyses simultaneously. In most of these hemodialysis units the nurses and technicians handle the entire procedure. A physician, usually a nephrologist, acts as director of the program and is responsible for diagnosing and prescribing the dialysis regimen for each patient. Since the physician is not usually present during the dialysis, it is essential for the dialysis nurse to have a thorough knowledge of the pathophysiology of renal failure, of the mechanical and technical aspects of the dialyzer, of the expected outcome and complications of hemodialysis, and particularly of the needs of the individual patient.

Nurse-Clinician

The nurse clinician develops a method of continuously evaluating or assessing each patient. The most effective tool is an assessment sheet devised by the nurse and filled out for each patient at each treatment. A sample assessment sheet appears in Appendix H. The information obtained from the assessment is used to devise nursing care plans, to assist the physician in diagnosis and treatment, to evaluate the effectiveness of dialysis, to monitor the patient's progress and provide information regarding his rehabilitation, and to assist the dialysis team and the patient in planning his future in the dialysis program.

Assessing the patient. The average dialysis patient comes to the hospital twice a week and is dialyzed for 6–12 hours. Assessment begins the minute the patient enters the unit. The nurse observes his gait, facial expression, tone of voice, dress and numerous other details of his physical appearance that provide information regarding his general condition. Since an accurate weight is of utmost importance the patient changes from street clothes to hospital pajamas and removes his shoes. The nurse weighs him, conducts a brief interview, and takes his blood pressure, pulse, and temperature. These data provide information regarding the patient's present condition and provide parameters that the nurse uses to evaluate him during dialysis. For example, an unusually high predialysis weight or blood pressure alerts the nurse to question the patient about his fluid and salt intake. Depending on his answer, the nurse makes a judgment and provides the appropriate therapy, i.e., increases the ultrafiltration pressure, reinforces the dietary regimen, schedules an appointment with the dietitian to review the diet with the patient, or perhaps supports and encourages the patient to follow the strict diet.

Next the nurse inspects the shunt site. In the case of a cannula, she removes the dressing and checks for signs of clotting or infection. Specifically she observes the color and pulsation, and inspects the insertion areas for redness, swelling, or drainage, and questions the patient regarding pain or tenderness. Prior to removing the dressing, the nurse takes notice of the condition of the dressing. Soiled outer bandages and poorly applied sterile dressings indicate a need for further questioning. A poorly kept shunt may occur for various reasons including lack of knowledge, lack of interest or acceptance, general depression, or physical inability to perform shunt care.

When the patient has a subcutaneous arteriovenous shunt the nurse inspects the arm for signs of thrombophlebitis. Specifically she observes for edema and cyanosis of the extremity and questions the patient regarding tenderness and pain.

The assessment continues as the nurse prepares the patient for dialysis. She obtains information regarding the general and specific aspects of his physical condition and his social and psychological well-being. The dialysis nurse who is adept at the art and skill of interviewing obtains most of this information through a relaxed informal conversation with the patient. The specific information that she must obtain prior to initiating dialysis, since it may influence the dialysis treatment, includes:

Data	*Effect on dialysis*
Temperature	An elevated temperature frequently indicates an inflammatory process. The dialysis time may be lengthened.
Blood pressure	An elevated blood pressure frequently accompanies circulatory overload. Ultrafiltration pressure may be increased.

Pulse	An irregular pulse may indicate a high serum potassium level. An EKG is indicated. Potassium may be reduced or eliminated in the dialysate.
Weight	An unusually high weight indicates excess fluid. Ultrafiltration pressure may be increased.
Date of previous dialysis and general dietary history	A prolonged interval between dialyses or increased consumption of protein food increases the BUN and predisposes the patient to convulsions. Anticonvulsants and a higher osmolality dialysate are utilized.
General physical condition	Malaise, lethargy, and nausea are symptoms of uremia. The dialysis time may be lengthened.
Condition of the shunt	An infected or clotted shunt requires immediate treatment.
History of bleeding	In the presence of a bleeding disorder, regional heparinization is used.

Initiating Dialysis

CANNULA. Using aseptic technique the nurse cleanses the shunt area. Alcohol, Zephiran or Betadine is frequently used to cleanse the cannula. Soap may be used on the skin but is never used on the cannula itself since it may cause the connections to slip apart. Both sides of the shunt are clamped and the Teflon connector is removed. Each clamp is briefly released to determine the arterial and venous sites. Blood samples for chemistry, hemoglobin, and hematocrit determinations are obtained from the arterial cannula. Next the clamped venous and arterial cannulas are attached to the corresponding clamped venous and arterial lines of the dialyzer. All clamps are removed and the dialysis is begun. The cannulas and tubings are secured to the patient's arm with nonallergenic adhesive or masking tape. The shunt site is covered with a sterile towel or a sterile dressing.

If a blood pump is used it is started at a low pumping rate initially, then gradually increased to the desired rate. The dialysate flow rate is adjusted and the ultrafiltration pressure regulated. The patient's vital signs, particularly the blood pressure, are monitored closely during the first 15 minutes of dialysis. If the patient shows signs of hypotension or shock the nurse puts him in supine position, slows the blood flow rate, and if necessary, adds saline to the arterial line, 500 ml per infusion until the blood pressure starts to rise.

It is also during the initiation that the nurse and technician monitor the dialyzer to insure proper functioning. Blood leaks occur most frequently in the first few minutes of dialysis and necessitate discontinuing the dialysis until the faulty membrane is replaced. A complete check list for monitoring the dialyzing machine can be found earlier in this chapter. If malfunctioning occurs at any time during the dialysis it is imperative not to alarm the patient. The knowledgeable nurse and technician calmly and efficiently correct the problem and reassure the patient.

As soon as blood begins to flow through the machine heparinization is begun. When total heparinization is used the nurse injects the calculated amount, usually 1 mg/kg of body weight, into the arterial line. When regional heparinization is used the infusion pumps are turned on and adjusted to the proper rate.

ARTERIOVENOUS FISTULA. The nurse inspects the limb for the best puncture site. An antiseptic such as Zephiran or Betadine is used to cleanse the area and 1 per cent lidocaine is injected intradermally to produce local anesthesia. A tourniquet is placed on the limb proximal to the puncture site and two 14- or 16-gauge metal or plastic needles are prepared. The afferent or "arterial" needle is placed distal to the efferent or "venous" needle with its tip pointing toward the fistula. The needle tip should be approximately 1 inch above the fistula to prevent injury to the fistula during insertion. The efferent or venous needle is inserted with its tip pointing toward the heart, the normal direction of venous blood flow (Fig. 41).

The venous needle may be inserted first and kept open with normal saline until the arterial needle is inserted. However, when the veins are prominent and the nurse is confident of her ability to insert the venous needle, she inserts the arterial needle and allows the dialyzer to slowly fill with blood while she inserts the venous needle. The tourniquet used during insertion may be removed. However, when a greater blood flow is desirable a tourniquet is placed on the limb between the two needles, i.e., proximal to the arterial needle and distal to the venous needle. Once both needles are inserted, connected to the dialyzer tubings, and secured, the initiation proceeds the same as that described for dialysis with the cannula.

When the machines and the patient are stabilized, the nurse makes the patient comfortable and continues her assessment. Some of the data are obtained by observation alone while other facts require questioning, listening, and providing information. The nurse continuously evaluates the patient's understanding and acceptance of his disease and treatment. She teaches, evaluates patient learning, provides encouragement and support, offers suggestions, and assists the patient in setting up schedules and establishing therapeutically sound patterns of behavior.

Monitoring. In units where technicians are available to monitor the dialyzers, the nurse is relieved of the task of constant checking. However, she is still responsible for periodically monitoring those functions of the machine that can be checked at the patient's bedside. The experienced dialysis nurse can do this in a minute or less. The parameters she checks include all or some of those listed previously in

Approved exception to SF 539

PATIENT'S NAME	AGE	SEX	RACE	CLAIM NO.	SOCIAL SECURITY NO.	NAME OF HOSPITAL
				C-		

PERTINENT HISTORY, CHIEF COMPLAINT, AND CONDITION ON ADMISSION

PERTINENT PHYSICAL FINDINGS

DOCTOR'S PROGRESS NOTES *(NOTE: Doctor's orders are on reverse)*

FINAL DIAGNOSIS *(Place the letter "X" before the one diagnosis responsible for the major part of the patient's stay. For discharge to nursing care, place the letter "N" before diagnosis(es) responsible for nursing care placement)*	ICDA CODE

OPERATION PERFORMED AT THIS HOSPITAL DURING CURRENT ADMISSION	DATE

ADMISSION DATE	DISCHARGE DATE	TYPE OF DISCHARGE	INPATIENT DAYS	WARD NO.	SIGNATURE OF PHYSICIAN

VA FORM DEC 1968 **10-1000a** **ABBREVIATED MEDICAL RECORD**

Figure 42. Hemodialysis log sheet used in Veterans Administration hospitals.

(*Figure 42 continued on opposite page.*)

this chapter. In units where the nurse is responsible for the total dialysis, she monitors the equipment continuously and periodically records her observations on a dialysis log sheet. Examples of log sheets appear in Figures 42 and 43.

In all units the nurse is responsible for monitoring the patient. Pa-

DOCTOR'S ORDERS *(Each entry must be dated and be signed by physician)*

DATE AND TIME WRITTEN	ORDERS *(Another brand of a generically equivalent product, identical in dosage form and content of active ingredient(s), may be administered UNLESS checked)* ➧	√	NURSE'S SIGNATURE
DIALYSIS	WEIGHT: Pre. Gain: Coil:		
#	Post. Loss: Bath:		

TEMPERATURE - PULSE - RESPIRATION						TEMP: NURSE'S NOTES
DATE AND TIME	B.P.	Bl.Flo.		Merc.		MEDICATION AND NURSE'S NOTES

Figure 42. *Continued.*

HEMODIALYSIS FLOW SHEET

DATE		Weight	Blood Pressure	Coil	Bath	Hct	Na	K	BUN	Creat.	Calcium	Phos.	Trans.	Saline	Other Bloodwork and Comments
	Pre														
	Post														
	Pre														
	Post														
	Pre														
	Post														
	Pre														
	Post														
	Pre														
	Post														
	Pre														
	Post														
	Pre														
	Post														
	Pre														
	Post														
	Pre														
	Post														

Figure 43. Nurse's hemodialysis log sheet.

tient variables that are measured and recorded at intervals during dialysis include:

1. Blood pressure
2. Pulse
3. Temperature
4. Weight
5. Shunt functioning
6. Clotting times
7. Clinical well being

In addition to these, she observes for all the mechanical and physiological complications discussed earlier in this chapter. The nurse's accurate diagnosis and prompt and effective intervention at the first sign of trouble can prevent or modify a complication.

The emotional reaction of a patient to the dialysis machine, to the dialysis procedure, and to the nurses is an important area of observation for the nurse. Since emotional reactions are difficult to measure, she bases her conclusions on her assessments of the patient's measurable behavioral manifestations. She records his actual behavior as well as her conclusion so that other team members can review the situation and make objective judgments. For example, instead of stating "patient withdrawn and uncooperative," the nurse records the following observations and patient behavior:

> Outer shunt bandage soiled and unraveling. Patient looked out the window while the nurse cleansed the shunt. Patient continued to look out window while nurse explained the steps in initiation of dialysis. While on dialysis the patient repeatedly used the cannulated arm in spite of nurse's repeated warning and instruction to use the opposite arm.

From this information another nurse can objectively conclude that the patient is not treating his shunt arm with the care and concern necessary to maintain proper function. The nurse then proceeds to interview the patient in an effort to find the cause of his behavior. Once the cause is determined the appropriate action is taken to overcome the problem. The problem and method of approach selected to solve it are written on the nursing care plan and evaluated at intervals.

Thus, the nurse is alert to the whole patient and his reactions to the treatment. Her knowledge of the physiology of dialysis enables her to monitor the patient for the desirable effects of dialysis. Her recorded observations are essential in planning future effective treatments.

Discontinuing dialysis. When the dialysis is complete the nurse clamps and disconnects the arterial line and infuses saline into the dialyzer, forcing the blood back into the patient. Postdialysis blood samples are obtained from the arterial shunt at this time. Next, she clamps and disconnects the venous line. If the patient has a cannula shunt the nurse, using sterile technique, reconnects the cannulas, cleanses the cannula site, and re-dresses the limb. In patients with arteriovenous fistulas, the nurse removes the needles and applies a secure pressure dressing to both puncture sites. These are removed by the patient several hours postdialysis.

Declotting cannula shunts. Along with infection, the most frequent complication of the cannula shunt is clotting. The expert dialysis nurse in many units is trained to declot shunts. Briefly, this involves attempting to remove visible clots by gentle traction and using a small syringe and a warm heparin and saline solution to irrigate the arterial and then the venous cannula.

Nurse-Teacher

The nurse begins teaching the dialysis patient at their first encounter, which is usually prior to the first dialysis when the patient is admitted for a medical evaluation. Ideally the patient is referred to the dialysis team when his renal function decreases to less than 10 per cent of normal and when his serum creatinine increases more than 10–12 per cent above normal.[68] He is evaluated as a prospective dialysis candidate at this time and if accepted has several months to adjust to the idea of dialysis and to begin learning about hemodialysis, shunt care, and diet. This also gives the patient time to review his job situation and make required changes or adjustments. If necessary he can begin a vocational retraining program.

Regardless of the program the patient is being trained for, all patients receive their instruction in a hospital or satellite unit. The nurse begins by evaluating the patient's acceptance of the program and his readiness to learn. Some patients are very eager to learn while others are frightened and act as if they were not interested. In addition to the patient's readiness to learn, the nurse evaluates his ability to learn. Some patients may never be capable of conducting their own dialyses. These facts must be determined early in the orientation so that the patient can be directed to the appropriate program.

The patient preparing for the hospital-based program must be knowledgeable concerning diet, shunt care, and activity and must have some understanding of the hemodialysis technique.

Diet. Diet is a familiar subject to start teaching since most patients with chronic renal failure have had to follow a restricted diet. The doctor prescribes the diet and the dietitian assumes responsibility for instructing both the patient and a family member. In situations in which the patient will not be preparing his own meals, the person responsible for cooking them is always instructed. Dietary restrictions vary from unit to unit and patient to patient; however, most patients are maintained on a low-protein, low-salt, low-potassium, and high-calorie diet with restricted fluid intake. Sample dietary regimens are available in Appendix D.

The nurse's teaching responsibility regarding diet is to reinforce and supplement the teaching of the dietitian. Due to her close continued relationship with the patient, the nurse is the person most qualified to evaluate his understanding and acceptance of the diet. She conducts periodic dietary reviews of all patients on maintenance hemodialysis. An effective way to check a patient's diet is for the nurse to ask him to recall everything he ate for two consecutive days, and record this information on his diet chart. The frequency of these reviews depends on the individual patient. Some patients require reinforcement and reinstruction continuously. Ordinarily, however, diet is reviewed once a month. The nurse is also responsible for referring patients to the dietitian when particular problems arise or when the patient needs intensive dietary teaching.

Cannula care. Since the shunt is the hemodialysis patient's "life line," it is crucial that he keep it functioning maximally. Prior to its insertion, the nurse explains the function and purpose of the shunt, shows the patient sample shunts, and arranges for him to see another patient's functioning shunt. The method and point of insertion are discussed. The patient is encouraged to ask questions and to verbalize his fears.

Daily washing and re-dressing techniques are explained, demonstrated, and supervised by the nurse. Since a clean cannula is essential to prevent shunt infection, the nurse spends many sessions on cannula care. Patients are asked to give return demonstrations of cannula care until the nurse is satisfied that he is adept at the procedure. Printed instructions on cannula care are given to the patient for home use. A sample cannula care instruction sheet is available in Appendix G. The patient is taught to inspect for and recognize the first signs of shunt infection, i.e., redness, pain, drainage, and swelling at the shunt site. Any of these signs are reported immediately to the physician.

The patient is instructed to observe the shunt for proper positioning to prevent kinking. He is also thoroughly schooled in recognizing and reporting the first signs of shunt clotting, i.e., pain, decreased pulsation of the shunt, change in color, and finally separation of the red blood cells and serum. He is instructed to call the dialysis unit or physician immediately.

Every patient is given two lightweight clamps that he wears on his person at all times, night and day. These clamps are to be used to occlude the cannula in case of accidental separation of the shunt.

Activity. Activity of the maintenance dialysis patient depends a great deal on his general physical condition and the type of shunt he has. The patient with an internal arteriovenous fistula is limited only by his energy and interest. He may resume all his normal daily activities once the incisional wound heals.

The patient with a cannula shunt is not as free to perform all his normal daily activities. The nurse teaches him to care for his shunt properly during certain activities and to avoid other activities altogether. The immersion of the cannulated limb in water without a waterproof covering is avoided since it may result in softening of the insertion sites or possibly introduction of an infection. The patient is taught to apply the waterproof plastic over the shunt dressing prior to showering, bathing, or swimming. If he is susceptible to infections, he may be advised to avoid swimming altogether. The patient is taught to avoid activities or sports that involve active use of the cannulated limb, i.e., golf, baseball, tennis (arm shunts) and bicycling, soccer, and skating (leg shunts).

The nurse cautions the patient to avoid extremes of heat or cold applied to the cannulated limb since this can cause venous spasms and result in clotting of the shunt. Flexion of the cannulated limb and pressure from tight clothing or sleeping and resting positions must also be avoided since they may cause clotting.

Dialysis technique. All patients are instructed in the technique of dialysis; however, the depth and extent of information imparted is dependent on the individual patient and the program in which he is involved. For example, it is not essential for the patient maintained on center dialysis to know every possible complication of the dialyzing machine, while the patient on home dialysis must comprehend this information. The home dialysis patient also needs practice in handling the various complications. The nurse evaluates the patient and the total situation and plans the content of the instruction program accordingly.

Each patient training for home dialysis selects a family member or friend to be his dialysis assistant. The dialysis assistant along with the patient is taught the technique of hemodialysis. When home dialysis began in 1964 the assistant assumed almost total responsibility for the procedure and the patient. However, this created feelings of dependence in many patients and led to frequent depression. Today the patient is trained to be the chief technician in performing the procedure while his assistant assumes a supportive role. The assistant, however, must be qualified to take over if at any time the patient is unable to carry out the procedure.

Nurse-Administrator

Administration is primarily a function of the nurse in the hospital and satellite units. The dialysis nurse in these settings is responsible for scheduling the time and days for each patient's treatment; for ordering meals, supplies, and equipment; for supervising staff; and for completing the hospital or center reports. The nurse may also be responsible for ordering equipment and supplies for home dialysis patients. Although some of these tasks are delegated to other members of the team, the nurse is ultimately responsible for them.

Nurse-Team Leader

The dialysis team consists of a physician, dietitian, social worker, psychologist, surgeon, technician, nurse, and patient. The nurse in charge, as leader of the team, is responsible for maintaining communication among the various members. She schedules regular multidisciplinary conferences to review patient progress and to coordinate team efforts. She supervises the care of all patients and makes appropriate referrals. The nurse team leader makes necessary arrangements for group instruction or discussion with patients and family and members of the other disciplines.

Nurse-Counselor

The dialysis nurse's most difficult and challenging role is that of a counselor. The long-term dialysis patient needs the nurse to be genuinely concerned and to listen to him. He needs her honest evaluation and advice. Family members are usually too personally involved to maintain an objective position regarding the patient, and he turns to the nurse for the support, encouragement, and guidance he needs.

In order to understand more fully and to assist the patient in this area, the nurse needs the help of the other disciplines, particularly the social worker and the psychologist. She evaluates the patient's adjustment to his situation and judges when to refer him to the social worker, psychologist, or physician for assistance.

Patients in chronic dialysis programs undergo changes in personality and frequently have psychological problems. The nurses find that continued relationships with demanding, suspicious, or hostile patients are emotionally draining. Group therapy sessions conducted by the psychologist for the nurses have been particularly successful in helping the nurses to maintain their morale and in giving them a release for their tensions and anger.

THE NURSE IN THE SATELLITE CLINIC

The nurse in the satellite clinic assumes many of the same roles as described for the nurse in a hospital unit including: nurse clinician, teacher, administrator, counselor, team leader, and team member. The difference in these functions lies mainly in degree. She spends considerably more time teaching the patient about the dialysis technique and encouraging him to assume as much responsibility for the procedure as he is able to. In many cases she assumes the role of the dialysis assistant and is merely available when the patient needs help or consultation.

Some satellite units are used as home dialysis training units, and in this situation the nurse acts as teacher and director of the training program. She also handles the administrative duties involved in setting up a dialysis machine in the patient's home.

THE NURSE AND HOME DIALYSIS

The nurse plays a major role in the home dialysis training program. This is the most economically desirable program for dialysis patients, the cost being less than half the cost of the hospital-based program for the same patient. The nurse involved in home dialysis training is initially a clinician, teacher, counselor, and administrator to the patient but later becomes primarily his clinical consultant. Home dialysis training programs are conducted either in hospital or satellite units. The nurse begins teaching the dialysis procedure to the patient and the family member who accompanies him from the first visit. She encourages the patient to be independent and to gradually assume full responsibility for his treatments, diet, and cannula.

The patient and family member learn to set up, test, monitor, and clean the machine in a few short weeks. The family member is also taught to determine blood pressures and clotting times during the dialysis. If the patient has a cannula, both he and the family member are taught to attach the arterial and venous lines to the machine. If he has a fistula the family member is taught to insert the needles; in some cases the patient may prefer to perform the venipuncture himself. The patient in home dialysis training is left alone with his family member for increasingly longer periods until they are functioning totally independently of the nurse. Most leaders of home dialysis training programs agree that the patient should be taught to do everything he possibly can for himself. The family member acts only as a back-up person. Some nurses prefer to teach the patient the procedures first and allow him to teach the family member under supervision.

The average length of time patients are involved in training for home dialysis is three months. During this time, the patient with the help of a technical consultant, makes all the necessary arrangements to set up a dialysis room at home. The nurse is present during the first home dialysis and may make a second visit if necessary. Patients are taught to handle all common complications such as coil leaks, a drop in blood pressure, or a bleeding shunt. However, if a problem arises

HOME HEMODIALYSIS RECORD

Name

Date		Weight	B.P.	Hours	Coil	Bath	Blood Flow	Venous Resistance	Saline	Comments
	Pre									
	Post									
	Pre									
	Post									
	Pre									
	Post									
	Pre									
	Post									
	Pre									
	Post									
	Pre									
	Post									
	Pre									
	Post									
	Pre									
	Post									
	Pre									
	Post									
	Pre									
	Post									
	Pre									
	Post									
	Pre									
	Post									
	Pre									
	Post									

Figure 44. Record to be kept by patient performing self-hemodialysis at home.

during dialysis that he can't handle quickly, the patient calls the nurse at the training center or discontinues dialysis. In some programs patients are taught to do laboratory procedures such as BUN, hematocrit, and chloride determinations at home; in other programs patients are asked to return to the hospital once a month for blood chemistry tests.

Once the patient is doing his own dialysis at home, the nurse's primary role is that of consultant. She makes visits to the patient's home as needed, evaluates the total situation, and offers advice and help if requested. She may act as counselor for both the patient and family and often refers them to other members of the dialysis team for assistance.

CASE STUDIES

I

Mr. B., a 31 year old cement worker was admitted because of a gunshot wound in the abdomen that injured the inferior vena cava and the small bowel. Surgery was performed immediately following Mr. B.'s admission to repair both the vessel and the bowel. Mr. B. received a total of 14 units of whole blood to correct severe hypotension. His systolic blood pressure was 40–50 mm Hg. Twenty-four hours after surgery, Mr. B. was in acute renal failure with a total urine output of 150 ml. Administration of furosemide (lasix), digoxin, and penicillin was started. Laboratory reports showed BUN 88 mg/100 ml, serum creatinine 11.2 mg/100 ml, and serum potassium 7.2 mEq/L. Kayexalate enemas were ordered and an arteriovenous shunt was inserted in his right forearm. Mr. B. remained oliguric; he was dialyzed every other day for 10 days. During this time he received nothing by mouth, had a nasogastric tube for continuous intermittent suctioning, and was receiving IV fluids to replace fluids lost. His fluid balance was monitored by a central venous pressure catheter. Mr. B.'s predialysis BUN level remained elevated at 100 mg/100 ml.

Sixteen days after the accident Mr. B. still had no urine output and was receiving hemodialysis treatments three times a week. His abdominal wounds were healing well, his bowels were functioning, and he was started on a low-protein diet by mouth. On the twentieth day he had a urine output of 580 ml and his BUN reached a plateau at 80 mg/100 ml. By the thirty-first day his BUN was down to 32 mg/100 ml and his urine output was up to 2000 ml/day. A renal scan showed bilateral renal function with no evidence of obstruction. Mr. B. was discharged 32 days after his accident in good condition on a low-protein diet and was followed in the renal clinic.

II

Mrs. G. a 21 year old college student was in good health until 1967 when she had infectious mononucleosis, after which she never felt like herself. She tired easily and seemed to have less energy. These symptoms were slow and progressive. Mrs. G. claimed she had had nocturia once each night as long as she could remember. In June 1969, she was married and took birth control pills until November 1970 when she stopped because of a positive pregnancy test. At this time she had 4+ proteinuria and hypertension (170/110) treated with salt restriction and diuretics. Her condition remained stable for two months and she was able to finish the semester at school. Then the weakness progressed markedly and she became severely anorectic, complaining of headaches, nausea, and vomiting, and was admitted to the hospital in January. Her weight had dropped from 90 to 76 lb in two months.

On admission Mrs. G. appeared frail, semistuporous, and acutely ill. She was afebrile, had dry mucous membranes, normal cardiac function and no edema. Her blood pressure was 150/100, pulse 100–120, and respirations 116. Laboratory tests revealed BUN 156 mg/100 ml, serum creatinine 14.4 mg/100 ml, serum potassium 4 mEq/L, and mild acidosis. The diagnosis of chronic renal failure of unknown etiology was made. It was determined that Mrs. G. was not pregnant and that her nausea and vomiting were due to azotemia. She and her husband were very disappointed about the pregnancy but were primarily concerned about Mrs. G.'s health and future.

Mrs. G. responded well to conservative therapy—a low-protein diet, IV fluids, and aluminum hydroxide gel (Amphogel). At discharge her BUN was stable at 60 mg/100 ml, and her creatinine clearance had increased from 8 to 10 ml per day. She was discharged to continue conservative therapy and did well until March when her symptoms recurred. At this time she started maintenance hemodialysis and was dialyzed three times a week in the hospital unit. Meanwhile, she held a part-time job. By July, Mr. and Mrs. G. were involved in the home dialysis training program. They had purchased a dialysis machine for their home and were confident that they could handle the routine dialyses. While receiving hemodialysis, Mrs. G.'s laboratory values remained stable and she felt better than she had felt in several years. She was steadily regaining the weight she had lost and seemed to be accepting the treatment well. She was planning to continue home dialysis until she could receive a transplant. In the meantime she planned to return to school to finish her requirements for a bachelor's degree.

References

1. Abel, J. J., Rowntree, L. G., and Turner, B. B.: The removal of diffusible substances from the circulating blood by dialysis. *Trans. Ass. Amer. Physicians, 28*:51, 1913.
2. Abram, H. S.: The psychiatrist, the treatment of chronic renal failure, and the prolongation of life. I. *Amer. J. Psychiat, 124*:1351, 1968.
3. Ackad, A., Haimov, M., Hering, A., and Schupak, E.: Subcutaneous arterial-venous fistula in home dialysis. *Trans. Amer. Soc. Artif, Intern. Organs, 16*:280, 1970.
4. Bailey, G. L., Hampers, C. L., and Merrill J. P.: Reversible uremic cardiomyopathy in uremia. *Trans. Amer. Soc. Artif. Intern. Organs, 13*:263, 1967.
5. Bailey, G. L., Hampers, C. L., Merrill, J. P., and Paine, P.: The artificial kidney at home. A look 5 years later. *J.A.M.A., 212*:850, 1970.
6. Beeson, P. B., and McDermott, W. (Eds.): *Cecil-Loeb Textbook of Medicine.* Thirteenth edition, W. B. Saunders Co., 1971.
7. Black, D. A. K. (Ed.): *Renal Disease.* Second edition, Philadelphia, F. A. Davis Co., 1967.
8. Blagg, C. R., Daly, S. M., Rosenquist, B. J., Jansen, W. M. and Eschbach, J. W.: The importance of patient training in home hemodialysis. *Ann. Intern. Med., 73*:841, 1970.
9. Blagg, C. R., Hickman, R. O., Eschbach, J. W., and Scribner, B. H.: Home dialysis: six years' experience. *New Eng. J. Med., 283*:1126, 1970.
10. Bluemle, L. W., Jr.: Current status of chronic hemodialysis. *Amer. J. Med., 44*:749, 1968.
11. Bluemle, L. W., Jr.: Dialysis. In Strauss, M. B., and Welt, L. G. (Eds.): *Diseases of the Kidney.* Second edition, Boston, Little, Brown and Co., 1971.
12. Brescia, M. J., Cimino, J. E., Appel, K., and Hurwick, B. J.: Chronic hemodialysis using venipuncture and a surgically created arteriovenous fistula. *New Eng. J. Med., 275*:1089, 1966.
13. Brest, A. N., and Moyer, J. H. (Eds.): *Renal Failure.* Philadelphia, J. B. Lippincott Co., 1968.
14. Byrne, J. P., Stevens, L. E., Weaver, D. H., Mazwell, J. G., and Reemtsma, K.: Advantages of surgical arteriovenous fistulas for hemodialysis. *Arch. Surg., 102*:359, 1971.
15. Chisholm, G. D.: The Scribner arteriovenous fistula for haemodialysis. *Brit. Med. J., 5243*:30, 1961.
16. Conn, J., Jr., Roguska, J., and Bergen, J. J.: Venous arterialization for hemodialysis. *Amer. J. Surg., 116*:813, 1968.

17. Cross, R. A., Tyson, W. H., Jr., and Cleveland, D. S.: Asymmetric hollow fiber membranes for dialysis. *Trans. Amer. Soc. Artif. Intern. Organs, 17*:279, 1971.
18. Cummings, J. W.: Hemodialysis, feelings, facts, fantasies. The pressures and how patients respond. *Amer. J. Nurs., 70*:70, 1970.
19. DeNour, A. K., and Czaczkes, J. W.: Emotional problems and reactions of the medical team in chronic haemodialysis. *Lancet,* 2:987, 1968.
20. Dunea, G.: Peritoneal dialysis and hemodialysis. *Med. Clin. N. Amer.* 55:155–175, 1971.
21. Epstein, F. H.: Calcium and the kidney. *J. Chron. Dis., 11*:255, 1960.
22. Epstein, F. H., and Merrill, J. P.: Chronic renal failure. In Wintrobe, M. M., Thorn, G. W., Adams, R. D., Bennett, I. L., Braunwald, E., Isselbacher, K. J., and Petersdorf, R. G. (Eds.): *Harrison's Principles of Internal Medicine.* Sixth edition. New York, McGraw-Hill Book Co., 1970.
23. Fellows, B. J.: The role of the nurse in a chronic dialysis unit. *Nurs. Clin. N. Amer., 1*:577, 1966.
24. Franzone, A. J., Tucker, B. L., Brennan, L. P., Fine, R. N., and Stiles, Q. R.: Hemodialysis in children: experience with arteriovenous shunts. *Arch. Surg., 102*:592, 1971.
25. Friedman, E. A., and Goodwin, J. J.: Expectations for maintenance hemodialysis. *Trans. N. Y. Acad. Sci., 30*:1093, 1968.
26. Friedman, E. A., and Thompson, G. E.: Hepatitis complicating chronic hemodialysis. *Lancet,* 2:675, 1966.
27. Gault, M. H., and Dossetor, J. B.: Kidney transplantation and long-term dialysis. *Amer. Heart J., 80*:439, 1970.
28. Ghantous, W. N., Bailey, G. L., Zschaeck, D., Hampers, C. L., and Merrill, J. P.: Long-term hemodialysis in the elderly. *Trans. Amer. Soc. Artif. Intern. Organs, 17*:125, 1971.
29. Girardet, R., Hacket, R. E., Goodwin, N. E., and Friedman, E. A.: Thirteen months' experience with the saphenous vein graft arteriovenous fistula for maintenance hemodialysis. *Trans. Amer. Soc. Artif. Intern. Organs, 16*:285, 1970.
30 Goldsmith, R. S., Furszyfer, J., Johnson, W. J., Fournier, A. E., and Arnaud, C. D.: Control of secondary hyperparathyroidism during long-term hemodialysis. *Amer. J. Med., 50*:692, 1971.
31. Gombos, E. A., Lee, T. H., Harton, M. R., and Cummings, J. W.: One year's experience with an intermittent dialysis program. *Ann. Intern. Med., 61*:462, 1964.
32. Halper, I. S.: Psychiatric observations in a chronic hemodialysis program. *Med. Clin. N. Amer., 55*:177, 1971.
33. Hampers, C. L., and Merrill, J. P.: Hemodialysis in the home – 13 months' experience. *Ann. Intern. Med., 64*:276, 1966.
34. Hampers, C. L., Merrill, J. P., and Cameron, E.: Hemodialysis in the home. A family affair. *Trans. Amer. Soc. Artif. Intern. Organs, 11*:3, 1965.
35. Hampers, C. L., and Shupak, E.: *Long-Term Hemodialysis.* New York, Grune & Stratton, 1967.
36. Hegstrom, R. M., Murray, J. S., Pendras, J. P., Burnell, J. M., and Scribner, B. H.: Hemodialysis in the treatment of chronic uremia. *Trans. Amer. Soc. Artif. Intern. Organs,* 7:136, 1961.
37. Hepinstall, R. H.: Pathology of end-stage kidney disease. *Amer. J. Med., 44*:656, 1968.
38. Husek, J. M.: *Psychological Aspects of Chronic Hemodialysis. A Summary and Review of the Literature, Suggestions for Future Research.* Los Angeles, University of California Press, 1966.
39. Jonasson, O.: Renal transplantation. Certain immunological considerations. *Med. Clin. N. Amer., 55*:193, 1971.
40. Kerr, D. N. S.: Chronic renal failure. In Beeson, P. B., and McDermott, W. (Eds.): *Cecil-Loeb Textbook of Medicine.* Thirteenth edition. Philadelphia, W. B. Saunders Co., 1971.
41. Kincaid-Smith, P.: Treatment of irreversible renal failure by dialysis and transplantation. In Beeson, P. B., and McDermott, W. (Eds.): *Cecil-Loeb Textbook of Medicine.* Thirteenth edition. Philadelphia, W. B. Saunders Co., 1971.
42. Kiil, F.: Artificial kidneys and renal transplantation. *Scand. J. Clin. Lab. Invest., 23*:281, 1969.

43. Kiil, F.: Development of a parallel flow artificial kidney in plastics. *Acta Chir. Scand., Suppl. 253*:142, 1960.
44. King, L. H., Jr., Bradley, K. P., and Shires, D. L., Jr.: Bacterial endocarditis in chronic hemodialysis patients. A complication more common than previously suspected. *Surgery, 69*:554, 1971.
45. Klinkman, H.: The disequilibrium syndrome in experimental dialysis. *Trans. Amer. Soc. Artif. Intern. Organs, 16*:523, 1970.
46. Kolff, W. J.: The artificial kidney. Past, present and future. *Circulation, 15*:285, 1957.
47. Kolff, W. J.: First clinical experience with the artificial kidney. *Ann. Intern. Med., 62*:608, 1965.
48. Kolff, W. J.: Kidney transplant or home dialysis. *Postgrad. Med., 44*:93, 1968.
49. Kolff, W. J.: Artificial organs in the seventies. *Trans. Amer. Soc. Artif. Intern. Organs, 16*:534, 1970.
50. Kolff, W. J., Nakomoto, S., and Studder, J. P.: Experiences with long-term intermittent dialysis. *Trans. Amer. Soc. Artif. Intern. Organs, 8*:292, 1962.
51. Kolff, W. J., and Watshinger, B.: Further development of a coil kidney: a disposable artificial kidney. *J. Lab. Clin. Med., 47*:969, 1956.
52. Kossoris, P.: Family therapy. An adjunct to hemodialysis and transplantation. *Amer. J. Nurs., 70*:1730, 1970.
53. Kuruvila, K. C., and Beven, E. G.: Arteriovenous shunts and fistulas for hemodialysis. *Surg. Clin. N. Amer., 51*:1219, 1971.
54. Lavender, A. R., Markley, F. W., and Forland, M.: A new pumpless parallel flow hemodialyzer. *Trans. Amer. Soc. Artif. Intern. Organs, 14*:92, 1968.
55. Merrill, J. P.: *The Treatment of Renal Failure. Therapeutic Principles in the Management of Acute and Chronic Uremia.* Second edition. New York, Grune & Stratton, 1965.
56. Merrill, J. P., and Hampers, C. L.: *Uremia. Progress to Pathophysiology and Treatment.* New York, Grune & Stratton, 1971.
57. Merrill, J. P., Schupak, E., Cameron, E., and Hampers, C. L.: Hemodialysis in the home. *J.A.M.A., 190*:468, 1964.
58. Merrill, J. P., Thorn, G. W., Walter, C. W., Callahan, E. J., III, and Smith, L. H., Jr.: Use of artificial kidney. Technique. *J. Clin. Invest., 29*:412, 1950.
59. Metheny, N. M., and Snively, W. D.: *Nurses' Handbook of Fluid Balance.* Philadelphia, J. B. Lippincott Co., 1967.
60. Muerche, R. C., Sheehan, M., Lawrence, A. G., Moles, J. B., and Mandal, A. K.: Home hemodialysis. *Med. Clin. N. Amer., 55*:1473, 1971.
61. Nakamoto, S., Brandon, J. M., Franklin, M., Rosenbaum, J., and Kolff, W. J.: Experience with A-V shunt cannulas for repeated dialysis. *Trans. Amer. Soc. Artif. Intern. Organs, 7*:57, 1961.
62. Nolph, K. D.: External shunts and internal fistulas. *Ann. Intern. Med., 74*:1008, 1971.
63. Nosé, Y.: *Manual on Artificial Organs.* Vol. I. The Artificial Kidney. St. Louis, C. V. Mosby Co., 1969.
64. Papadimitriou, M., Carroll, R. N. P., and Kutatilake, A. E.: Clotting problems with the Teflon-Silastic arteriovenous shunt in patients on regular hemodialysis. *Brit. Med. J., 2*:15, 1969.
65. Papper, S.: Renal failure. *Med. Clin. N. Amer., 55*:335, 1971.
66. Pendras, J. P., and Erickson, R. V.: Hemodialysis. A successful therapy for chronic uremia. *Ann. Intern. Med., 64*:293, 1966.
67. Pendras, J. P., and Pollard, T. J.: Eight years' experience with a community dialysis center. The Northwest Kidney Center. *Trans. Amer. Soc. Artif. Intern. Organs, 16*:78, 1970.
68. Pendras, J. P. and Stinson, G. W. (Eds.): *The Hemodialysis Manual.* Seattle, Wash., Edmark Corp., 1970.
69. Platt, R. D.: Co-operation for hemodialysis programs. *New Eng. J. Med., 284*:335, 1971.
70. Potter, D., Larsen, D., Leumann, E., Perin, D., Simmons, J., Piel, C. F., and Holliday, M. A.: Treatment of chronic uremia in childhood. II. Hemodialysis, *Pediatrics, 46*:678, 1970.

71. Quinton, W., Dillard, D., and Scribner, B. H.: Cannulation of blood vessels for prolonged hemodialysis. *Trans. Amer. Soc. Artif. Intern. Organs,* 6:104, 1960.
72. Ramirez, O.: Artificial kidneys. Relative merits of available types. In Brest, A. N., and Moyer, J. H.: *Renal Failure.* Philadelphia, J. B. Lippincott Co., 1967.
73. Relman, A. S.: The acidosis of renal disease. *Amer. J. Med., 44:*706, 1968.
74. Remmers, A. R., Sailes, H. E., Fish, J. C., Smith, G. H., Thomas, F. D., and Lindley, J. D.: Unexpected complications of unattended dialysis in the home. *Trans. Amer. Soc. Artif. Intern. Organs, 16:*85, 1970.
75. Rosen, S. M., O'Connor, K., and Shaldon, S.: Hemodialysis disequilibrium. *Brit. Med. J.,* 2:672, 1964.
76. Sand, P., Livingston, G., and Wright, R. G.: Psychological assessment of candidates for a hemodialysis program. *Ann. Intern. Med., 64*:602, 1966.
77. Schreiner, G. E.: The role of hemodialysis (artificial kidney) in acute poisoning. *Arch. Intern. Med., 102*:896, 1958.
78. Schreiner, G. E.: Current problems in the delivery of dialysis and renal transplantation. *Arch. Intern. Med., 123*:558, 1969.
79. Schreiner, G. E., and Maher, J. F.: *Uremia; Biochemistry, Pathogenesis and Treatment.* Springfield, Ill. Charles C Thomas, 1961.
80. Schreiner, G. E., and Maher, J. F.: Hemodialysis for chronic renal failure. III. Medical, moral, and ethical and socio-economic problems. *Ann. Intern. Med., 62*:551, 1965.
81. Schreiner, G. and Teehan, B. P.: Dialysis of poisons and drugs—annual review. *Trans. Amer. Soc. Artif. Intern. Organs, 17*:513–544, 1971.
82. Schreiner, G. E., Maher, J. F., Freeman, R. B., and O'Connell, J. M. B.: Problems of hemodialysis. In *Proceedings of the Third International Congress of Nephrology,* Washington, D.C., 1967.
83. Schupak, E., and Merrill, J. P.: Experience with long-term intermittent hemodialysis. *Ann. Intern. Med., 62*:509, 1965.
84. Schwartz, W. B., and Kassiren J. P.: Medical management of chronic renal failure. *Amer. J. Med., 44*:786, 1968.
85. Scribner, B. H., and Blagg, C. R.: Maintenance dialysis. In Rapaport, F. T., and Dausset, J. (Eds.): *Human Transplantation.* New York, Grune & Stratton, 1968.
86. Shaldon, S.: Independence in maintenance hemodialysis. *Lancet, 1*:520, 1968.
87. Shambough, P. W., Hampers, C. L., Bailey, G. L., Snyder, D., and Merrill, J. P.: Hemodialysis in the home. Emotional impact on the spouse. *Trans. Amer. Soc. Artif. Intern. Organs, 13*:41, 1967.
88. Shea, E. J., Brogden, D. F., Freeman, R. B., and Schreiner, G. E.: Hemodialysis for chronic renal failure. IV. Psychological considerations. *Ann. Intern. Med., 62*;558, 1965.
89. Shimizu, A., Triedi, H., Fay, W. P., and Thompson, G. D.: Straight arteriovenous shunt for long-term hemodialysis. *J.A.M.A., 216*:245, 1971.
90. Smith, E. K. M., MacDonald, S. J., Curtis, J. R., and De Wardener, H. E.: Hemodialysis in the home. Problems and frustrations. *Lancet, 1*:614, 1969.
91. Strauss, M. B., and Welt, L. G. (Eds.): *Diseases of the Kidney.* Second edition. Boston, Little, Brown and Co., 1971.
92. Swartz, C. D.: Indications for chronic hemodialysis. In Brest, A. N., and Moyer, J. H. (Eds.): *Renal Failure.* Philadelphia, J. B. Lippincott Co., 1967.
93. Teschan, P. E., Baxter, C. R., O'Brian, T. F., Freyhof, J. N., and Hall, W. H.: Prophylactic hemodialysis in the treatment of acute renal failure. *Ann. Intern. Med., 53:*992, 1960.
94. Travenol Laboratories: *Ultra-Flo 145 Dialyzer.* Morton Grove, Ill. Travenol Laboratories, 1971.
95. Travenol Laboratories: *Ultra-Flo 100 Dialyzer with Cuprophane Membranes.* Morton Grove, Ill., Travenol Laboratories, 1968.
96. Wintrobe, M. M., Thorn, G. W., Adams, R. D., Bennett, I. L., Braunwald, E., Isselbacher, K. J., and Petersdorf, R. G. (Eds.): *Harrison's Principles of Internal Medicine.* Sixth edition. New York, McGraw-Hill Book Co., 1970.
97. Wright, R. G., Sand, P., Livingston, G.: Psychological stress during hemodialysis for chronic renal failure. *Ann. Intern. Med., 64*:611, 1966.

CHAPTER 8

Renal Transplantation

In the latter part of the 1800's a young Swiss surgeon, Reverdin, began to transplant small pieces of healthy skin onto open ulcers to speed healing. This technique is practiced today under the name "pinch grafts." From that time until the early 1900's, transplantation was confined primarily to skin grafts. Other organ transplants could not be performed because of limitations in the surgical techniques of blood vessel anastomosis.

At the turn of this century, however, two American physiologists, Drs. Carrel and Guthrie developed a successful technique for anastomosis of blood vessels that is still used by vascular surgeons today.[160] Soon afterward they conducted an extensive series of experiments to study organ transplantation in animals. Their work included grafting an entire head of a puppy to the cervical vessels of a larger dog and transplantation of kidneys, livers, hearts, and limbs of dogs. These grafts functioned well for a few days but then were sloughed by the host. A successful kidney transplantation was eventually accomplished by reimplanting the organ into the neck of the same animal (autograft). Thus, it was clearly demonstrated that the failure of organ transplantation from one animal to another was not related to the surgical technique of anastomosis. At the same time, a series of investigators in a different field showed that tumor transplantation imparted an "immunity" in animals. In 1903 Dr. Jensen, a Danish biologist, noted that mice that temporarily supported a first transplant tumor immediately rejected a second transplant of the same tumor.[2] This "immunity" was attributed to previous exposure of the recipient to live tumor cells. Pertinent information about the transplantation of normal tissues was slower to evolve. Holman noted in 1924 that an initial skin graft sensitized the patient to further skin grafts.[61] Although he did not use the word immunity, he proposed that this phenomenon appeared to be an allergic response.

It was not until the 1940's, however, that Medawar demonstrated that allografts of normal tissue (skin) confer a specific systemic sensitivity on the recipient, which he described as acquired immunity.[83] He also showed that second grafts were rejected more quickly, indicating that antigens were present not only on the cells of skin grafts but also on the leukocytes. As a result, blood lymphocytes, which are easily accessible, have been used for detection of these antigens. In 1952 Dausset described leukocyte antibodies in man, thus introducing serological identification of these antigens with specific antibodies. With the introduction of immunosuppressive techniques to prevent rejection, in the late 1950's and early 1960's, the stage was set for organ transplantation as a clinical treatment. Further development in histocompatibility testing in the 1960's led to longer transplant survival, especially in kidney transplants.

The terminology concerned with transplantation has developed and evolved during this century also. The term "autograft" is used for a transplant in which the donor also serves as the recipient. "Isograft" refers to a graft exchanged between two individuals of identical genetic background, such as identical twins. The term "allograft" has largely replaced the older "homograft" and refers to transplants in individuals of the same species but of different genetic background. The term "xenograft" has largely replaced the older term "heterograft," referring to transplantation between two animals of different species.

Renal Transplants

As was noted earlier, Alexis Carrel and others performed successful autotransplantation of the kidney more than 70 years ago. They demonstrated that the kidney could be totally removed and implanted elsewhere in the body and would resume normal functioning as long as the blood supply was re-established. These studies showed that innervation and immediate lymphatic drainage were not necessary to allow adequate renal function.

The first attempt to transplant a kidney in man was made by Voronoy in 1936; this was followed in the 1940's by sporadic attempts in the United States and Paris, all of which failed.[127] It was not until 1951 that a series of human kidney transplants was reported in Paris, and not until 1953 that Dr. Hamburger of Paris reported one patient who lived 23 days with a live donor kidney from his mother.[160] In the early 1950's Drs. Hume, Murray, and Merrill at Peter Bent Brigham Hospital performed a series of 15 transplantations of kidneys from unrelated donors—without immunosuppressive therapy—to patients dying of uremia. The length of function of these transplants ranged up to six months. Four patients produced measurable function and experienced temporary clinical improvement lasting 37–180 days. The development of effective hemodialysis in the 1950's increased the interest in and investigation of transplants, since a patient could be maintained indefinitely until a kidney was available.

In 1954 Dr. Merrill and his associates performed the first successful human kidney transplant between monozygotic (identical) twins.[87] It had been known for many years that monozygotic twins were immunologically identical, hence successful transplants were expected. Since that time large numbers of transplants between identical twins have been successful without the use of immunosuppressive agents. Unfortunately, in some instances, the transplanted kidney has developed the same disease that afflicted the patient's own kidneys, resulting in ultimate loss of the transplant. A significant cause of death among monozygotic twin recipients has been recurrence of glomerulonephritis in the transplant, but at the present time, proper diagnosis and early treatment can control this problem without loss of renal function.

In spite of the success of renal transplantation in identical twins, the primary problem remained in totally unrelated persons or persons not genetically identical. In 1959 Schwartz and Dameshek described a state of "drug-induced immunological tolerance," thus paving the way for the current series of renal transplants.[128] They found that the antigen-antibody immune response was blocked in rabbits receiving 6-mercaptopurine. Between 1959 and 1968 the usual immunosuppressive program following renal transplantation included azathioprine, corticosteroids, and actinomycin C. Local x-ray therapy, extracorporeal x-irradiation, splenectomy, thymectomy, and thoracic duct drainage were used by various teams to control rejection but have largely been abandoned as general practice since long-term results have not supported their value. Antilymphocyte globulin (ALG), under investigation in the early 1960's, was introduced clinically in 1967 and has proved successful in controlling rejection in many transplant patients. There is great hope that, with further research, ALG and accurate tissue typing will eliminate most rejection crises following transplantation. A complete discussion of immunosuppressive therapy can be found later in this chapter.

Together with immunosuppression, tissue typing or histocompatibility has made possible the tremendous improvement in transplant survival in the past decade. Tissue typing involves the identification of antigens in the leukocytes. Compatibility is then predicted according to the presence or absence of antigens in both the donor and recipient. Terasaki and his associates have made the greatest contribution to tissue typing.

In addition to typing, another technique aimed at improving tissue matching has been developed. Bach and Hirschhorn first suggested a method of testing compatibility of prospective donors and recipients by using a mixed lymphocyte culture.[8] This technique can, however, only be used with live donors, and most kidneys for transplant come from cadavers.

Organ preservation is another area in which improvements have made transplantation more successful. In 1938 Carrel, in cooperation with Charles Lindbergh, developed an extracorporeal pump to preserve human organs outside the body. Later attempts were made to freeze organs as a method of preservation. Whole organs were, however, found to be seriously damaged by freezing. At present organs are preserved for as long as 72 hours by using cooling techniques and perfusion pumps.

One of the most important advances in transplantation has been the development in the field of tissue typing. Future improvements in transplant survival will no doubt result from further advances in our understanding of histocompatibility.

Histocompatibility

Probably the single most important factor affecting kidney transplant survival is tissue matching or histocompatibility. Dr. Paul I. Terasaki's group reported in the *New England Journal of Medicine* in September, 1968, that of the patients who received matched kidneys 34 per cent had no rejection crisis, while of the patients who received unmatched donor kidneys 92 per cent had rejection crises. Survival rates of the kidneys were also significantly different. Almost 40 per cent of the unmatched kidney transplants failed in two years while only 11 per cent of the matched kidneys failed.

Histocompatibility testing may be defined as the detection on or in cells of antigens (proteins) that determine the segment of an individual's genetic composition that is responsible for that person's tissue being accepted or rejected by another individual.[21] The antigens involved are called transplant or histocompatibility antigens.

GENETICS

Antigens are inherited and, like other inherited attributes, are determined by the units of inheritance called genes. Each gene occupies a single position called a locus on the chromosomes. Chromosomes are located in the nucleus of the cell and in man consist of 23 pairs or 46 autosomes and two sex chromosomes. Thus, the individual inherits from each parent one of every pair of autosomes and one sex chromosome.

The genes at the same locus of the two chromosomes of a pair are called alleles and dictate the attributes of a single characteristic. "Homozygous" refers to like genes at the same locus and "heterozygous" to unlike genes at a locus.

It is believed that only a few loci are involved in histocompatibility; however, each locus may have many alleles. The estimate of the number of genes in man ranges between 10,000 and 100,000; therefore the chance of two people other than identical twins having completely identical genetic make-up is nearly impossible. Since an individual inherits half his genes from each parent he must share half his antigenic makeup with each. For this reason many parent-child transplants have been genetically good matches with good survival rates. Considering a single locus, let us examine the genetic possibilities when a heterozygous father, AB, is mated with a heterozygous mother, CD. Figure 45 represents the inheritance of the human leukocyte antigen (HL-A) factors. Each child inherits one genetic unit from each of his parents. Parental units are designated A and B and C and D for convenience. A child will inherit A or B from the father and C or D from the mother, so only the combinations AC, AD, BC, or BD are possible. Within a given family therefore, there is a 1 in 4 chance that two siblings have identical HL-A alleles. The greater the difference in genetic make-up of the parents, the greater the range of differences in the children. It is possible to produce two

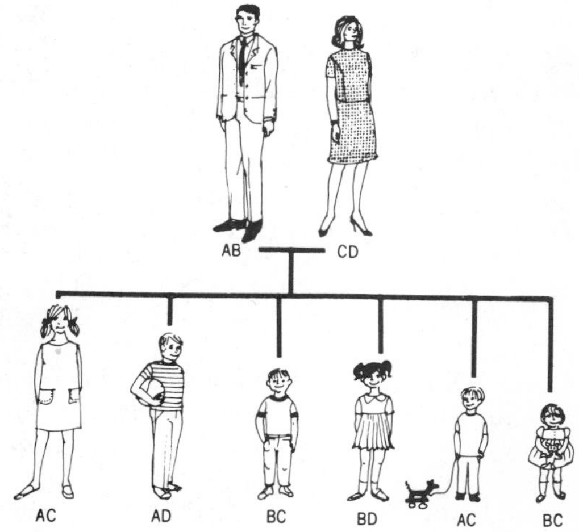

Figure 45. Inheritance of the human leukocyte antigen (HL-A) factors. (From Amos, D. B.: Immunologic and genetic aspects of kidney transplantation. In Strauss, M. B., and Welt, L. G. (Eds.): *Diseases of the Kidney.* Second edition. Boston, Little, Brown, and Co., 1971.)

children having the same genetic make-up for one locus. Thus the fewer loci and alleles involved, the greater the chances of two children having like genetic make-up for several loci. This is the basis of success in sibling kidney transplantation.

Antigen Systems

Two major antigenic systems, the blood group ABO antigens and the leukocyte and tissue antigens of the human leukocyte antigen system, have been recognized as important in determining rejection in humans. Research is currently being carried on in order to identify the antigens involved in histocompatibility. The role of ABO blood groups in compatibility has been disputed. However, when the records of kidney transplantations are reviewed, it is apparent that the prognosis for allografts in ABO incompatible individuals is poor.

Leukocyte antibodies reactive with specific human antigens were first described by Dausset in the sera of individuals who had received multiple blood transfusions. Shortly thereafter, van Rood found antibodies capable of agglutinating human leukocytes in the sera of multiparous women. These antibodies make up "typing antisera" and can be produced during normal pregnancy, after blood transfusions, following rejection of a kidney or skin allograft, or after intentional immunization of a volunteer with foreign leukocytes. The usefulness of these sera as tissue typing reagents was a result of the work of van Rood who devised a method for elucidation of human white blood cell antigenic groups. Terasaki, as well as Dausset and Payne, described additional leukocyte antigens. Progress was rapid and by 1968 The Third International Workshop for Histocompatibility Testing agreed upon an international nomenclature for these histocompatibility antigens.[103] The system was called HL-A, standing for human leukocyte antigen. More than 24 histocompatible antigens have been isolated in this complex, but only 11 are internationally accepted.

The model proposed for the HL-A antigens is represented by a single complex locus having two series of antigens. The first series has six and the second series five internationally accepted HL-A antigens.

1 series	1, 2, 3, 9, 10, 11
2 series	5, 7, 8, 12, 13

It has been shown that when all the antigens are detected, an individual has a total of four; two from the first series and two from the second series. Significant differences in the frequency of the various antigens occur in the various races. For example, HL-A 1, 2, 8, and 11 occur less frequently in the American Negro than in the Caucasian.

GRADING

Grading the donor-recipient match is a serious problem. The A, B, C, D classification described by Terasaki was based only on antigens detected. For example, if only two and the same two antigens were found in both donor and recipient, the match was graded A. However, it was not proved that only two antigens were present and the rejection rates of some A matches indicate that the failure was caused by undetected antigens. A single mismatched recipient antigen reduces the grade to B, and one and two mismatched donor antigens reduce the match to C and D respectively (Table 5). Research now under way into the clinical results of parent-child transplants will provide complete and accurate typing data correlated with the clinical results so that the success of future mismatched grafts can be predicted. In order to overcome the problem of undetected antigens, many investigators are grading donor-recipient matches according to the number of mismatched antigens (0, 1, or 2) without attempting to weigh the specific antigens.

TECHNIQUES OF HISTOCOMPATIBILITY TESTING

In the early 1960's, prior to serological identification of histocompatibility antigens, other techniques were introduced for matching donor-recipient pairs. These included skin grafts, the normal lymphocyte transfer test (NLT), and the mixed lymphocyte culture (MLC).

Skin grafts. The observed cross reactions and the differences in individual rejections suggested to early researchers that unrelated human subjects may share tissue transplant antigens. The transplant recipient received skin grafts from all the possible living donors. The

*TABLE 5. Donor-Recipient Match Grading**

A match:	HL-A identity
B match:	All the HL-A antigens of the donor are present in the recipient. The recipient has antigens not present in the donor.
C match:	The donor has one HL-A antigen not present in the recipient.
D match:	The donor has two HL-A antigens not present in the recipient.
E match:	The donor has three HL-A antigens not present in the recipient.
F match:	The recipient has antibodies active against the donor's HL-A antigen(s).

*From Falk, J. A., and Falk, R. E.: HL-A antigens in clinical transplantation. *Med. Clin. N. Amer.*, 56:403, 1972.

donor was then selected according to the graft survival time. The donor of the longest surviving graft was the first choice since it was believed that this donor-recipient match shared the most antigens. This test has been abandoned since it was shown that skin transplantation antigens caused presensitization (preformed antibodies) in the recipient that resulted in hyperacute rejection and immediate allograft failure of the transplanted kidney.

Another skin graft test was called the "third-man test" and consisted of grafting skin from the potential recipient of a kidney transplant to an unrelated volunteer. Later skin grafts from potential donors were placed on the "third man." The interpretation of the test was that the more antigens a certain donor had in common with the recipient, the more rapidly the graft could be rejected. Although this test gave information about the shared donor-recipient antigens, it failed to test for unshared antigens; therefore, it is no longer used.

Normal leukocyte transfer test. The normal leukocyte transfer test developed by Brent and Medawar consisted of injecting leukocytes of the graft recipient intradermally into possible donors. The reaction was interpreted to represent the reactivity of the recipient against the potential donor graft. Since the test lacked sensitivity and the correlation between skin and kidney graft survival was poor, it was discarded.

Mixed lymphocyte culture (MLC). In the mixed lymphocyte culture test, one set of cells is treated with the drug mitomycin-C, which prevents them from responding to but allows them to stimulate the other set of cells. Stimulation is indicative of compatibility; thus it provides a physiological indication of the donor-recipient cellular reaction. The mixed lymphocyte culture measures HL-A antigens and correlates with other histocompatibility tests currently used and is thought to detect mismatches not detected by other serological tests. This test is also referred to as the mixed leukocyte culture since it is actually the leukocyte cells in the lymph that produce the reaction. The lymph is used as a test medium since it is an easily accessible source of leukocytes.

Cytotoxicity tests. The primary tests used in clinical tissue typings are the cytotoxicity tests in which specific antibodies kill cells containing related antigens. The most frequently used cytotoxicity test is that developed by Terasaki in 1967 in which lymphocytes from the prospective recipient and each of the possible donors are exposed to a panel of standard sera containing all the known HL-A antibodies. These sera are obtained from individuals who have had multiple pregnancies or blood transfusions or have had several allografts. The reactions of the donor and recipient cells to each of these sera are compared. The most favorable donor is assumed to be the one whose lymphocytes react to the test antisera in a manner most similar to that

TABLE 6. Procedures for Histocompatibility Testing

1. Blood typing
2. Cytotoxicity
   lymphocytotoxic technique
3. Mixed lymphocyte culture (MLC)
4. Agglutination
   leukocyte agglutination technique

of the lymphocytes of the recipient. The Terasaki method of serotyping is rapid, taking less than three hours, and simple to perform.

Agglutination reactions. The several techniques available for demonstrating leukocyte agglutination differ only slightly. Basically the leukocytes of the prospective recipient and donors are exposed to a panel of sera containing high-titer leukocyte agglutinating antibodies. Agglutination reactions between the potential donors and the recipient are compared. Results of the leukocyte agglutination test show a direct relationship between the leukocyte incompatibilities and the number and severity of rejection crises in a series of renal transplants. Another technique, the mixed leukocyte agglutination test is used to detect human tissue isoantigens. The two tests together have been effective in determining isoantigenic patterns. Table 6 shows the routine procedures currently recommended for histocompatibility testing.

NURSING IMPLICATIONS OF HISTOCOMPATIBILITY TESTING

Since the nurse is the professional person in closest and most constant contact with the patient, she is responsible for answering questions concerning histocompatibility testing and reinforcing the information. In order to observe the patients intelligently after the individual tests, she familiarizes herself with the techniques involved in testing. Since family members are frequently tested as possible donors, the nurse makes sure that they understand the tests. She is frequently called upon to explain the implications of the results to prospective donors. Both the patient and family look to the nurse for support in difficult donor selection cases. For example, a relative who is a poor match may suffer depression and have guilt feelings when he is rejected as a potential donor. The nurse can be instrumental in relieving these feelings. The details of donor selection related to emotional factors are discussed later in this chapter.

The nurse's understanding of the grading system for donor-recipient matches allows her to arrive at realistic expectations regarding postoperative rejection crises. For example, the nurse can expect the grade "D" or "4" transplant to have a greater antibody reaction than the grade "A" or "0" and thus to require more immunosuppressive therapy.

Selection of Candidates

RECIPIENT SELECTION

Approximately 30,000 persons die each year of chronic progressive renal failure. In spite of the advances and growth in long-term hemodialysis and transplantation, in the early 1970's it is estimated that 9 out of 10 of the prime candidates for either of these treatments are doomed to die. The criteria for selection of candidates vary at the different centers; there are, however, some requirements basic to most programs. Since the outcome of transplantation is still somewhat uncertain, the only patients selected are those with advanced symptomatic renal failure unresponsive to all available conservative therapy.

Disease. Patients having systemic diseases, particularly those that may involve the kidney, are usually rejected. Patients are examined for the presence of life-threatening diseases involving other organs. Diabetes mellitus, primary gout, systemic lupus erythematosus, malignant tumors, and polyarteritis, which may interfere with the transplanted kidney's functioning, are contraindications. Vascular, cardiac, and neurological changes that are secondary to chronic uremia are not contraindications but may limit the degree of rehabilitation of the patient following transplantation.

If renal failure is the result of glomerulonephritis, transplantation is delayed until the "active" disease is controlled, since it can be transferred to the kidney transplant. The prospective recipient is evaluated to determine his ability to withstand the trauma of major surgery. Frequently, daily dialysis is used to reduce the patient's uremic state.

Age. Age is an important factor in patient selection, since many older patients have other related illnesses that may compromise the success of the transplant. In addition, the health status of siblings, whose age is close to that of the patient, is often so similar that the chance of finding an acceptable living donor is restricted. The usual cut-off point is 50 years of age. In the younger recipient, body size and emotional maturity are major considerations. Statistics show that the best survival rate for transplanted kidneys occurs in the 20–40 year old recipients. However, successful transplants have been recorded in infants and children as well as in one patient over 80 years of age.

Urological evaluation. A complete examination of the urinary system is conducted in order to rule out or correct any abnormality that may endanger the success of the transplantation. Any surgical correction or medical treatment is begun immediately. In the past, patients who had severe bladder malfunctions were rejected; recently, however, successful transplantation into ileal conduits has been reported.[81]

Psychiatric evaluation. The physician primarily responsible for the patient offers the initial evaluation. The nurses who have extensive contact with the patient are also involved in the psychiatric assessment. If he has been receiving maintenance dialysis, the nurse and physician in the unit have ample time to judge his adjustment to the program, his maturity, and his emotional stability, as do the social worker and psychiatrist working with the patient in the dialysis unit. In addition to these early observations, a psychiatric examination is conducted at the time of his selection for kidney transplantation. At this time, the psychiatrist evaluates the patient's maturity, emotional stability, cooperation, and genuine desire for a transplant. The patient is informed of the high cost of the procedure, the need for follow-up dialysis, the need for continued medication, and the possibility of rejection.

The nurse plays an important role reinforcing the information and determining the patient's level of understanding and acceptance. She can arrange for the prospective transplant recipient to talk with other patients who have had transplants. The patient needs to be aware of both the positive and the negative aspects of transplantation.

Medical preparation. The recipient's preparation for renal transplantation may begin in the outpatient clinic long before his condition is terminal. Patients with progressive renal failure are given the facts and statistics concerning their disease so they can plan for the future. In these cases gradual introduction of the idea of dialysis and transplantation allows the patient considerable time to accept the possibility.

The nurse begins formal preoperative preparation and teaching the moment the patient is considered for transplant. Although at present most patients who are candidates for kidney transplantation are participating in chronic dialysis programs that have access to transplantation programs, some are referred for transplantation in a state of advanced uremia. In addition to increased BUN, such patients frequently have fluid retention, heart failure, hyperkalemia, hyponatremia, and acidosis. These complications can be readily corrected by dialysis. Repeated hemodialysis for a few days will produce a rapid improvement in the patient's well-being and responsiveness. Only when he is thinking clearly can he be psychiatrically evaluated for transplantation.

The patient's metabolic state is brought as close to normal as possible by dialysis and dietary measures. Limitation of protein, sodium, potassium, and fluid intake is necessary. In general, the treatment and nursing care follows the course of that for patients in acute renal failure who are receiving hemodialysis—with a few additions. Many transplant teams routinely perform bilateral nephrectomies on prospective transplant recipients to prevent the possible spread of disease and to control the patient's blood pressure.

Since large doses of steroids are necessary postoperatively to prevent rejection, any suggestion of peptic ulcer or other possible complicating factor is evaluated. Infections of any kind are vigorously treated in order to prevent their spread due to immunosuppressive therapy. Complications caused by hypertension, cardiac failure, infection, secondary hyperparathyroidism, and peripheral neuropathy must be controlled prior to the bilateral nephrectomy or transplantation. These treatments are described in the chapters on medical management and hemodialysis.

Laboratory tests. In addition to meeting the foregoing criteria, prospective recipients must undergo a series of laboratory studies prior to transplantation. These routinely include a complete blood count with differential count, reticulocyte count, ABO blood typing, LE cell preparation, urinalysis, urine culture, liver function studies, EKG, and x-rays of the chest, abdomen, and long bones. Serial creatinine clearance tests are done, and determinations of BUN and alkaline phosphatase are made. Measurements of fasting blood sugar and plasma concentrations of sodium, potassium, chloride, bicarbonate, uric acid, cholesterol, calcium, and phosphorus are performed. Other diagnostic studies that may be included are nerve conduction studies, renal angiography, and tissue biopsies of bone, skin, muscle, and kidney.

When the patient is officially accepted as a transplant recipient the nurse begins a specific program of instruction including a description of the transplant procedure, postoperative expectations, drugs, and follow-up treatment and care.

Donor selection

Living Donors

A kidney can come from either a living or a nonliving donor. At present only human kidneys are being transplanted in humans (allograft). Duration of function of living donor transplants is approximately 70 per cent for one year and 72 per cent for two years. This exceeds the functioning of nonliving donor transplants by about 30 per cent. Functioning of all related donor transplants, including identical twins, is nearly 85 per cent for one year.[3] The greater survival rates in related donor grafts are attributed to the genetic relationship, which increases the chance of graft acceptance.

Related donor. Donor kidneys are usually obtained from normal related family members who, because of their close emotional relationship to the patient, volunteer to donate a kidney. The potential recipient is asked for information concerning living related donors when he enters the transplant program.

In discussing kidney donation with those who wish to volunteer, an objective account is given, not only regarding the risks to themselves, but also concerning the prognosis of the potential recipient. The potential benefits and limitations of transplantation, the risks and morbidity surrounding organ donation, and the necessary expense and time commitment required of all prospective donors for immunological and medical evaluation are discussed. All family members who wish to volunteer undergo preliminary blood testing without any commitment to the program. Those who are compatible are given a few days to rethink their position, and anyone who decides to continue is scheduled for further immunological and medical evaluation.

The general health and ABO blood type of the potential donors is determined, and a series of specific immunological tests is performed. The initial medical examination of a compatible donor can be performed on an outpatient basis. This usually includes a complete history and physical examination, hemogram, urinalysis, urine culture, LE cell preparation, glucose tolerance test, EKG, chest x-ray, and serial creatinine clearance tests. In addition, BUN concentrations and serum levels of electrolytes, total protein, albumin, calcium, phosphorus, and uric acid are determined. Urological consultation, intravenous urography, and psychiatric interviews and tests are conducted. If the results of these and appropriate follow-up studies are within normal limits, the potential donor is hospitalized for renal angiography.

Only at the end of this evaluation and after intensive and repeated briefing on the risks involved and the chances for success is the potential donor asked to make a final decision and permitted to give his consent to the transplantation of his organ. The medical team assures the potential donor that if at any time prior to the surgery he decides not to donate, they will supply a plausible medical excuse to the recipient and family.

Unrelated donor. There is still much controversy concerning unrelated living donors. Although about half the transplant centers approve of them in particular cases, only one fourth of the centers routinely use unrelated living donors.

Statistics show that the one and two year survival rates of cadaver kidneys is somewhat better than that of those from the living unrelated donor. In light of these statistics and with the continued efforts toward educating the public regarding cadaver organ donation, it appears that use of the unrelated living donor will eventually be abandoned. At present only 2 per cent of the total transplants done per year use kidneys from unrelated living donors; 1 per cent of these donors are the patient's spouse.

Psychological aspects of donor selection. Finding a suitable donor is sometimes a very stressful situation. Rejected donors with strong emotional attachment to the patient may experience guilt and depression, but this is usually relieved when a suitable donor is found. The selected donor must be mature, stable, and highly motivated, as determined by observation, interview, and the psychological tests. In some cases the spouse of the recipient is so anxious to obtain a suitable donor that he puts pressure on a potential donor. In other cases family members have been excluded from testing by the family member who controls the situation. Occasionally a willing potential donor is persuaded against the operation by his spouse or by another potential donor who wishes to be chosen himself.

In general, when a willing related donor is found there will have been little conflict in the initial decision-making process. Throughout the long period of waiting and the extensive tissue typing, however, the potential donor must defend his decision to family, friends, and medical staff. Potential donors who undergo extensive waiting periods with postponements show signs of greater tension related to their decision than do those whose surgery is closer to the initial decision.

Donors cite two predominant rewards for the sacrifice; the satisfaction of seeing the recipient improve rapidly; and, regardless of the survival rate of the transplant, an increase in self-esteem and a more positive self-identity.[47]

Role of the nurse. The nurse in the kidney transplantation program establishes an important relationship with the potential donor. She explains medical tests and examinations and reinforces teaching concerning them. Since the donor is usually a close relative, he may spend a considerable amount of time visiting the hospitalized patient recipient. During this time the nurse is able to observe the potential donor and may detect beginning problems of understanding, motivation, or anxiety that she may resolve or refer to another team member. She is also able to observe the dynamics of the family relationship and evaluate the situation. Donors as well as patients need the nurse's constant reinforcement and support. Preoperative teaching of donor patients is one of the nurse's important functions. She arranges for potential donors to meet and talk with other donors who have successfully recovered from their surgery.

Cadaver Donors

Although the overall duration of function of transplants from live donors, related and unrelated, exceeds that of kidneys from cadaver donors, a suitable live donor is not always available. Additional advantages of the cadaver donor are that it provides two kidneys at once and eliminates the risk involved in using a live donor. Unfortunately, however, even with all the available histocompatibility tests, the duration of function of cadaver kidney transplants is only 46 per cent in one year.

The chief sources of cadaver kidneys are accident victims whose deaths result from cerebral trauma, young patients with massive cerebral hemorrhage, victims of massive myocardial infarctions, or cardiovascular surgical deaths. Death of the donor is declared by the donor's attending physician for ethical reasons. However, when death appears imminent the family is approached for consent to remove the kidneys at death. If consent is given, immunological testing of the donor's and potential recipient's tissue is carried out.

Transplantation centers in the various areas of the United States work together to find the best possible match for the cadaver kidney. Computers make it possible for the histocompatibility test data on the cadaver donor and all possible recipients in that geographic area to be tabulated and the best match selected. Kidneys are distributed to patients within the center where the kidneys are found if there is a compatible match or are transported by car or plane to the best recipient. In addition to patient-recipient selection according to ideal match, consideration is given to the length of time a patient has been waiting for a transplant. During transport the kidney is cooled and perfused to prevent ischemia. Details of perfusion appear later in this chapter.

Surgery

SURGICAL TECHNIQUE

The recipient is hospitalized and, if necessary, dialysis is performed immediately prior to transplantation, and immunosuppressive therapy is begun. If the donor kidney has not yet been removed the donor and recipient are taken to surgery simultaneously and the operative procedures are conducted in adjoining suites. The donor

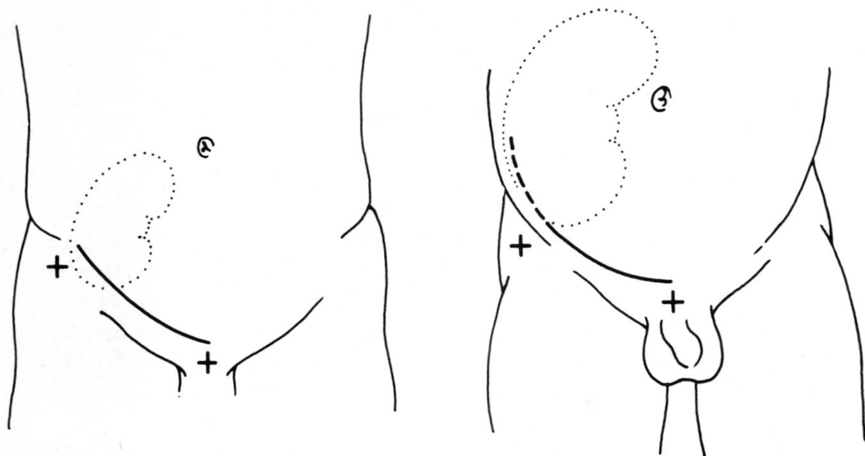

Figure 46. The incisions used for nephrectomy in transplantation. The incision begins below the iliac crest and parallels the inguinal ligament. In children the upper limit of the incision is carried a little higher than in adults. (From Rapaport, F. T., and Dausset, J. (Eds.): *Human Transplantation.* New York, Grune & Stratton, 1968. Reprinted by permission.)

kidney is not removed until the recipient is ready to receive it. Then the donor kidney is placed in the recipient retroperitoneally in the iliac fossa through a lower quadrant incision (Fig. 46). The renal vein is anastomosed end-to-side with the external iliac vein, and the renal artery either end-to-end with the hypogastric artery or end-to-side with the common iliac or external iliac artery (Fig. 47). When two or more renal arteries are present (found in 20 per cent of kidneys) an on-lay patch graft anastomosis is performed (Fig. 48).

The ureter is implanted into the bladder by a submucosal tunnel technique. Care is taken to avoid angulation and undue tension on the ureter so that the urine flow will not be impeded. The bladder incision is closed tightly to prevent leakage, the abdominal incision is closed, and a Foley catheter is connected to closed drainage. The patient is returned to his own room where a specially trained transplant nurse cares for him in reverse isolation.

Postoperative care

Postoperative nursing care is essentially the same as that for any nephrectomy patient—with a few exceptions. The unique aspect of postoperative therapy involves prevention of infection and homograft rejection, which is discussed in detail later. First we will examine the physiological response and surgical complications following kidney transplantation and the related nursing care.

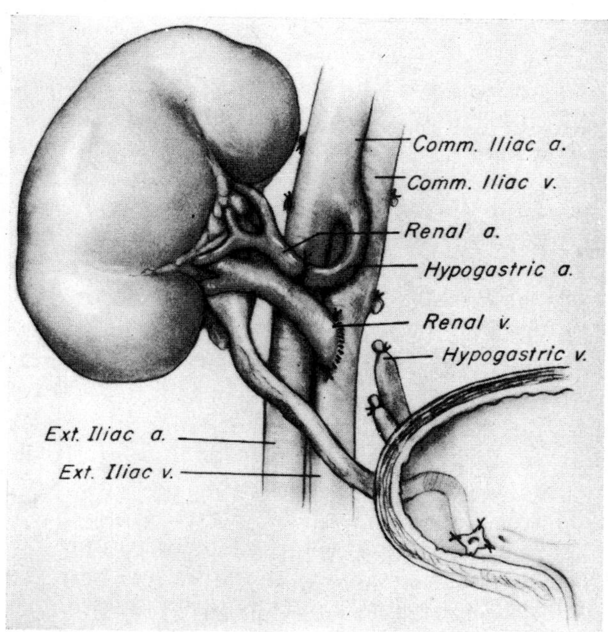

Figure 47. The usual surgical technique used in the adult. The renal artery is anastomosed to the hypogastric artery and all branches of the iliac vein are ligated and tied. The periureteral tissue is left intact and the ureter is placed into the bladder through a tunnel. (From Rapaport, F. T., and Dausset, J. (Eds.): *Human Transplantation.* New York, Grune & Stratton, 1968. Reprinted by permission.)

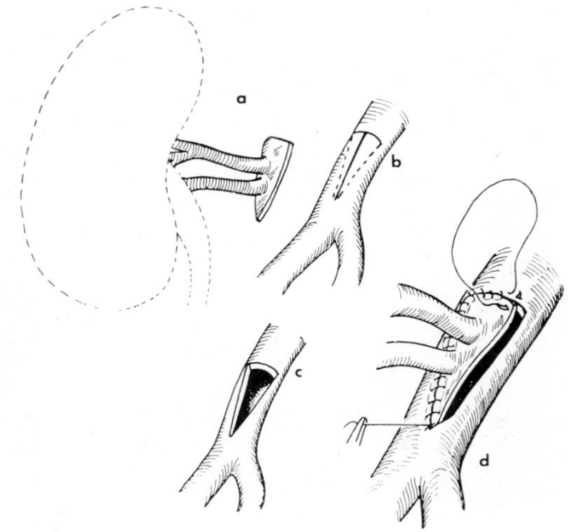

Figure 48. When the donor kidney has two renal arteries, a patch graft is used. a. An aortic cuff is taken for an on-lay patch graft anastomosis. b. A T-shaped incision is made in the wall of the common or external iliac artery. c. Edges are trimmed to enlarge the opening. d. The patch is stitched in place with arterial silk. (From Stewart, B. H.: The surgery of renal transplantation. *Surg. Clin. N. Amer.*, *51*:5:1128, 1971.)

Physiological Response

Following successful kidney transplantation surgery, urine output from massive diuresis to total anuria or anything in between these two extremes can be observed.

Massive diuresis. With successful transplantation many of the symptoms of uremia are reversed with such abruptness that homeostatic alterations may threaten the patient's life. Massive diuresis begins in most patients receiving kidneys from live donors. Weight losses ranging from 5–50 lb have been recorded. Therefore the patient is placed on an accurate weighing bed such as the Brookline Metabolic scale (Fig. 49). This bed scale provides a constant record of the patient's weight and the comfort of a regular bed. Patients have been reported to excrete volumes of dilute urine up to 2000 ml/hour. The nurse accurately records the output of urine and the total amount of fluids administered. These amounts are totaled hourly and the fluid deficit or excess determined and corrected.

Serum electrolytes are determined frequently to monitor the patient's chemical balance. Intravenous fluids are ordered according to the electrolyte levels. The nurse watches the laboratory reports carefully, anticipates the type of IV fluids to be administered, and keeps a supply available.

If losses are not replaced adequately, hyponatremia, hypokalemia, and even hypotension may occur. The patient's electrocardio-

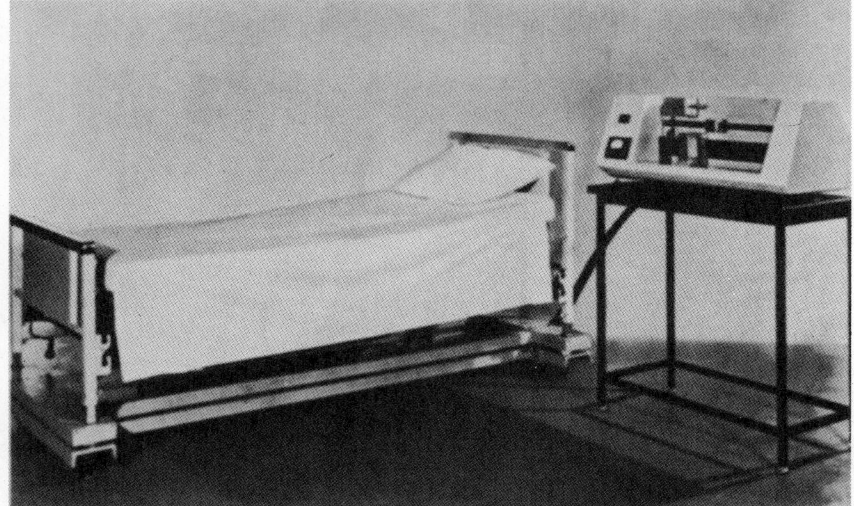

Figure 49. Metabolic bed scale. (From Roe, F. C.: New equipment for metabolic studies. *Nurs. Clin. N. Amer.*, *1*:4:622, 1966.)

gram is monitored at least every four hours during the diuretic phase. A rapid decrease in serum potassium as a result of diuresis may precipitate cardiac arrhythmias, particularly in the digitalized patient (see Fig. 4 for sample EKG). Emergency equipment and drugs for cardiopulmonary resuscitation are kept available. The principles of medical management of the diuretic phase following transplantation are similar to those of the diuretic phase of acute renal failure from other causes (see Chapter 5 for more detail).

Central venous pressure (CVP) equipment is inserted into the patient's left atrium in order to monitor the effect of fluid loss on his circulating volume of blood and to determine replacement therapy. For a detailed discussion of CVP the reader is referred to Metheny or Betson.[17, 90] Marked changes in the patient's circulating volume of blood are indicated by a CVP below 8 cm H_2O or above 20 cm H_2O. The nurse observes and records the CVP hourly or more frequently if necessary.

Anuria. Representing the other extreme response to renal transplantation are the patients who are anuric or severely oliguric in the immediate postoperative period. This occurs most frequently with cadaver kidneys for which the ischemic period is long. Anuria or severe oliguria may follow one of two courses. It may be irreversible and result in cortical necrosis and death of the kidney or it may be due to renal ischemia and reversible tubular necrosis. Anuria due to rejection is discussed later in this chapter. The reversibility of the ischemic disease is difficult to predict, and anuria may persist up to five weeks before adequate renal function begins. The length of postoperative anuria does not seem to affect the graft survival rate.

During the oliguric phase patients continue to receive immunosuppressive agents and antibiotics if necessary; however, careful regulation of dosage is required with those drugs normally excreted by the kidney. The patient is maintained in good health with intermittent hemodialysis. Continuity of nursing care is very important in order to reduce the patient's anxiety during the tense period. The patient is kept informed of his progress and is encouraged to verbalize his fears. His level of anxiety may be directly related to the number of transplants he has received. A patient receiving a second or third transplant can be expected to be more tense when renal function is poor.

Partial function. Last, there is the patient whose transplant is functioning but whose output is inadequate. This may occur either immediately or after several days of good urine output. This inadequate functioning is most frequently due to rejection. The general treatment whenever rejection is suspected consists of immediate and vigorous administration of steroids. However, microscopic examination of a renal biopsy will confirm the diagnosis and dictate the course of action.

Complications

THE EARLY POSTOPERATIVE PERIOD

Infection. Reverse isolation is used the first postoperative week, and sterile technique is carried out continuously to avoid contamination. Although the value of reverse isolation is unproved, the practice is continued in most centers because 85 per cent of the patients who die following transplantation have active infections that frequently are the cause of death. Since the patients receive large doses of immunosuppressive drugs in the early postoperative period, they are more susceptible to all infections. In cases of life-threatening infections the dosage of immunosuppressive agents is decreased to the minimum necessary for graft survival.

Although gram-positive staphylococcal infections occur, gram-negative organisms, which may arise from the patient's own intestinal tract, occur more frequently. The most persistent of these are Proteus, *Aerobacter aerogenes,* and *Pseudomonas aeruginosa.* Treatment consists of prompt and vigorous administration of antibiotics effective against the specific bacteria.

Pneumonias are the most common and the most devastating infections encountered. The nurse instructs all persons who are in contact with the patient in the principles and techniques of reverse isolation. Written instructions are posted on the patient's door and at the nurses' station. Individuals with colds are kept away from the patient and the total number of people who do come in contact with him during the early postoperative period is kept to a minimum. The nurse is responsible for restricting visitors and explaining the importance of this to the patient and his family. Turning, coughing, and deep breathing are essential postoperative techniques in light of the incidence of pneumonia. Blow-bottles may be used to encourage the patient to expand his lungs.

Delayed wound healing as a result of steroid therapy makes it necessary to continue to use aseptic technique for dressing changes longer than is required for the average nephrectomy patient.

Vascular complications. Vascular complications of the graft itself are attributed to technical errors during the operation and can be eliminated by extremely careful dissection and complete hemostasis. Signs of vascular complications include severe flank pain, anuria, and frank bleeding at the incisional site. The nurse observes for these signs in the early postoperative period.

Postoperative thromboembolic complications are not unusual and frequently take the form of thrombophlebitis of the lower extremity on the side of the allograft. It may be due to trauma to the vessels during surgery or to muscular inactivity of the patient coupled with excessive weight loss postoperatively. The nurse performs passive exercises on the patient's lower extremities immediately postoperatively and assists him with active exercises as soon as he is awake. Elastic stockings are applied to the patient's legs to further enhance circulation and decrease the pooling of venous blood. Early ambulation—for most patients on the second postoperative day—is also helpful in increasing muscle tone and maintaining adequate circulation.

Gastrointestinal disturbance. Vomiting and ileus are frequent postoperative complications and are partly due to the surgery itself or to hypokalemia, which causes muscle weakness. Diarrhea and intestinal colic may result from hyperkalemia. The patient has a nasogastric tube connected to Gomco suction for the first few days after surgery until bowel function returns. Fluid and electrolyte loss through gastrointestinal suction is measured accurately and recorded.

Genitourinary complications. The most frequently seen genitourinary complications are urinary fistulas and urethral strictures. Fistulas resulting from technical failure at the cystotomy site are detected by urography or by efflux of urine through the skin incision. The nurse inspects the dressing regularly in the early postoperative period for urine as well as bloody drainage.

Urethral strictures, which occurred frequently in the past, have been greatly reduced since the introduction of the Silastic Foley catheter. It is believed that the rubber catheter caused a high percentage of strictures. Foley catheters are routinely kept in place from three to seven days, but sometimes may be removed earlier. Since the danger of infection is so great in these patients, efforts are made to remove all drainage tubes as soon as possible.

Hypertension. Severe hypertension may occur immediately after surgery and may not respond to ordinary forms of therapy. It may be an early sign of rejection and, unlike other types of hypertension, may respond to large doses of corticosteroids. For acute hypertensive crisis, intravenous diazoxide (Mutabase) 5 mg/kg may be effective. Occasionally patients in severe hypertensive crises may respond only to intravenous sodium nitroprusside. Milder forms of hypertension can be treated with reserpine, hydralazine (Apresoline), and oral phenoxybenzamine (Dibenzyline). Prognosis for graft survival is poor for patients with unresponsive persistent hypertension.

Massive diuresis. Massive diuresis in the first few postoperative days may cause dehydration or hyponatremia and hypokalemia. Dehydration is a more serious problem in children and occurs very rapidly. Keeping accurate fluid balance sheets as well as monitoring weight changes and obtaining laboratory electrolyte studies is essential in this period.

Acute tubular necrosis (ATN). The incidence of ATN is greatest in transplanted cadaver kidneys; however, it is seen less frequently since the advent of perfusion and preservation techniques. It is characterized by oliguria and anuria. Treatment is basically the same as for ATN from other causes, i.e., early dialysis. Hemodialysis is used in transplant patients.

Hepatitis. Hepatitis may occur as a result of multiple blood transfusions received during dialysis or may be transmitted directly from a cadaver kidney. Azathioprine (Imuran) has also been reported as causing liver damage that mimics hepatitis. Corticosteroids are used to treat hepatitis.

Hyperparathyroidism. Hyperparathyroidism associated with chronic renal failure ordinarily subsides following transplantation when the calcium and phosphorus levels return to normal. Occasionally, however, the parathyroid hyperfunction continues and parathyroidectomy is indicated.

"Transplant lung." The term "transplant lung" refers to a syndrome consisting of alveolar-capillary block with absence of or minimal lung findings on physical examination, i.e., no cough and no sputum. It frequently accompanies kidney graft rejection. X-rays show changes resembling pneumonia, pneumonitis, or miliary tuberculosis. Blood gas studies show a low arterial pO_2 with a normal pCO_2. In severe cases cyanosis, leukopenia, and very low oxygen saturation are seen. Treatment consists of administering large doses of corticosteroids unless contraindicated by the presence of infection.

Glomerulonephritis. Recurring glomerulonephritis is most frequently seen in identical twin kidney transplants and may occur within days after the surgery. Glomerulonephritis is most likely to occur in transplants in patients who have antiglomerular basement membrane antibodies. It is difficult to differentiate between allograft rejection and glomerulonephritis unless a renal biopsy is performed. Immunosuppression is the treatment of choice.

REJECTION

At present, there are no clinical signs or symptoms that permit the accurate diagnosis of allograft rejection. However, advances in the area of immunopathological mechanisms of allograft rejection have made it possible to use allograft microscopy to diagnose rejection specifically. Microscopic examination of renal biopsies, particularly following cadaver kidney transplantation, prevents the unnecessary increase of immunosuppressive drugs in those patients whose grafts do not show the morphological changes of rejection.

Immunological Factors of Rejection

Although knowledge of the immunological response of rejection is far from complete, it is believed that the basic mechanism involved in allograft rejection is composed of an immunological arc with afferent and efferent pathways.

Afferent arc. The afferent arc represents the recipient's recognition of a foreign tissue, or more specifically the sensitization of the recipient by the antigens from the living cells of the donor. These antigens are located on various tissue cells including lymphocytes, which, it is theorized, play a major part in the sensitization. Sensitization occurs in one of three ways: (1) lymphocytes of the recipient pass through the allograft, pick up antigens, and return to the lymph node to initiate immune response; (2) antigens are released from the venous circulation of the organ; or (3) passenger lymphocytes in the transplanted organ provide the major antigenic stimulus.[44]

Many methods (irradiation, freezing, heating) have been tried clinically to block this afferent immunological response—all without success. The only successful method of altering the afferent response has been the establishment of acquired immunological tolerance in laboratory animals. Acquired tolerance is established by introducing antigens into host animals either in utero or during neonatal life prior to their developing an immune response. As pure, soluble transplantation antigens are developed and used in conjunction with immunosuppressive drug therapy, it is believed, tolerance to specific tissues may be developed in man.

Efferent arc. The efferent arc represents the recipient's response to the foreign tissue. The recipient reacts to the foreign tissue either by the formation of immunologically competent lymphocytes or by the formation of antibodies against the foreign tissue. In the usual type of rejection, cellular immune injury (lymphocyte response) probably plays the more important role. However, in the very violent and rapid type of rejection, as seen in ABO blood group incompatibility or in patients who have had multiple pregnancies or whole blood transfusions, the humoral antibody is mainly responsible for rejection. Figure 50 schematically summarizes the usual type of rejection.

Patterns of Rejection

ABO blood incompatibility. A rapid, violent rejection occurs within hours or days after transplantation when donor and recipient are ABO incompatible. This type of rejection is characterized morphologically by massive thrombosis of the renal artery and necrosis of the

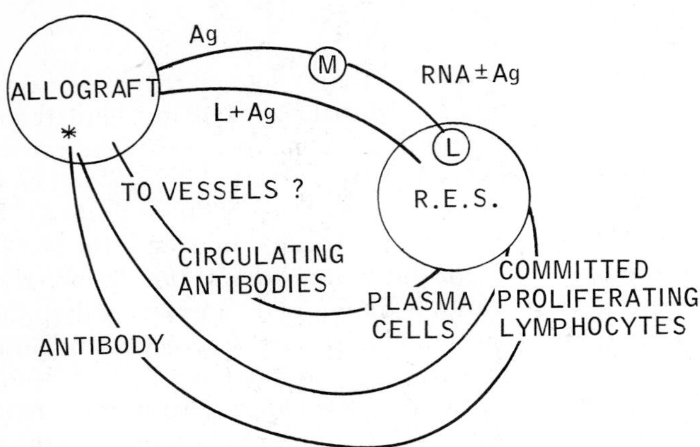

Figure 50. Sensitization of the recipient by the donor antigens from the living cells of the donor. Lymphocytes (L) may pass through the allograft and become informed of the foreign tissue. On returning to the reticuloendothelial system (R.E.S.) of the recipient some lymphocytes may return to the allograft covered with antibody and cause the classic homograft rejection. It is possible that antigen (Ag) is released from the graft, is processed by macrophages (M) and with or without RNA is delivered to the R.E.S. as the form of stimulus for the pictured reaction. (From Hardy, J. D. (Ed.): *Human Organ Support and Replacement.* Springfield, Ill., Charles C Thomas, 1971.)

entire kidney pelvis. Clinically the nurse observes a rapid and dramatic decrease in urine output owing to the decrease or absence of blood flow. The patient may complain of severe flank pain due to ischemia on the side of the allograft. Because of disastrous allograft failures due to ABO incompatibility in the early 1960's, ABO matching has become an absolute requirement in selecting donor-recipient pairs; consequently, this severe type of rejection is no longer observed.

Hyperacute rejection. This pattern of early graft rejection is observed in patients who have preformed cytotoxic antibodies directed against donor lymphocyte antigens as a result of previous whole blood transfusions, previous pregnancies, or a previous allograft. This rapid, violent rejection occurring within hours or the first two days after transplantation is caused by the circulating humoral lymphocytotoxic antibody. Morphologically it is characterized by fibrin thrombi in small arteries and arterioles with extensive cortical necrosis. The clinical picture is nearly identical to that of ABO incompatibility rejection. Advances in histocompatibility testing, in particular the cytotoxicity tests, will decrease the frequency of the hyperacute form of rejection.

Acute rejection. The term "acute" pertains more to the morphological changes that occur with this type of rejection than to the time span in which they occur. Acute rejection can occur from one or two weeks to up to months after transplantation. Morphologically the kidney is grossly large, swollen, edematous, often weighing two to four times normal, with a tense capsule and areas of cortical necrosis (Fig. 51).

The characteristics most important in diagnosing this type of rejection are: (1) infiltration of mononuclear cells in the interstitial and perivascular areas; and (2) fibrinoid necrosis of small arteries, arterioles, and glomerular capillaries.[44] The degree of these changes as determined by microscopic examination of a renal biopsy indicates the prognosis and dictates the course of action. A severe reaction indicates an irreversible process, hence the removal of the allograft. A slight reaction indicates a reversible process that requires increased immunosuppressive therapy.

The most common functional manifestations of acute rejection include: (1) decreased rates of glomerular filtration, renal blood flow, and urine flow; (2) increased urine osmolality; and (3) decreased urine sodium concentration. The blood urea nitrogen and the serum creatinine concentrations begin to rise in response to the decrease in filtration rate. Although all these changes can be attributed to renal ischemia from any cause, when manifested at any time following transplantation, even during later periods, they signal danger and warrant close follow-up examination of the patient. The nurse caring for

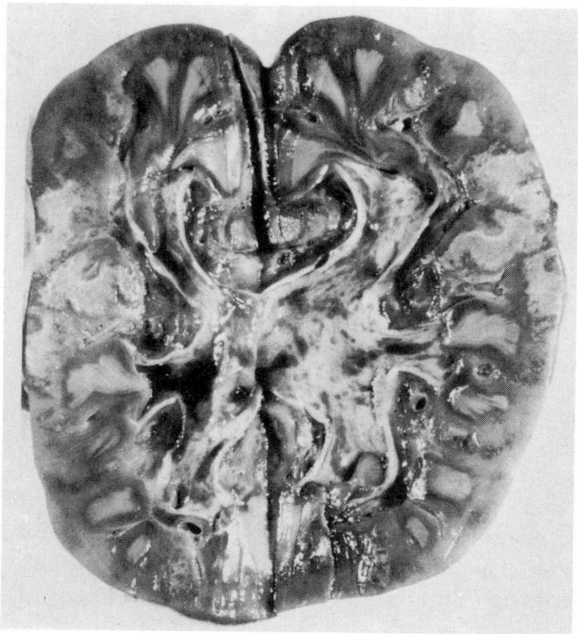

Figure 51. Gross view of acute rejection. Note the extensive cortical necrosis. (From Deodhar, S. D., and Benjamin, S. P.: Pathology of human renal allograft rejection. *Surg. Clin. N. Amer.*, *51*:5, 1148, 1971.)

the patient in the hospital or follow-up clinic is alert to these laboratory signs of rejection and immediately reports any abnormality to the attending physician.

In the immediate postoperative period, a classic rejection episode generally appears with sudden oliguria, swelling of the kidney, fever, and perhaps hypertension. The nurse observes the patient closely for any of these symptoms and reports them immediately. The patient may complain of acute tenderness, which may be difficult to differentiate from incisional pain. The tenderness of rejection is caused by the acute pericapsular inflammatory process, which stimulates the somatic nerves in the body wall. The nurse accurately observes, records, and evaluates the specific aspects of the patient's pain and general condition. However, rejection is a complex phenomenon that is at best difficult to detect clinically. All the symptoms just mentioned may result from complications other than rejection and all may be completely masked by steroid therapy. Since there is no single physical sign, symptom, or laboratory or radiological test that is diagnostic of rejection, the diagnosis is made first by excluding other causes of allograft failure and then is confirmed by renal biopsy.

Laboratory signs of rejection include increased blood urea nitrogen (BUN) and creatinine levels, proteinuria, and decreased creatinine clearance. The BUN value alone is unreliable, however, since it is susceptible to changes in total body catabolism and may rise as a direct result of fever, diet, and steroid therapy. A more sensitive indicator of renal function is serial determination of serum creatinine. An elevation of more than 50 per cent above the base line indicates a significant decline in function. Creatinine clearance rates are also of value, but the degree of fluctuation is greater than that for serum creatinine.

The nurse is familiar with the patient's latest laboratory values as well as the biopsy results. She anticipates the medical therapy on the basis of the patient's clinical appearance, the biopsy, and laboratory tests, and plans her nursing care accordingly. For example, if all data suggest a rejection crisis, the nurse assumes that the patient will receive intensive immunosuppressive therapy; consequently, she prepares to resume or continue reverse isolation.

Chronic rejection. The term "chronic rejection" also pertains to morphological changes in the transplanted kidney rather than to the time span in which they occur. Chronic rejection occurs at any time from weeks to months to years after transplantation. Grossly, the outer surface of a chronically rejected kidney appears irregular as a result of old infarcts and in severe cases it may have a nodular appearance with marked scalloping (Fig. 52). Morphologically, the hallmark of chronic rejection is obliterative vascular disease with subintimal fibroplasia (Fig. 53).

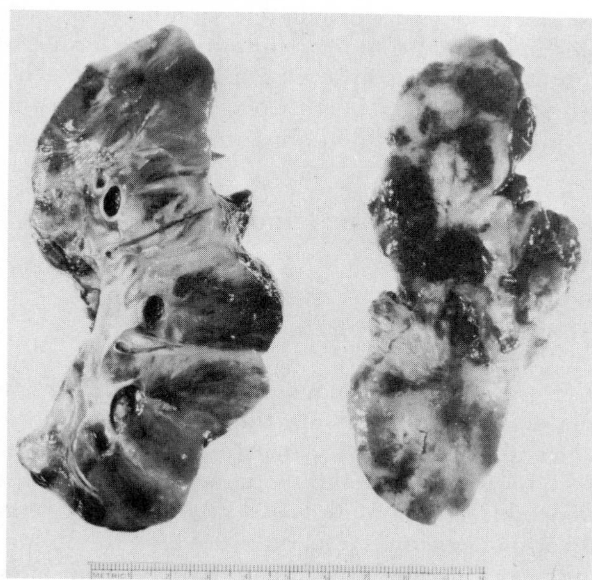

Figure 52. Chronic rejection, gross view (18 months after transplant). Note the irregular scalloped appearance. (From Deodhar, S. D., and Benjamin, S. P.: Pathology of human renal allograft rejection. *Surg. Clin. N. Amer., 51*:5, 1153, 1971.)

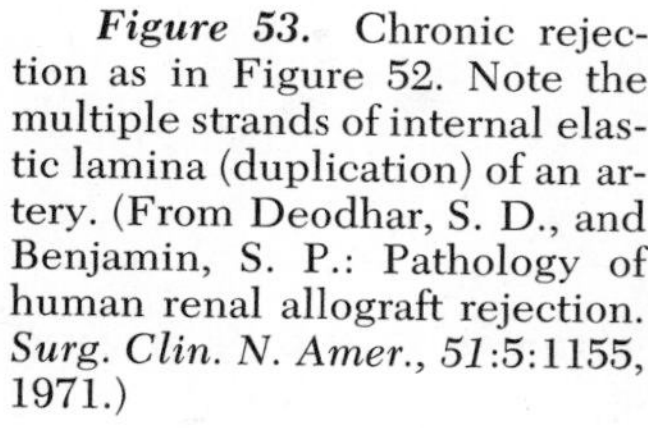

Figure 53. Chronic rejection as in Figure 52. Note the multiple strands of internal elastic lamina (duplication) of an artery. (From Deodhar, S. D., and Benjamin, S. P.: Pathology of human renal allograft rejection. *Surg. Clin. N. Amer., 51*:5:1155, 1971.)

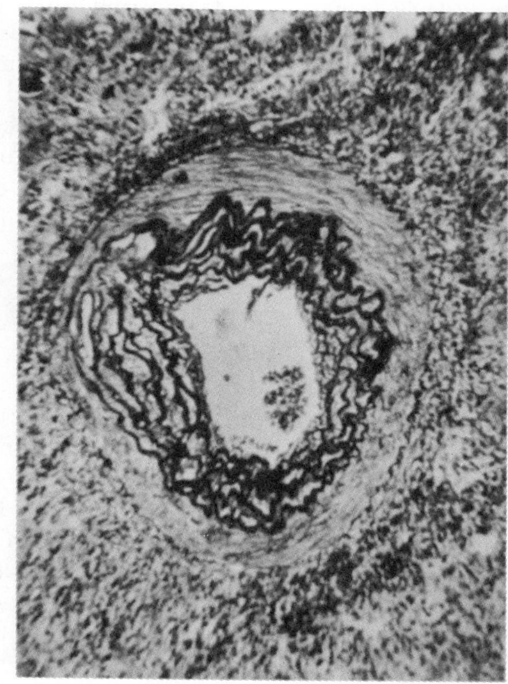

The vascular disease of chronic rejection is believed to be the irreversible end stage resulting from immunological injury due to both cellular and humoral factors in acute rejection. It is also theorized that these chronic changes may be the result of a slow, low-grade immunological injury that in time ends in rejection.

LONG-TERM COMPLICATIONS OF KIDNEY TRANSPLANTATION

Late Failure of Renal Allografts

Acceptance of renal transplantation as an effective mode of therapy depends on the ability of the transplanted kidney to maintain good function and a useful life for an extended period of time. The use of serological tissue typing and immunosuppressive therapy have greatly increased the allograft survival rate. The most common long-term complication is chronic rejection in which the kidney gradually loses its ability to function. Late rejection may occur after as long as five years, as is more completely described later in this chapter. Recurring renal disease is another long-term complication that results in allograft failure. Glomerulonephritis and pyelonephritis are frequently found to have caused transplant failure after several years of normal functioning. Interstitial and arterial lesions in the allograft are also seen in late allograft failure. It is not known what factors determine the precise mode of failure. Hamburger and Dormont postulate that the various lesions correspond to a specific pattern of histocompatibility or antigenic difference between donor and recipient.[56] Thus various parts of the same kidney may carry different antigenic determinants, which may or may not elicit an immune response, depending on the antigenic make-up of the host. This theory is at present under laboratory investigation.

Drug Related Complications

Transplant patients receive long-term corticosteroid therapy and are thus subject to all the complications of maintenance steroid usage. A detailed description of steroid complications can be found later in this chapter. Withdrawal of corticosteroids may lead to arthralgia, joint effusions, fever, and malaise. In addition, some transplant patients develop "transplant lung" upon withdrawal. It may occur in a period of steroid withdrawal or may be associated with rejection of the allograft. It has been found that increasing the steroid dose reverses this condition.

Medical Complications

Infectious diseases. The long-term use of azathioprine along with corticosteroids increases the risk of lethal infections, particularly in patients with deteriorating kidney function. Organisms that do not ordinarily cause clinical disease as well as a variety of bacteria and viruses have been causative agents of multiple infections in transplant patients.

Transmission of cancer. When the transplant kidney is obtained from a donor with cancer, there is always a possibility of transmitting the cancer to the recipient. Cancer cells are more easily transplanted than normal cells and will grow under the influence of immunosuppressive drugs. Thus, kidneys of cadavers or living persons who have a history of cancer are rejected as donor organs.

Other complications. Medical complications resulting from drug therapy are frequently seen. For example, gastroenteritis associated with steroid therapy presents mild to severe medical problems in some patients. Hepatitis and hyperparathyroidism are also seen as long-term complications of kidney transplantation.

Treatment of Rejection

Rejection of the transplanted kidney is a major problem with transplantation. Several forms of therapy are used to slow or stop the rejection process: azathioprine, corticosteroids, antilymphocyte globulin, Actinomycin C, thoracic duct drainage, irradiation of the kidney, and irradiation of the blood.

AZATHIOPRINE

Azathioprine (Imuran) is one of the basic drugs for treating rejection. An antimetabolite, it inhibits the synthesis of DNA and RNA and, thereby, inhibits cell division. Azathioprine inhibits cell division in all tissues, but its effects are particularly felt in those in which cells are dividing rapidly. The cells of lymphoid tissue, which play an active role in causing rejection, divide and proliferate rapidly during the rejection process. Because azathioprine slows this division, it therefore slows or inhibits rejection.

Azathioprine administration, and the entire immunosuppressive regimen, vary somewhat from one transplant center to another. Sometimes begun one to five days preoperatively, it is almost always started within 24 hours postoperatively. The dose during the early postoperative period usually ranges between 3 and 5 mg/kg/day. The dose is gradually reduced over a period of three months or so to a maintenance dose of 1–2 mg/kg/day. Patients usually continue the maintenance dose indefinitely. The dose of azathioprine usually remains stable during a rejection crisis; other medications are added to treat the crisis.

Azathioprine dosage is gauged by the patient's white blood cell count, the desirable dose being the greatest amount that does not cause bone marrow depression. (Bone marrow depression is considered present when the WBC is about 4000/ml or less.) The patient's sensitivity to azathioprine, as reflected by the WBC, can vary significantly during his course of treatment. The dosage is altered to suit this sensitivity. The dose of azathioprine is reduced when the urine output is low, as the drug is partially eliminated by the kidneys. The dosage is reduced by two thirds to three fourths when the patient is receiving allopurinol (Zyloprim) concomitantly.

A specific example of azathioprine administration, from the University of Utah College of Medicine, Salt Lake City, is as follows. Patients who are to receive living donor kidneys begin azathioprine two days preoperatively. Patients receiving cadaver kidneys begin azathioprine immediately postoperatively. The initial dose is 4 mg/kg/day for five days. The dose is decreased thereafter as freedom from rejection permits.[140]

Azathioprine is given orally, in 50 mg tablets, or intravenously. For intravenous administration, it is dissolved in normal saline that has been made alkaline by the addition of sodium hydroxide. A typical IV solution contains 400 mg azathioprine, 1.4 ml normal sodium hydroxide, and 200 ml normal saline.

Azathioprine has several side effects. These are:

Bone marrow depression. Bone marrow depression was reported to have an 11 per cent incidence in centers participating in the Human Kidney Transplant Registry.[7] The white cell counts were depressed most often; platelet counts were depressed next most often. To guard against this side effect, a complete blood count is usually taken daily when the dosage is being adjusted, and at regular, usually weekly, intervals thereafter. The effects of a dose of azathioprine are reflected in the white count in about five to seven days. Conversely, the white cell count begins to recover a few days after azathioprine is withdrawn. The drug is stopped or given in decreased amounts when bone marrow depression appears.

Infection. The incidence of infection was 7 per cent in the aforementioned series.[7] The infections are secondary to the immunosuppressive effects of the drug and are sometimes fatal.

Hepatitis. The incidence of hepatitis was 3 per cent in this series.[7] The hepatitis is caused by the toxic effects of azathioprine on the liver.

Other side effects. These include anorexia, nausea, vomiting, diarrhea, oral lesions, skin rashes, fever, alopecia, pancreatitis, negative nitrogen balance with weight loss, and possible teratogenic effects.

Nursing care. The nurse gives the azathioprine as ordered daily. If she is responsible for drawing blood, she obtains CBC's as ordered. This will be daily at first, and less frequently after the dosage is adjusted. In some centers the blood work is done in the morning, the results are analyzed, and the azathioprine is given in the evening in a single dose. The nurse must be aware of the patient's serial CBC's, particularly his WBC's and platelet counts, as she bases some of her nursing care on his hematological status.

When the patient's WBC is low and infection is a serious threat, the nurse helps guard him from infection. The patient is often placed in reverse isolation if his WBC is about 1000/ml or less. When he is in reverse isolation, the nurse carries out the isolation technique herself, and sees that visitors and others also do so. When isolation is discontinued, the nurse places the patient in a single room if possible. If a single room is not available, he should be in a room with patients who do not have infectious diseases. Only healthy persons, without infections such as colds and sore throats, are assigned to care for the patient. The nurse avoids unnecessary venipunctures, catheterizations, nasotracheal suctioning, and other instrumentation, as this increases chances of infection. She uses proper sterile technique with procedures such as dressing changes, and she observes for and reports any signs of infection such as fever, tachycardia, local heat, swelling, redness, and pain.

The nurse protects the patient from unnecessary trauma that may cause bleeding due to a low platelet count. For example, when inserting a nasogastric tube, she lubricates the tip well with surgical jelly. She teaches the patient to use a soft toothbrush for dental hygiene.

As most patients will continue to take azathioprine after discharge, the nurse teaches the patient self-administration of the drug—the dosage and the important side effects, i.e., infection and bleeding. She stresses the importance of keeping appointments for blood counts, avoiding unnecessary exposure to infection, and reporting signs of developing infection promptly.

Adrenal corticosteroids

Adrenal corticosteroids are the second drugs used in most immunosuppressive regimens. The drugs act by suppressing the inflammatory response.

Corticosteroids are sometimes given preoperatively. In the immediate postoperative period they are given in large doses of about 1–2

*TABLE 7. Relative Anti-inflammatory Potencies of Corticosteroids**

Compound	Relative Anti-inflammatory Potency
Tetrahydrocortisol	0
Cortisone	0.8
Hydrocortisone	1
Prednisone	4
Prednisolone	4
6 α-methylprednisolone ((Medrol)	5
Triamcinolone (Aristocort)	5
Dexamethasone (Decadron)	25

*Adapted from Goodman, L. S., and Gilman, A. (Eds.): *The Pharmacological Basis of Therapeutics*. Fourth edition. New York, Macmillan Co., 1970.

mg prednisolone (or its equivalent) /kg/day. The dosage is gradually reduced over a period of two to three months to about 10 mg/day. Eventually the drug may be discontinued completely. During a rejection crisis, the dosage is greatly increased—corticosteroids are the prime agents for treating these crises. During rejection, the dose is about 100–200 mg prednisolone/day.

Corticosteroids are available in a variety of preparations. A list of commonly used preparations and their relative anti-inflammatory potencies are given in Table 7.

A specific example of steroid administration, from the University of Utah, is as follows: Patients receiving kidneys from living donors begin prednisolone two days preoperatively. Patients receiving cadaver kidneys begin prednisolone immediately postoperatively. Initially the dose is 1 mg/kg/day for four weeks. This is gradually decreased to 0.67 mg/kg/day in one to two weeks. It is then further decreased gradually. If signs of rejection appear, the dose is doubled for several weeks and again gradually reduced.[140]

There are numerous side effects from corticosteroid therapy, most of which occur with prolonged administration and high dosage. Some of these side effects, and their treatment, are as follows:

Increased susceptibility to infection. Care is taken to avoid infection. Established infections are treated vigorously.

Reactivation of tuberculosis. If the patient has had tuberculosis, he is given an antituberculosis drug along with the corticosteroids.

Reactivation or formation of an ulcer. The patient is given milk and alkalies, such as Amphogel, to prevent ulcer formation. During a rejection crisis, when the steroid doses are quite large, the patient is given milk or alkali every hour.

Fluid and electrolyte disturbance. Corticosteroids promote sodium and water retention and potassium loss. The patient's fluid and electrolyte status is monitored, fluid and sodium intake are restricted, potassium supplements are given, and diuretics are given as needed.

Hyperglycemia and diabetes mellitus. Because hyperglycemia may develop and diabetes mellitus may be precipitated, blood and urine glucose is monitored. Insulin is given if needed.

Cosmetic effects. Patients may develop darkened skin, striae, and acne; they may gain weight and develop the characteristic "moon facies"; women may develop facial hair. These developments are treated symptomatically. For example, the darkened skin and striae can be covered with make-up. Acne is treated with regular thorough cleansing. Women can bleach facial hair so that it is less noticeable.

Psychological changes. The patient's behavior may be abnormal, ranging from mildly depressed to psychotic, although severe changes are rare. These changes are usually reversed when the drug is withdrawn or the dosage reduced.

Nursing care. The nurse administers the drug as ordered. She makes certain that it is, indeed, given regularly because if it is stopped suddenly, as by accidental omission, the patient can become quite ill. Symptoms of sudden steroid withdrawal are: decreased blood pressure, fever, weakness, abdominal pain, vomiting, and diarrhea. Omissions are particularly likely to occur before a test or preoperatively, when the patient is receiving nothing by mouth. In such cases, the steroids are given parenterally. Omissions are also likely to occur when the patient changes services. The nurse is careful to prevent such errors of omission.

The nurse observes for the development of any side effects, reports such development to the doctor, and aids in the treatment of these effects. She helps the patient avoid infection, as described earlier. She checks to see that each patient receiving steroids has had a chest x-ray and tuberculin skin test to detect old or active tuberculosis, and that patients with positive findings are receiving antituberculosis drugs. She administers the ordered milk and alkalies to prevent ulcer formation. She weighs the patient at regular intervals, every one to three days, to help determine fluid balance. She tests the urine of all patients for glucose—daily as a screening measure, and more often if it is ordered or if the patient has glucosuria. She helps the patient manage cosmetic problems and reassures him that these effects disappear as the dosage is decreased. She explains to the patient and his family that the psychological changes are temporary, and that he will return to his usual mental state as the dose is decreased.

The drug is usually taken at home, so the nurse instructs the patient regarding self-administration.

ANTILYMPHOCYTE GLOBULIN

Antilymphocyte globulin (ALG) is the third medication used in most immunosuppressive regimens. ALG contains antibodies against human lymphocytes, which are active in causing rejection. The exact mode of action of ALG is not known: it may alter the lymphocytes that cause rejection and render them inactive, or it may reduce the number of these lymphocytes. ALG usually causes a reduction of circulating lymphocytes, but this reduction can be temporary; the lymphocyte count can return to normal, yet the ALG will still be effective.

Antilymphocyte globulin is prepared by injecting a horse or other animal with a preparation of human lymphocytes, usually derived from spleen or thymus glands. The horse develops a high antibody titer to the human lymphocytes. Blood is taken from the horse, and the fraction of the horse serum containing the lymphocyte antibodies is purified and processed to yield ALG.

At present there are no standard methods of quantitating ALG, although there are tests for measuring the activity of ALG in the laboratory. According to the method of Stevens, one unit of ALG activity is, "the amount of antibody required to agglutinate or cause to clump more than half of 5000 fresh lymphocytes in 0.1 ml of buffer solution. . . ."[140] There are, however, no standard tests that measure the ability of ALG to prolong the survival of a transplant. Such methods are needed and are the subject of current research.[13, 80, 123, 126]

Administration of ALG usually begins on the day of transplantation and continues for three to four weeks thereafter. It is given by intramuscular or subcutaneous injection. A specific example of ALG administration, from the University of Utah, is as follows:[140]

Days from transplantation	*Units of ALG, according to the method of Stevens*
0	41,000
1	82,000
2,3,4,5,6	123,000
8,10,12	123,000
15,19,22,26	123,000

Possible side effects from ALG include:

Serum sickness and anaphylaxis. Severe systemic reactions to the foreign animal antigen, including serum sickness and anaphylaxis, can occur. Symptoms of serum sickness include fever, chills, pruritus, hematuria, and joint pains. Anaphylaxis is characterized by rapidly developing shock—a falling blood pressure and a weak, thready pulse. Patients should have skin tests for sensitivity to horse (or other animal) serum before ALG is given, to help avoid these reactions.

Elevated temperature. The patient often develops a temperature 1–2° F above normal following ALG injection. The temperature returns to normal within a few hours.

Local inflammatory reaction. Many patients experience moderate to severe pain at the injection site. The pain typically lasts 3–12 hours and occasionally radiates down the leg. Swelling, redness, and hyperthermia also occur at the injection site.

Thrombocytopenia. Some patients show a reduction in the number of platelets. For example, one patient developed a platelet count of 3000/ml (normal 150,000–300,000/ml).[140] It seems that the thrombocytopenia is due to an antiplatelet factor in the ALG, and that this factor can be removed with better methods of purification.[140]

Nursing care. The nurse checks to see that the patient has had skin tests for sensitivity to horse (or other animal) serum before administering the ALG. She has medication readily available for the treatment of serum sickness and anaphylaxis—diphenhydramine (Benadryl), epinephrine, and corticosteroids. She observes and records the patient's reaction to the ALG and immediately reports to the physician any symptoms of serum reaction or anaphylaxis.

The nurse explains to the patient beforehand that he may experience some pain and swelling at the injection site, and that this will be relieved with symptomatic measures. She gives the patient a systemic analgesic about one half hour before the ALG. She alternates injection sites and applies warm soaks to the area after the injection. Procaine can be given with the injection, but this relieves the pain for a short time only. The nurse should give the ALG in the morning in order to allow the pain to subside as much as possible before the patient's sleeping hours.

The nurse is aware of the patient's platelet count. If he develops thrombocytopenia, she helps him avoid trauma, particularly to the delicate mucous membranes.

Actinomycin C

Actinomycin C is a drug used in many immunosuppressive regimens. It is a mixture of three related antibiotics isolated from the fungus *Streptomyces chorysomallus*. The drug inhibits the synthesis of nucleic acids, which are essential for cell reproduction. The effects of actinomycin C are especially pronounced on lymphoid tissue, the cells of which divide rapidly, especially during a rejection crisis.

Actinomycin C is sometimes used as primary immunosuppressive therapy, but it is most often used during a rejection crisis. For example, at the University of Utah, during a severe rejection crisis, actinomycin C is given in a dosage of 200 micrograms intravenously per day for several days.[140]

Side effects of actinomycin C are:

Bone marrow depression. Leukopenia and thrombocytopenia occur.

Ulceration of mucosa. Superficial ulcerations of the gastrointestinal mucosa occur fairly often.

Other side effects. Other side effects are anorexia, nausea, vomiting, alopecia, liver damage, and polyneuritis.

Nursing care. The nurse observes for and helps treat any side effects. She follows the patient's blood counts and protects him from infection in the presence of leukopenia, and from trauma in the presence of thrombocytopenia. If mucosal ulceration is present, the nurse teaches the patient to avoid mucosal irritation such as constipation and vigorous nose blowing. She treats lesions with topical medications such as glycerin for oral ulcers.

THORACIC DUCT DRAINAGE

Drainage of lymph and lymphocytes from the thoracic duct is used in some immunosuppressive regimens. For example, it is used as part of the primary immunosuppressive therapy at the Peter Bent Brigham Hospital in Boston.[101] Under local anesthesia, an indwelling Silastic catheter is placed in the thoracic duct. A short drainage tube connects the catheter to a plastic collecting bag (Fig. 54). The lymph drains from the duct to the bag by gravity. This procedure is performed three to seven days before transplantation. The drainage is maintained for as long as possible, up to 21–30 days, after which the fistula is closed. Between 25×10^9 and 150×10^9 lymphocytes in 10–83 L of lymph have been removed from patients.[101]

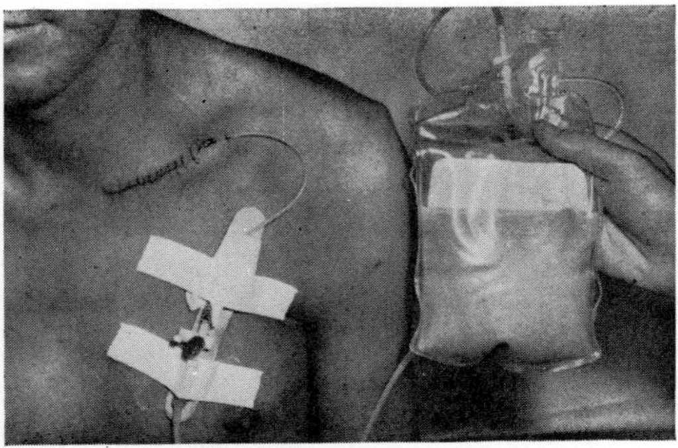

Figure 54. A thoracic duct fistula in situ in a patient, draining lymph through short connecting tubing into a collecting bag. (From Tilney, N. L., and Murray, J. E.: Chronic thoracic duct fistula: operative technique and physiologic effects in man. *Ann. Surg.*, *167*:1:3, 1968.)

Major side effects of a thoracic duct fistula are systemic infection and local infection of the neck wound.

Nursing care. The nurse explains the procedure to the patient and protects him from systemic infection. In caring for the fistula wound, she uses sterile technique to clean and dress it, and she changes the tubing and drainage bag at intervals to maintain sterility. She observes the fistula for patency. The fistula is especially likely to become clotted during the first 48 hours after transplantation, but clotting occurs at other times also. The nurse milks the tubing, changes the tubing, and irrigates the fistula with saline as needed to maintain patency. She keeps the drainage bag below the level of the fistula—at the waist or lower—to allow for gravity drainage of the lymph. The patient can ambulate with a draining fistula, but the nurse must instruct him regarding the position of the bag.

LOCAL IRRADIATION THERAPY

Local external radiation over the transplanted kidney is used in some immunosuppressive regimens. The radiation inactivates lymphocytes and lymphatic tissue and is used either as primary immunosuppressive therapy or as part of the therapy for a rejection crisis. At the University of Utah, where it is used during a rejection crisis, a total dosage of 600 rads in four divided treatments is given every other day.[140]

Side effects of radiation therapy include bone marrow depression, skin changes, and possible teratogenic effects.

Nursing care. The nurse explains the procedure to the patient. If bone marrow depression occurs, she helps guard him from infection. She gives special care to the irradiated skin: she washes the area with water only, as soap can be drying and irritating, and uses a bland oil or cream on the area if it becomes dry. She cautions the patient to avoid exposing the irradiated area to the sun, as this can cause further drying and irritation.

EXTRACORPOREAL IRRADIATION OF THE BLOOD

Extracorporeal irradiation of the blood is used in some immunosuppressive regimens for primary therapy or for treatment of a rejection crisis. It is not, however, used widely. As with external radiation, the immunosuppressive effect of this therapy is due to inactivation of lymphocytes, which are radiosensitive. To administer the treatment, an arteriovenous shunt, like one used for hemodialysis, is created. Via the shunt, the blood is diverted out of the body and through a coil placed in a specially constructed adapter, which permits exposure of the blood to the radiation. The blood then returns to the body via the A-V shunt. The capacity of the coil is about 175 ml. Doses from 1000–3000 rads/day have been given up to 20 times during 9–40 days. The lymphocyte count is usually not reduced markedly, but there are morphological and functional changes in these cells. Infection is the most serious side effect of this treatment.[111]

Nursing care. The nurse explains the procedure to the patient and assists with administering the treatment. Nursing care during extracorporeal circulation is discussed in detail in Chapter 6. The nurse is careful to protect the patient from infection.

OTHER THERAPY

Immunosuppressive measures that were used in the past but are now used infrequently include: thymectomy, splenectomy, total body irradiation, and azaserine.

Organ Preservation

Short-term methods of organ preservation became essential as the use of cadaver organs for transplantation increased in the late 1960's. The techniques used to preserve organs include use of hyperbaric oxygen, metabolic inhibitors, flushing solutions, and artificial perfusion. The most successful preservation has been achieved by combining all these techniques and was first described by Belzer and his associates in 1967.[15]

PERFUSION

The most commonly used perfusion solution is cryoprecipitated plasma. Several liters of plasma of the specific blood group common to both donor and recipient are pooled. Medications added to the plasma commonly include penicillin, magnesium sulfate, insulin, and cortisone. The plasma is frozen until needed, when it is thawed in a water bath and filtered through a microfilter to remove lipoprotein precipitates.

PRESERVATION TECHNIQUE

The preservation system most commonly used is the LI–400 unit, which consists of a pulsatile pump adjustable for rate and stroke vol-

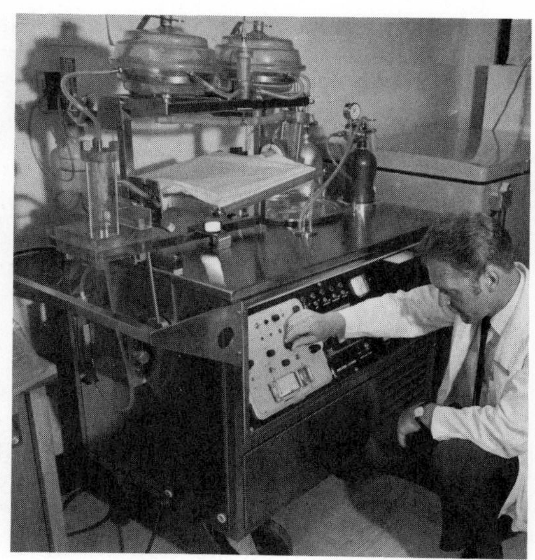

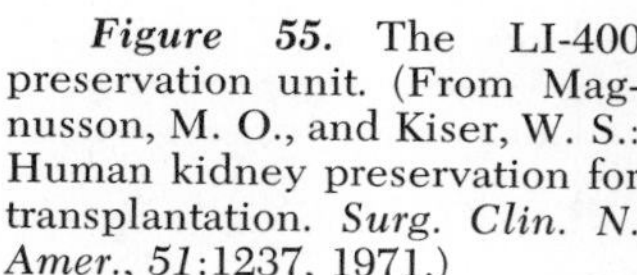

Figure 55. The LI-400 preservation unit. (From Magnusson, M. O., and Kiser, W. S.: Human kidney preservation for transplantation. *Surg. Clin. N. Amer.*, *51*:1237, 1971.)

ume, a disposable membrane oxygenator, two kidney chambers, arterial and venous reservoirs, and a heat exchanger (Fig. 55). A control panel contains pressure and temperature monitors and cooling and oxygenation systems. The machine is electrically operated and can be run by batteries for transportation.

When a kidney becomes available the perfusion circuit is primed with 700 ml of plasma; a Teflon cannula is inserted into the renal artery under aseptic conditions; the renal vein and ureter are left free; and all the air is removed from the arterial line before perfusion is begun. A temperature probe is placed under the kidney to insure that the kidney is maintained between 8° and 10° C during perfusion. Perfusion pulse rate is between 60 and 70 beats per minute at a pressure of 60 mm Hg systolic.

While the kidney is being perfused it is evaluated for its viability. In general a viable kidney is one that is tan in color and pulses rhythmically during perfusion and easily tolerates perfusion pressures of 50–60 mm Hg systolic. Kidneys of good quality ordinarily show an increase in pH of the perfusate during the first hour of perfusion and a minimum release of potassium and enzymes. In contrast the nonviable kidney is characteristically mottled during perfusion, shows signs of progressive swelling, registers a persistently elevated perfusion pressure with a reduced flow rate. Poor kidneys show a lowered pH indicative of tissue hypoxia and acidosis, and increased enzyme and potassium levels indicative of tissue destruction. It is essential that

*TABLE 8. Advantages of Human Cadaver Kidney Preservation**

Allows prospective tissue typing to be performed.
Allows assessment of kidney viability.
Allows postmortem examination of questionable donors.
Prospective recipients can live at a distance from the transplantation center.
Selected recipients can be prepared by dialysis preoperatively.
Source of cadaver kidneys is increased.
The transplant operation becomes an elective procedure.

*From Magnusson, M. O., and Kiser, W. S.: Human kidney preservation for transplantation. *Surg. Clin. N. Amer.*, *51*:5:1241, 1971.

the history of the cadaver kidney be known and taken into consideration before it is accepted or rejected for transplantation.

Human kidneys have been preserved up to 50 hours by this system and have been successfully transplanted. The advantages of human cadaver kidney preservation are listed in Table 8. With the successful clinical introduction of the preservation systems, regional transplant societies have developed programs that provide histocompatibility testing, optimal donor selection, and if necessary, transportation of either the recipient or the preserved cadaver kidney (Fig. 56).

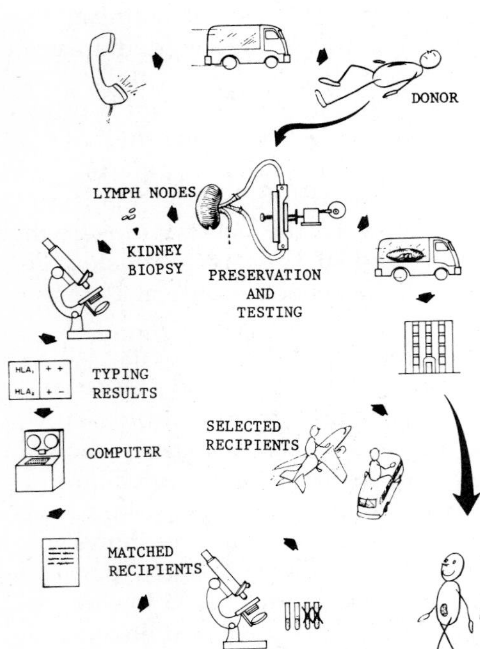

Figure 56. Schematic outline of cadaver procurement, tissue typing, and transplantation program. (From Belzer, F. O., and Kountz, S. L.: Preservation and transplantation of human cadaver kidneys. A two-year experience. *Ann. Surg.*, *172*:402, 1970.)

Survival Rates

TRANSPLANT REGISTRY

In 1963 the Kidney Transplant Registry was established with headquarters in Boston. Data from kidney transplants performed all over the world were sent to the registry for correlation. In 1971 the physical equipment and files of the registry were transferred to its present location in the headquarters of the American College of Surgeons in Chicago. This merged the activities of the Renal Transplant Registry with the other organ transplant registries funded by the National Institutes of Health. The annual reports of the Renal Transplant Registry are published in the *Journal of The American Medical Association*. The following statistics are summarized from the ninth and tenth reports published in April 1972 and September 1972 and based on the data accumulated until 1972. The Tenth Report of the Human Renal Transplant Registry includes data from 8332 kidney transplants in 7675 patients reported to the registry since 1951.

Overview. There has been little variation in patient survival and duration of function of the transplanted kidneys since 1967. Renal transplant results as a whole have reached a plateau of success at this time. The statistics will most probably remain constant until a major break-through occurs in the area of immunology. As of September 1972, 62 per cent of all renal transplant patients were alive. Seventy-five per cent of these have functioning grafts while the other 25 per cent are maintained with dialysis therapy. Of the patients dying following transplantation, 60 per cent had functioning grafts. These figures include all but 1.7 per cent of the transplant patients since 1951.

Diseases. The renal diseases most frequently responsible for renal failure that have been treated by transplantation are glomerulonephritis, pyelonephritis, and polycystic disease. A complete list of diagnoses of transplant patients appears in Table 9.

Related donor kidneys. The data show that among monozygotic twins who receive transplants from each other 100 per cent of the recipients and grafts survive for a two-year period and more than 60 per cent survive 10 years. One transplant from a monozygotic twin has been functioning for 16 years. The survival of recipients receiving sibling and parent grafts, collectively, in 1971 was nearly 85 per cent at one year, 83 per cent at two years, and 73 per cent at three years. The functioning of the grafts in the same group was 69 per cent at one year, 72 per cent at two years, and 63 per cent at three years. One graft from a parent has functioned for nine years. In all cases the duration and function of familial grafts were superior to those of the cadaver grafts.

*TABLE 9. Diagnoses Submitted to Transplant Registry**

Disease	No. Reported	Per Cent of Total
Glomerulonephritis	3,403	59.8
Pyelonephritis	892	15.7
More than one primary disease	301	5.3
Polycystic kidneys	259	4.6
Malignant hypertension	160	2.8
Renal disease, unspecified	137	2.4
Glomerulonephritis and pyelonephritis	100	1.8
Familial nephropathy	83	1.5
Congenital, nonobstructive	79	1.4
Nephritis, secondary to drugs	39	0.7
Medullary cystic disease	31	0.5
Obstructive uropathy	24	0.4
Diabetic glomerulosclerosis	19	0.3
Cortical necrosis	19	0.3
Lupus nephritis	16	0.3
Traumatic loss or removal	16	0.3
Cancer of kidney	13	0.2
Goodpasture's syndrome	11	0.2
Congenital, obstructive	10	0.2
Gout	10	0.2
Tuberculosis	9	0.2
Amyloidosis	8	0.1
Cystinosis	8	0.1
Nephrocalcinosis	8	0.1
Oxalosis-oxaluria	8	0.1
Tubular necrosis	8	0.1
Calculus disease	4	0.1
Radiation nephritis	4	0.1
Hyperparathyroid	2	0
Angiokeratoma corporis diffusum (Fabry's)	2	0
Periarteritis nodosa	1	0
Subacute bacterial endocarditis	1	0
Collagen disease	1	0
Nail-patella syndrome	1	0
Endocarditis	1	0

*From The Advisory Committee to the Renal Transplant Registry: The ninth report of the human renal transplant registry. J.A.M.A. *220*:255, 1972. Copyright 1972, The American Medical Association.

Cadaver donor kidneys. The continually improving survival statistics and availability have led to an increase in the use of cadavers as a donor source and a decrease in the use of living donors. Figure 57 shows the trend and distribution of the source of renal donors since 1953. Survival rates for recipients of cadaver kidneys are reported to be 68 per cent at one year, 64 per cent at two years, and 54 per cent at three years. Graft functioning for this group is 46 per cent at one year, 46 per cent at two years, and 40 per cent at three years. Table 10 shows the survival rates of patients and duration of function of transplants performed in the years 1951 to 1966 as compared with the years 1967, 1968, 1969, 1970, and 1971.

Age. The ages of the recipient and donor seem to have little effect on the success of the graft. Only two transplants have been reported in the over 80 age group and neither patient survived. Ten

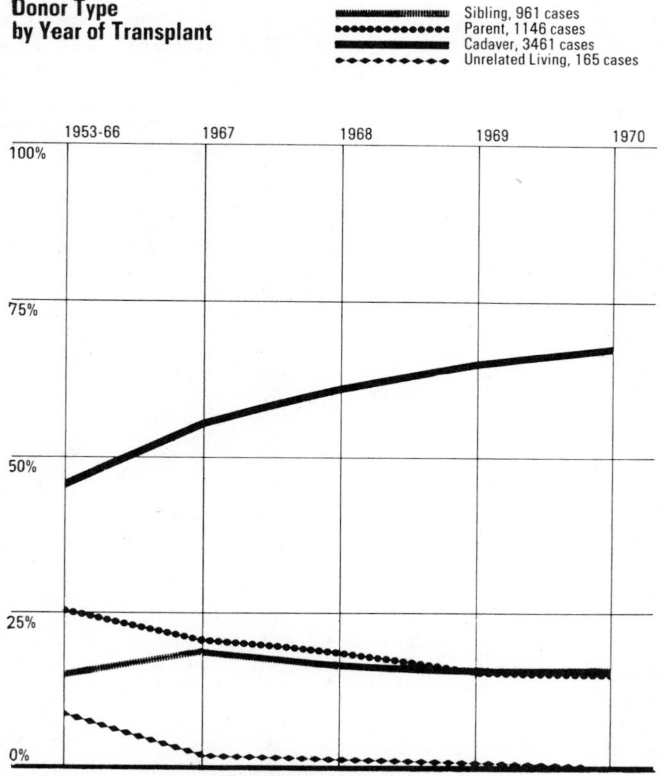

Figure 57. The trend and distribution of the source of renal donors from 1953 to 1970. (From The Advisory Committee to the Renal Transplant Registry: The ninth report of the human renal transplant registry. *J.A.M.A.*, *220*:254, 1972. Copyright 1972, The American Medical Association.)

TABLE 10. *Calculated Patient Survival and Transplant Function: First Transplant Only by Donor Source and Year of Transplant**

Donor Type	Year of Transplant	Sample Size	One Year: Per Cent Living†	One Year: Per Cent Functioning†	Two Year: Per Cent Living†	Two Year: Per Cent Functioning†	Three Year: Per Cent Living†	Three Year: Per Cent Functioning†
Sibling	1951–1966	240	69	64	62	58	59	53
	1967	138	85	79	77	71	72	66
	1968	185	89	81	84	75	81	71
	1969	195	83	77	79	72	79	70
	1970	207	87	82	86	80	...	...
	1971	109	82	73	...	...	...	...
Parent	1951–1966	403	61	57	57	50	53	46
	1967	145	74	71	69	63	64	57
	1968	190	79	73	75	68	71	60
	1969	199	80	71	74	64	68	59
	1970	199	85	71	83	67	...	...
	1971	102	89	66	...	...	...	...
Cadaver	1951–1966	663	41	35	34	28	29	22
	1967	365	56	45	48	38	44	33
	1968	584	58	47	51	39	44	33
	1969	737	66	55	59	46	54	40
	1970	858	70	54	64	46	...	...
	1971	466	68	46	...	...	...	...
Monozygotic twin	1951–1966	41	90	90	85	85	83	83
	1967	3	100	100	100	100	100	100
	1968	5	100	100	100	100	100	100
	1969	3	100	100	100	100	100	100
	1970	2	100	100	...	...	...	...
	1971	1	100	100	...	...	...	...
Dizygotic twin	1951–1966	14	64	64	57	57	43	43
	1967	3	67	67	67	67	67	67
	1968	5	100	100	100	100	100	100
	1969	0	...	...	...	...	...	...
	1970	1	100	100	...	...	...	...
	1971	1	...	...	...	...	...	...
Son or Daughter	1951–1966	0	...	...	...	...	...	...
	1967	1	100	100	100	100	100	100
	1968	2	100	100	100	100	100	100
	1969	12	74	74	74	63	74	63
	1970	17	68	59	53	46	...	...
	1971	13	86	61	...	...	...	...
Other related	1951–1966	20	63	60	63	60	57	54
	1967	16	66	56	66	56	59	50
	1968	11	91	91	82	82	70	70
	1969	11	79	54	79	54	79	54
	1970	5	100	80	100	80	...	...
	1971	5	...	...	...	...	...	...
Unrelated living	1951–1966	123	29	24	25	21	19	15
	1967	9	71	44	71	44	54	33
	1968	9	87	78	62	56	62	44
	1969	6	58	33	58	33	58	33
	1970	6	67	67	67	67	...	...
	1971	8	87	74	...	...	...	...
Spouse	1951–1966	18	20	19	13	13	13	6
	1967	4	25	25	25	25	...	...
	1968	6	67	50	67	50	67	50
	1969	3	33	33	33	33	33	33
	1970	0	...	...	...	...	...	...
	1971	1	...	...	...	...	...	...

*Adapted from The Advisory Committee to the Renal Transplant Registry: The tenth report of the human renal transplant registry. J.A.M.A., *221*:1495, 1972. Copyright 1972, The American Medical Association.

†Rounded off to the nearest whole number.

patients under age 3 have received grafts. The youngest patient with a functioning graft is 10 years old, while the oldest is 63. In the former patient, the same graft has been functioning for more than seven years, and, in the latter, four years.

Frequency. Of the 8332 transplant cases recorded as of 1972, 7614 cases are first transplants, 648 are second, 61 are third, 8 are fourth, and one is a fifth graft. Figure 58 shows the frequency of repetitive transplants by year.

Rehabilitation. Figure 59 depicts the status of rehabilitation of recipients of renal transplants. The data suggest that more cadaveric and unrelated grafts have a "chronic-in-hospital" course than familial transplants. Conversely more familial transplants reach a state of normalcy than patients with unrelated grafts.

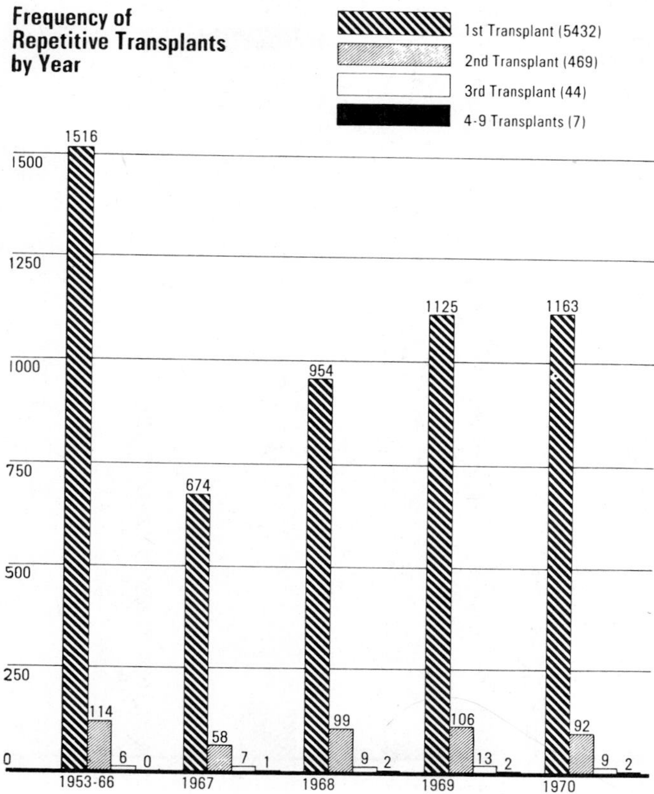

Figure 58. (From The Advisory Committee to the Renal Transplant Registry: The ninth report of the human renal transplant registry. *J.A.M.A., 220*:254, 1972. Copyright 1972, The American Medical Association.)

Cause of death. Although a single cause of death in renal transplant patients is difficult to determine, the data available in the Ninth Report of the Human Renal Transplant Registry are given in Table 11. The Tenth Report states that there has been a slight increase in the incidence of sepsis, cardiac arrest, and myocardial infarction. There have also been decreases in technical causes of death and deaths related to immunosuppression.

The information just summarized represents data from all the transplants reported from centers around the world. The advantage of collective analysis is that greater numbers are achieved. The disadvantage is that these statistics are not applicable to individual centers with greater or lesser experience. Thus these statistics represent the average performance achieved by all groups. Specific reports by

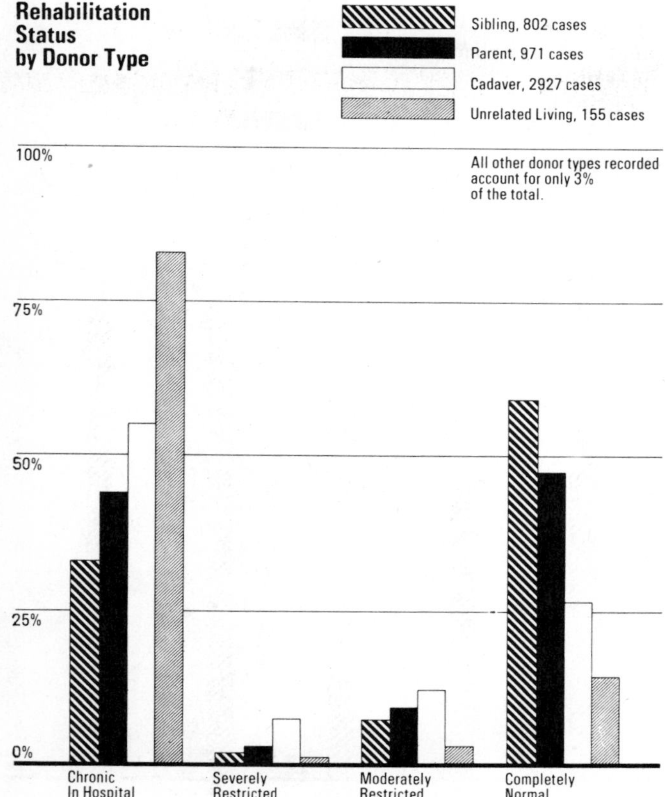

Figure 59. (From The Advisory Committee to the Renal Transplant Registry: The ninth report of the human renal transplant registry. *J.A.M.A., 220*:257, 1972. Copyright 1972, The American Medical Association.)

*TABLE 11. Results of Renal Transplantation: Causes of Renal Recipient Death**

Cause of Death	Frequency	Per Cent of Total
Sepsis	792	31.1
Unknown	325	12.8
Rejection	235	9.2
Rejection and Sepsis	221	8.7
Technical	145	5.7
Unrelated to transplant	141	5.5
Gastrointestinal hemorrhage and ulceration	96	3.8
Myocardial infarction	96	3.8
Technical and sepsis	74	2.9
Cardiac arrest	58	2.3
Cerebrovascular accident	54	2.1
Immunosuppression	49	1.9
Pulmonary embolus	34	1.3
Cancer	32	1.3
Immunosuppression and sepsis	29	1.1
Pancreatitis	27	1.0
Rejection, technical, and sepsis	23	0.9
Tubular necrosis	21	0.8
Rejection and technical	16	0.6
Rejection, immunosuppression, and sepsis	16	0.6
Diffuse vasculitis	14	0.5
Hepatitis	13	0.5
Immunosuppression and technical	8	0.3
Immunosuppression, technical, and sepsis	8	0.3
Rejection, immunosuppression, technical, and sepsis	5	0.2
Rejection and immunosuppression	5	0.2
Subdural hematoma	3	0.1
Rejection, immunosuppression, and technical	2	0.1
Liver failure	1	0.1

*From The Advisory Committee to the Renal Transplant Registry: The tenth report of the human renal transplant registry. J.A.M.A., *221*:1495, 1972. Copyright 1972, The American Medical Association.

physicians from the individual centers are available and contain survival statistics at each center.

Future of Renal Transplantation

Renal transplantation has evolved from experimental investigation to a clinical reality. Progressive increases in the survival of both the recipient and the graft have advanced renal transplantation to a feasible, acceptable method of treatment for chronic renal failure. Advances in tissue typing and immunosuppressive therapy as well as continued research and development in these areas are expected to further increase the host and graft survival rates.

RESEARCH

At present, research is being done to produce immunological tolerance. Researchers have produced specific immunological tolerance to allografts by administering living lymphoid cells from the prospective donor to animals still in utero. Tolerance is believed to result from exposure of the mammalian host to foreign antigens while it is still immunologically immature and incapable of producing an immune response. Recognizing the injected antigens as self rather than non-self, the animal's maturing immune system therefore fails to develop antibodies against them. Some investigators are continuing this research on mature laboratory mice in order to develop a method that may be used for humans.

Specific immunological tolerance appears to be the ideal solution to the problem of graft rejection in human organ transplantation. Specific tolerance allows unresponsiveness to transplanted tissue yet permits normal immune responsiveness against other foreign antigens. The specific immunological tolerance is not yet easily transferable to man, since injection of lymphoid tissue produces a graft-versus-host reaction in which the injected tissue forms antibodies that attack the antigens of the host. In addition, it is difficult to obtain from the lymphoid tissue of one donor, the large quantities of transplantation antigen necessary to produce a significant degree of immunological tolerance. Nevertheless, it seems logical to pursue this avenue of research in striving to achieve immunological tolerance to kidney transplants. Suppression of immune response to transplant tissue and maintenance of normal immune response to other foreign antigens are essential for transplantation to be a safe and effective routine method of treatment for kidney failure.

ADVANCES

Advances in organ preservation, computer analysis of tissue typing data, and regional transplantation programs are making it possible to ascertain the optimum recipient to match a prospective donor. Transportation of donor or recipient to another city for transplantation is increasing the availability of organs to all victims of renal failure regardless of location.

LIMITATIONS

One problem that the transplanters will continue to face is the limited availability of donor material. Although healthy donor kidneys are not a rarity, the supply is far from adequate to meet the demands of the potential recipients. Criteria are established by the transplant teams to insure maximum success. For example, transplantation may be restricted by a poor tissue match, by systemic disease within the donor, and by possible harm to a live donor. These criteria eliminate a great many potential donors. The number of cadaver kidneys available is limited, and selection of only the best reduces their number. The available good kidneys are obtained primarily from victims of head injuries who maintain good perfusion to the kidneys until the moment of death.

Another factor limiting the number of transplantations that are done is the cost of performing such an operation. Estimated costs are as high as $40,000, which is beyond the financial limits of many patients, most of whom have been paying $7000 to $14,000 a year to maintain their lives by dialysis. Subsidized programs other than those of the Veterans Administration hospitals are not readily available.

Outlook

Since transplantation is not possible on a large scale in the immediate future, regional transplant programs must include back-up dialysis facilities and the manpower to staff a nationwide network of dialysis units.

In general, the future of transplantation is very bright. It seems likely that within our lifetime continued research will make it possible to transplant most of the major organs with a high success rate.

CASE STUDIES

I

Mrs. N., a 26 year old homemaker and mother of one, had been maintained by intermittent hemodialysis for two years before receiving a kidney transplant. When she was nine, Mrs. N.'s disease was diagnosed as acute glomerulonephritis and she was treated for a prolonged period of time with steroids for nephrotic syndrome. When she was 16, Mrs. N. had an exploratory laparotomy for an upper quadrant mass. A splenectomy was done and the diagnosis of bilateral polycystic kidneys was made. At this time, she was treated for hypertension. Her renal function was relatively stable until she became pregnant at the age of 22. At this time she had a marked exacerbation with decreased renal function. The following year she developed a ureteral obstruction secondary to a blood clot, and a left ureterostomy was performed. Following this surgery, her renal function progressively deteriorated and she began home dialysis every third day via an A-V fistula. She was able to continue her household duties and work part time in a bank.

Mrs. N. continued to have hypertension in spite of good control of fluids and dialysis. Therefore, after a year of dialysis, a bilateral nephrectomy was performed to control the hypertension. Her continuing problems included repeated infections, pneumonia and cellulitis, anemia and mild cardiomegaly. While receiving dialysis, she took the following medications: Basaljel, ferrous sulfate, Berocca tablets, and methyldopa (Aldomet). She followed an 80 g. protein, 2 g. salt diet with 100 ml of fluid per day.

In July 1972, Mrs. N. was admitted to the hospital for a transplant. An A match cadaver kidney was available and was perfused for 15 hours prior to being transplanted into Mrs. N.'s right iliac fossa. Immediately postoperatively there was no urine output for 45 minutes. However, within two hours after surgery Mrs. N.'s urine output was 200–250 ml/hr. Following a diuretic phase that lasted three days with an average urine output of 3800 ml, Mrs. N.'s output stabilized at approximately 2000 ml/day. Routine immunosuppressive medications included methylprednisolone (Solu-Medrol) and azathioprine (Imuran).

Mrs. N.'s laboratory tests prior to surgery showed a BUN level of 38 and a serum creatinine level of 8.4 mg/100 ml. On the second postoperative day the BUN was 18 and the serum creatinine 1.6 mg/100 ml. Mrs. N.'s postoperative course was smooth until the sixth postoperative day when rejection threatened. This was evidenced by a BUN of 49 and serum creatinine of 2.2 mg/100 ml, a decreased urine output, and a slightly elevated temperature. During this threatened rejection Mrs. N. received a daily "cocktail" of methylprednisolone 1 gm, actinomycin D 0.5 mg, and heparin 5000 units intravenously. Three radiation treatments to both kidneys were done on alternate days. After four days of "cocktails" and radiation treatment Mrs. N.'s BUN was reduced to 26 and her serum creatinine to 1.3 mg/100 ml. Fifteen days after surgery Mrs. N. was discharged in good condition. She continues to take methylprednisolone (Medrol) and azathioprine (Imuran) twice daily and has resumed her normal life style as wife, homemaker, and part-time employee.

II

Mr. W. is a 43 year old man with a history of hypertension for five years that led to renal failure. His hypertension was diagnosed as primary or "essential" hypertension. Mr. W. had, for one year prior to his transplant, been treated with hemodialysis, on which he did well except for fluid overload and severe pruritus. In March 1972 he received an E match cadaver kidney. Immediately postoperatively diuresis commenced, and in 24 hours his urine output was 30,000 ml. Diuresis gradually decreased, and Mr. W. followed a routine postoperative course until the sixth day when rejection threatened. This was evidenced by fever, decreased urine output, 2+ proteinuria, and cells in the urine compatible with the transplant. Mr. W. received nine rejection "cocktails" of methylprednisolone (Solu-Medrol) 1 gm, actinomycin D 0.5 mg, and heparin 5000 units. However by the eleventh postoperative day there was no urine output and an arteriogram showed severe changes of rejection. Mr. W.'s BUN was 175 mg/100 ml by the fifteenth postoperative day, and he was hemodialyzed three times a week.

Thirty days after transplant Mr. W.'s BUN was stabilized at 84 mg/100 ml, his urine output was up to 1000 ml/day, and his renal scan showed improvement. Mr. W.'s blood pressure remained high at 170/100 and methyldopa (Aldomet) was continued. Thirty-eight days postoperatively, Mr. W. was discharged with poor but fairly stable renal function. He continued to take azathioprine (Imuran) and prednisone.

Ten days after discharge Mr. W. was readmitted with chills, fever, nausea, vomiting, and a BUN value of 140 mg/100 ml. Intensive immunosuppressive therapy was administered and blood cultures were made. The blood cultures were positive for gram-negative organisms, including *Enterobactor aerogenes*. The following week Mr. W. developed rales and wheezing due to pulmonary congestion. The kidney was removed and he returned to the long-term intermittent hemodialysis program, where he will remain until a suitable cadaver kidney is available for a second transplant.

References

1. Aach, R., and Kissane, J. (Eds.): Renal transplantation. *Amer. J. Med., 48*:93, 1970.
2. Abram, H. S., and Ackermann, J. R.: The nature of the kidney donor. *New Eng. J. Med., 285*:56, 1971.
3. Advisory Committee to the Renal Transplant Registry: The ninth report of the human renal transplant registry. *J.A.M.A., 220*:253, 1972.
4. Al-Askari, S.: Urologic aspects of renal transplantation. In Rapaport, F. T., and Dausset, J. (Eds.): *Human Transplantation.* New York, Grune & Stratton, 1968.
5. Amos, D. B.: Immunologic factors in organ transplantation. *Amer. J. Med., 44*:767, 1968.
6. Amos, D. B.: Immunologic and genetic aspects of kidney transplantation. In Strauss, M. B., and Welt, L. G. (Eds.): *Diseases of the Kidney.* Second edition, Boston, Little, Brown and Company, 1971.
7. Azathioprine (Imuran), official literature on new drugs. *Clin. Pharmacol. Ther., 10*:136–141, 1969.
8. Bach, F., and Hirschhorn, K.: Lymphocyte interaction: A potential histocompatibility test in vitro. *Science, 143*:813, 1964.
9. Back, J. F., Dormant, J., Dardenne, M., and Balner, H.: In vitro rosette inhibition by antihuman, antilymphocyte serum: correlation with skin graft prolongation in subhuman primates. *Transplantation, 8*:265–280, 1969.
10. Balner, H., van Bekkum, D. W., and Rapaport, F. T.: (Eds.): *Transplantation Today. Proceedings of the Third International Congress of the Transplantation Society.* New York, Grune & Stratton, 1971.
11. Batchelor, J. R., and Joysey, V.: Influence of HL-A incompatibility on cadaveric renal transplantation. *Lancet, 1*:790, 1969.
12. Beard, B. H.: The quality of life before and after renal transplantation. *Dis. Nerv. Syst., 32*:24, 1971.
13. Begemann, H.: Clinical experience with actinomycin C. *Ann. Acad. Sci., 289*:454–462, 1960.
14. Belzer, F. O., and Kountz, S. L.: Preservation and transplantation of human cadaver kidneys. A two-year experience. *Ann. Surg., 172*:394, 1970.
15. Belzer, F. O., Ashby, B. S., and Dunphy, J. E.: Twenty-four and 72-hour preservation of canine kidneys. *Lancet, 2*:536, 1967.
16. Bertelli, M., Monaco, A. P., and Donati, L. (Eds.): *Pharmacological Treatment in Organ and Tissue Transplantation. Proceedings of an International Symposium.* Milan, 1969.
17. Betson, C., and Ude, L.: Central venous pressure. *Amer. J. Nurs., 69*:1466, 1969.
18. Billingham, R. E., and Silvers, W.: *The Immunology of Transplantation.* Englewood Cliffs, N.J., Prentice-Hall, 1971.
19. Billingham, R. E., Brent, L., and Medawar, R. B.: Actively acquired tolerance to foreign cells. *Nature* (London), *172*:603, 1953.
20. Bowers, E.: Organs for transplantation. *Lancet, 1*:707, 1971.

21. Braun, W. E.: Immunologic aspects of renal transplantation. *Surg. Clin. N. Amer., 51*:1161, 1971.
22. Braun, W. E., Grecek, D. R., and Murphy, J. J.: Histocompatibility testing. *Surg. Clin. N. Amer., 51*:1175, 1971.
23. Brent, L., and Medawar, P. B.: Tissue transplantation. A new approach to the typing problem. *Brit. Med. J., 2*:269, 1963.
24. Burkholder, P. M.: Ultrastructural demonstration of injury and perforation of glomerular basement membrane in acute glomerulonephritis. *Amer. J. Path., 56*:261, 1969.
25. Calne, R. Y.: Renal Transplantation. London, Edward Arnold Publishers, Ltd., 1967.
26. Calne, R. Y.: *A Gift of Life. Observations on Organ Transplantation.* New York, Basic Books, 1970.
27. Calne, R. Y. (Ed.): *Clinical Organ Transplantation.* Oxford, Blackwell Scientific, 1971.
28. Campbell, M. P., and Harrison, J. H. (Eds.): *Urology.* Third edition, Philadelphia, W. B. Saunders Co., 1970.
29. Carpenter, C. B., and Austen, K. F.: The early diagnosis of renal allograft rejection. In Rapaport, F. T., and Dausset, J.: *Human Transplantation.* New York, Grune & Stratton, 1968.
30. Carpenter, C. B., and Merrill, J. P.: Modifications in renal allograft rejection in man. *Arch. Intern. Med., 123*:501, 1969.
31. Castelnuovo-Tedesco, P. (Ed.): *Psychiatric Aspects of Organ Transplantation.* New York, Grune & Stratton, 1971.
32. Ceppellini, R.: The genetic basis of transplantation. In Rapaport, F. T., and Dausset, J. (Ed.): *Human Transplantation.* New York, Grune & Stratton, 1968.
33. Clapp, J. R., and Robinson, R. R.: Functional characteristics of the transplanted kidney. *Arch. Intern. Med., 123*:531, 1969.
34. Collins, G. V., Bravo-Shugarman, M., and Terasaki, P. I.: Kidney preservation for transplantation. *Lancet, 2*:1219, 1969.
35. Converse, J. M., and Casson, P. R.: The historical background of transplantation. In Rapaport, F. T., and Dausset, J. (Eds.): *Human Transplantation.* New York, Grune & Stratton, 1968.
36. Daguillard, F.: Immunologic significance of in vitro lymphocyte responses. *Med. Clin. N. Amer., 56*:293, 1972.
37. Dammin, G. J.: The pathology of human renal transplantation. In Rapaport, F. T., and Dausset, J. (Eds.): *Human Transplantation.* New York, Grune & Stratton, 1968.
38. Dausset, J.: Technique for demonstrating leukocyte agglutination. In Russell, P. S., Winn, H. J., and Amos, D. B. (Eds.): *Histocompatibility Testing.* Washington, D.C., National Academy of Sciences, 1965.
39. Dausset, J., and Rapaport, F. T.: The Hu-1 system of human histocompatibility. In Rapaport, F. T., and Dausset, J. (Eds.): *Human Transplantation.* New York, Grune & Stratton, 1968.
40. Dausset, J., and Rapaport, F. T.: Blood group determinants of human histocompatibility. In Rapaport, F. T., and Dausset, J. (Eds.): *Human Transplantation.* New York, Grune & Stratton, 1968.
41. Dausset, J., Hamburger, J., and Matthe, G. (Eds.): *Advances in Transplantation.* Copenhagen, Williams & Wilkins Co., 1968.
42. Davies, D. A. L.: Transplantation antigens. In Rapaport, F. T., and Dausset, J. (Eds.): *Human Transplantation.* New York, Grune & Stratton, 1968.
43. De Planque, B., Williams, G. M., Siegel, A., and Alvarez, C.: Comparative typing of human kidney cells and lymphocytes by immune adherence. *Transplantation, 8*:852, 1969.
44. Deodhar, S. D., and Benjamin, S. P.: Pathology of human renal allograft rejection. *Surg. Clin. N. Amer., 51*:5:1141, 1971.
45. Eilert, J. B., Eggert, D. E., Derlacki, D. J., and Bergan, J. J.: Kidney graft storage after surface cooling. *Arch. Surg., 102*:197, 1971.
46. Falk, J. A., and Falk, R. E.: HL-A antigens in clinical transplantation. *Med. Clin. N. Amer., 56*:403, 1972.

47. Fellner,C. H.: Selection of living kidney donors and the problem of informed consent. In Castelnuovo-Tedesco, P. (Ed.): *Psychiatric Aspects of Organ Transplantation.* New York, Grune & Stratton, 1971.
48. Fellner, C. H., and Marshall, J. R.: Kidney donors—the myth of informed consent. *Amer. J. Psychiat. 126*:1245, 1970.
49. Fine, R. N., Edelbrock, H. H., Brennan, L. P., Korsch, B. M., Riddell, H., Stiles, Q., and Lieberman, E.: Cadaveric renal transplantation in children. *Lancet, 1*:1087, 1971.
50. Flannigan, W. J., Caldwell, F. T., Williams, G. D., Brewer, T. E., Glenn, W. E., Headstream, J. W., and Campbell, G. S.: Clinical patterns of renal autograft rejection. *Ann. Surg., 173*:733, 1971.
51. Goodman, L. S., and Gilman, A.: *The Pharmacological Basis of Therapeutics.* Fourth edition. New York, The Macmillan Co., 1970.
52. Goodwin, W. E., and Martin, D. C.: Renal transplantation. In Campbell, M. F., and Harrison, J. H. (Eds.): *Urology.* Third edition. Philadelphia, W. B. Saunders Co., 1970.
53. Gordon, J.: The mixed leukocyte culture rejection. *Med. Clin. N. Amer., 56*:337, 1972.
54. Hamburger, J.: Professor Hamburger on renal transplantation. *J.A.M.A., 215*:494, 1971.
55. Hamburger, J., and Crosnier, J.: Moral and ethical problems in transplantation. In Rapaport, F. T., and Dausset, J. (Eds.): *Human Transplantation.* New York, Grune & Stratton, 1968.
56. Hamburger, J., and Dormont, J.: Functional and morphologic alterations in long-term kidney transplants. In Rapaport, F. T., and Dausset, J. (Eds.): *Human Transplantation.* New York, Grune & Stratton, 1968.
57. Hardy, J. D. (Ed.): *Human Organ Support and Replacement. Transplantation and Artificial Prosthesis.* Springfield, Ill., Charles C Thomas, 1971.
58. Harris, R., Wentzel, J., Orr, W. McN., Mallick, N. P., and Mainwaring, A. R.: Value of tissue-typing in cadaveric renal transplantation. *Lancet, 1*:544, 1971.
59. Hill, R. B., Jr., Dahrling, B. E., II., Starzl, T. E., and Rifkind, D.: Death after transplantation. *Amer. J. Med., 42*:327, 1967.
60. Hirschhorn, K.: In vitro histocompatibility testing. In Rapaport, F. T., and Dausset, J. (Eds.): *Human Transplantation.* New York, Grune & Stratton, 1968.
61. Holman, E.: Protein sensitization in isoskingrafting. Is the latter of practical value? *Surg. Gynec. Obstet., 38*:100, 1924.
62. Hors, J., Fradelizi, D., Feingold, N., and Dausset, J.: Critical evaluation of histocompatibility in 179 renal transplants. *Lancet, 1*:609, 1971.
63. Hume, D. M.: Kidney transplantation. In Rapaport, F. T., and Dausset, J. (Eds.): *Human Transplantation.* New York, Grune & Stratton, 1968.
64. Hume, D. M., Merrill, J. P., Miller, B. J., and Thorn, G. W.: Experience with the renal homotransplantation in the human. *J. Clin. Invest., 34*:327, 1955.
65. Johnson, J. W., Hattner, R. S., Hampers, C. L., Bernstein, D. S., Merrill, J. P., and Sherwood, L. M.: Secondary hyperparathyroidism in chronic renal failure. Effects of homotransplantation. *J.A.M.A., 215*:479, 1971.
66. Jonasson, O.: Renal transplantation. Certain immunological considerations. *Med. Clin. N. Amer., 55*:193, 1971.
67. Jonasson, O., Lichter, E. A., Hamby, W. B., Smith, R. D., Gantt, C. L., and Nyhus, L. M.: Donor selection for renal transplantation based on genotypic analysis of HL-A in a family. *Arch. Surg., 101*:219, 1970.
68. Kashiwagi, N., Brantigan, C. O., Brettschneider, L., Groth, C. G., Starzl, T. E.: Clinical reactions and serologic changes after the administration of heterologous antilymphocyte globulin to human recipients of renal homografts. *Ann. Intern. Med., 68*:275, 1968.
69. Kincaid-Smith, P.: Histological diagnosis of rejection of renal homografts in man. *Lancet, 2*:849, 1967.
70. Kincaid-Smith, P.: Treatment of irreversible renal failure by dialysis and transplantation. In Beeson, P. B., and McDermott, W. (Eds.): *Cecil-Loeb Textbook of Medicine.* Thirteenth edition. Philadelphia, W. B. Saunders Co., 1971.
71. Kincaid-Smith, P., Morris, P. J., Saker, B. M., Ting, A., and Marshall, V. C.: Immediate renal-graft biopsy and subsequent rejection. *Lancet, 2*:748, 1968.

72. Kiser, W. S., Magnusson, M. O., McLaughlin, T. C., Hewitt, C. B., and Straffon, R. A.: Preservation of human cadaver kidneys for transplantation. *J. Urol., 105*:779, 1971.
73. Lawrence, H. S.: Immunological considerations in transplantation. In Rapaport, F. T., and Dausset, J. (Eds.): Human Transplantation. New York, Grune & Stratton, 1968.
74. Liu, W. P., Humphries, A. L., Jr., Russell, R., Stoddard, L. D., and Maretz, W. H.: 48-hour storage of canine kidneys after brief perfusion with Collins' solution. *Ann. Surg., 173*:748, 1971.
75. McDonald, J. C., Ritchey, R. J., Fuselier, P. F., and McCracken, B. H.: Sepsis in human renal transplantation. *Surgery, 69*:189, 1971.
76. MacLean, L. D., MacKinnon, K. J., and Dossetor, J. B.: Transplantation of the kidney. In Hardy, J. D. (Ed.): *Human Organ Support and Replacement.* Springfield, Ill., Charles C Thomas, 1971.
77. Magnusson, M. O., and Kiser, W. S.: Human kidney preservation for transplantation. *Surg. Clin. N. Amer., 51*:1235, 1971.
78. Manax, W. G.: Human renal transplantation. Progress in organ preservation in vitro. *Med. Clin. N. Amer., 55*:205, 1971.
79. Mannick, J. A., and Egdahl, R. H.: Kidney transplantation. In Strauss, M. B., and Welt, L. G. (Eds.): *Diseases of the Kidney.* Second edition, Boston, Little, Brown and Co., 1971.
80. Mannick, J. A., Davis, R. C., Cooperbrand, S. R., Glasgow, A. H., Williams, F., Harrington, J. T., Cavallo, T., Schmitt, G. W., Idelson, B. A., Olsson, C. A., and Nabseth, D. C.: Clinical use of rabbit antihuman lymphocyte globulin in cadaver-kidney transplantation. *New Eng. J. Med., 284*:1109–1115, 1971.
81. Marhland, J., Najarian, J., Fraley, E., and Kelly, W.: Survival of four patients after renal homotransplantation into iliac urinary conduits. *Amer. Soc. Nephrology Abstr.,* 1970.
82. Martin, W. J., and Miller, J. F.: Site of action of antilymphocyte globulin. *Lancet, 2*:1285–1287, 1967.
83. Medawar, P. B.: The behavior and fate of skin autografts and skin homografts in rabbits. *J. Anat., 78*:176, 1944.
84. Medawar, P. B.: The immunology of transplantation. Harvey Lect., *52*:144, 1968.
85. Merrill, J. P.: Medical management of the transplant patient. In Rapaport, F. T., and Dausset, J. (Eds.): *Human Transplantation.* New York, Grune & Stratton, 1968.
86. Merrill, J. P.: The clinical transplant unit. In Rapaport, F. T., and Dausset, J. (Eds.): *Human Transplantation.* New York, Grune & Stratton, 1968.
87. Merrill, J. P., Murray, J. E., Harrison, J. H., and Guild, W. R.: Successful homotransplantation of the human kidney between identical twins. *J.A.M.A., 160*:277, 1956.
88. Merrill, J. P., Murray, J. E., Harrison, J. H., Friedman, E. A., Dealy, J. B., and Dammin, G.: Successful homotransplantation of the kidney between nonidentical twins. *New Eng. J. Med., 262*:1251, 1960.
89. Metcoff, J. (Ed.): *Homotransplantation: Kidney and Other Tissues.* New York, National Kidney Foundation, 1966.
90. Metheny, N. M., and Snively, W. D., Jr.: *Nurses' Handbook of Fluid Balance.* Philadelphia, J. B. Lippincott Co., 1967.
91. Mittal, K. K., Mickey, M. R., Singal, D. P., and Terasaki, P. I.: Serotyping for homotransplantation, XVIII. Refinement of microdroplet lymphocyte cytotoxicity test. *Transplantation, 6*:913, 1968.
92. Moore, F. D.: *Give and Take. The Development of Tissue Transplantation.* Philadelphia, W. B. Saunders Co., 1964.
93. Moore, F. D.: *Transplant. The Give and Take of Tissue Transplantation.* New York, Simon and Schuster, 1972.
94. Morris, B. J., Kincaid-Smith, P., McKinzie, I. F. C., Marshall, V. C., and Ting, A.: Leukocyte antigens in renal transplantation. Immediate allograft rejection with a negative crossmatch. *Med. J. Aust., 2*:379, 1969.
95. Moynihan, P. C., and Jackson, J. F.: Histocompatibility testing. In Hardy, J. D. (Ed.): *Human Organ Support and Replacement.* Springfield, Ill., Charles C Thomas, 1971.

96. Movat, H. Z.: Chemical mediators of the vascular phenomena of the acute inflammatory reaction of immediate hypersensitivity. *Med. Clin. N. Amer., 56*:541, 1972.
97. Murray, J. E., and Barnes, B. A.: The world-wide status of kidney transplantation. In Rapaport, F. T., and Dausset, J. (Eds.): *Human Transplantation.* New York, Grune & Stratton, 1968.
98. Murray, J. E., Barnes, B. A., and Atkinson, J. C.: Eighth report of the human kidney transplant registry. *Transplantation, 11*:328, 1971.
99. Murray, J. E., Merrill, J. P., and Harrison, J. H.: Kidney transplantation between seven pairs of identical twins. *Ann. Surg., 148*:343, 1958.
100. Murray, J. E., Merrill, J. P., and Harrison, J. H.: Renal transplantation between identical twins. *Surg. Forum, 6*:432, 1968.
101. Murray, J. E., Wilson, R. E., Tilney, N. L., Merrill, J. P., Cooper, W. C., Birtch, A. G., Carpenter, C. B., Hager, E. B., Dammin, G. J., and Harrison, J. H.: Five years' experience in renal transplantation with immunosuppressive drugs. *Ann. Surg., 168*:416, 1968.
102. Nelson, S. D., and Russell, P. S.: In vivo histocompatibility testing. In Rapaport, F. T., and Dausset, J. (Eds.): *Human Transplantation.* New York, Grune & Stratton, 1968.
103. Nomenclature for factors of HL-A system. *Bull. Wld. Hlth. Org., 39*:483, 1968.
104. Nossal, G. J. V.: Immunologic tolerance. In Rapaport, F. T., and Dausset, J. (Eds.): *Human Transplantation.* New York, Grune & Stratton, 1968.
105. Ogden, D. H., and Holmes, J. H.: Urinary solute excretion as an index of renal homograft rejection. *Ann. Intern. Med., 64*:804, 1966.
106. Patel, R., and Mocelin, A.: Tissue typing in human kidney transplantation. A review. *J. Urol., 107*:684, 1972.
107. Patel, R., and Terasaki, P. I.: Significance of the positive crossmatch in kidney transplantation. *New Eng. J. Med., 280*:735, 1969.
108. Patel, R., Merrill, J. P., and Briggs, W. A.: Analysis of results of kidney transplantation. Comparison in recipients with and without preformed antileukocyte antibodies. *New Eng. J. Med., 285*:274, 1971.
109. Patel, R., Mickey, M. R., and Terasaki, P. I.: Serotyping for homotransplantation. *New Eng. J. Med., 279*:501, 1968.
110. Perper, R. J., Lyster, S. C., Monovich, R. E., and Bowersox, B. E.: Analysis of the biological activity of antilymphocyte serum. *Transplantation, 9*:447–456, 1970.
111. Persson, B., Rosengren, B., Bergenty, S. E., and Hood, B.: Evaluation of preoperative extracorporeal irradiation of the blood in human renal transplantation. *Transplantation, 7*:534–544, 1969.
112. Popowniak, K. L., and Nakamoto, S.: Immunosuppressive therapy in renal transplantation. *Surg. Clin. N. Amer., 51*:1191, 1971.
113. Potter, D.: More on renal transplantation. *J. Pediat., 78*:369, 1971.
114. Potter, D., Belzer, F. O., Rames, L., Holliday, M., Kountz, S. L., and Najarian, J. S.: The treatment of chronic uremia in childhood. I. Transplantation. *Pediatrics, 45*:432, 1970.
115. Potter, K. A., Dossetor, J. B., Marchioro, T. L., Peart, W. S., Rendall, J. M., Starzl, T. E., and Terasaki, P. I.: Human renal transplants. I. Glomerular changes. *Lab. Invest., 16*:153, 1967.
116. Rapaport, F. T., and Dausset, J. (Eds.): *Human Transplantation.* New York, Grune & Stratton, 1968.
117. Rapaport, F. T., and Dausset, J. (Eds.): *Tissue Typing Today.* New York, Grune & Stratton, 1971.
118. Rapaport, F. J., Dausset, J., Hamburger, J., Hume, M., Kano, K., Williams, M. G., and Milgrom, F.: Serologic factors in human transplantation. *Ann. Surg., 166*:596–608, 1967.
119. Renal transplantation. *Lancet, 2*:249, 1971.
120. Rosenberg, J. C., Broersma, R. J., Bullemer, G., Mammen, E. F., Lenaghan, R., and Rosenberg, B. F.: Relationship of platelets, blood coagulation, and fibrinolysis to hyperacute rejection of renal allografts. *Transplantation, 8*:152, 1969.
121. Rowlands, D. T., and Bossen, E. H.: Immunological mechanisms of allograft rejection. *Arch. Intern. Med., 123*:491, 1969.
122. Russell, P. S.: Kidney transplantation. *Amer. J. Med., 44*:776, 1968.

123. Russell, P. S.: Antilymphocyte serum as an immunosuppressive agent. Editorial. *Ann. Intern. Med., 68*:483–486, 1968.
124. Russell, P. S., and Monaco, A. P.: *The Biology of Tissue Transplantation.* Boston, Little, Brown and Co., 1964.
125. Salaman, J. R., Calne, R. Y., Pena, J., Sells, R. A., White, H. J. O., and Yoffa, O.: Surgical aspects of renal transplantation. *Brit. J. Surg., 56*:413, 1969.
126. Saleh, W. S., MacLean, L. D., Gordon, J., and Lamoureaux, G.: A test to measure the immunosuppressive potency of antilymphocyte sera. *Transplantation, 8*:524–526, 1969.
127. Schreiner, G. E.: Current problems in the delivery of dialysis and renal transplantation. *Arch. Intern. Med., 123*:558, 1969.
128. Schwartz, R., and Dameshek, W.: Drug-induced immunological tolerance. *Nature, 183*:1682, 1959.
129. Simmons, R. G., Hickey, K., Kjellstrand, C. M., and Simmons, R. L.: Family tension in the search for a kidney donor. *J.A.M.A., 215*:909, 1971.
130. Snell, G. D.: The terminology of tissue transplantation. *Transplantation, 2*:655, 1964.
131. Starzl, T. E.: *Experience in Renal Transplantation.* Philadelphia, W. B. Saunders Co., 1964.
132. Starzl, T. E.: A look ahead at transplantation. *J. Surg. Res., 10*:291, 1970.
133. Starzl, T. E., and Porter, K. A.: Autolymphocytic globulin. Clinical use. In Rapaport, F. T., and Dausset, J. (Eds.): *Human Transplantation.* New York, Grune & Stratton, 1968.
134. Starzl, T. E., Penn, I., and Halgrimson, C. G.: Immunosuppression and malignant neoplasms. *New Eng. J. Med., 283*:934, 1970.
135. Starzl, T. E., Marchioro, T. L., Porter, K. A., Moore, C. A., Ritkind, D., and Waddell, W. R.: Renal homotransplantation. Late functions and complications. *Ann. Intern. Med., 61*:470, 1964.
136. Starzl, T. E., Penn, I., Schroter, G., Putnam, C. W., Halgrimson, C. G., Martineau, G., Amemiya, H., and Groth, C. G.: Cyclophosphamide and human organ transplantation. *Lancet, 2*:70–74, 1971.
137. Starzl, T. E., Groth, C. G., Putnam, C. W., Penn, I., Halgrimson, G. G., Flatmark, A., Gecelter, L., Brettschneider, L., and Stonington, O. G.: Urological complications in 216 human recipients of renal transplants. *Ann. Surg., 172*:1, 1970.
138. Starzl, T. E., Porter, K. A., Andres, G., Groth, C. G., Putnam, C. W., Penn, I., Halgrimson, C. G., Starkie, S. J., and Brettschneider, L.: Thymectomy and renal homotransplantation. *Clin. Exp. Immun., 6*:803–804, 1970.
139. Starzl, T. E., Porter, K. A., Andres, G., Halgrimson, C. G., Hurwitz, R., Giles, G., Terasaki, P. I., Penn, I., Schroter, G. T., Lilly, J., Starkie, S. J., and Putnam, C. W.: Long-term survival after renal transplantation in humans. *Ann. Surg., 172*:437–472, 1970.
140. Stevens, L. E., Freeman, T. S., Kentel, H., and Reemtsma, K.: Preparation and clinical use of antilymphocyte globulin. *Amer. J. Surg., 116*:795–799, 1968.
141. Stevens, L. E., Terasaki, P. I., Ricks, D., and Reemtsma, K.: Successful preservation and transportation of human kidneys between distant dialysis centers. *The Transplantation Society Proceedings,* 1970.
142. Stewart, B. H.: The surgery of renal transplantation. *Surg. Clin. N. Amer., 51*:1123, 1971.
143. Straffon, R. A.: Current status of renal transplantation. *Surg. Clin. N. Amer., 55*:1105, 1971.
144. Surgery Training Committee of the National Institute of General Medical Sciences: *Statistics of Transplantation 1968.* Washington, D.C., National Institutes of Health, 1968.
145. Swartz, R. S.: Immunosuppressive drug therapy. In Rapaport, F. T., and Dausset, J. (Eds.): *Human Transplantation.* New York, Grune & Stratton, 1968.
146. Swenson, O., Given, G., King, R., Indriss, F. S., and Ahmadian, Y.: Kidney transplants in children. *J. Pediat. Surg., 6*:245, 1971.
147. Taylor, H. E.: The clinical application of antilymphocyte globulin. *Med. Clin. N. Amer., 56*:419, 1972.

148. Terasaki, P. I. (Ed.): *Histocompatibility Testing, 1970.* Copenhagen, Munksgaard, 1970.
149. Terasaki, P. I., Kreisler, M., and Mickey, R. M.: Presensitization and kidney transplant failure. *Postgrad. Med., 47*:89, 1971.
150. Terasaki, P. I., Vredevoe, D. L., and Mickey, M. R.: X. Survival of 196 grafted kidneys, subsequent to typing. *Transplantation* (Suppl.), 5:1057, 1967.
151. Terasaki, P. I., Mickey, M. R., Singal, D. P., Mittal, K. K., and Patel, R.: Serotyping for homotransplantation. XX. Selection of recipients for cadaver donor transplants. *New Eng. J. Med., 279*:1101, 1968.
152. Tilney, N. L., and Murray, J. E.: Chronic thoracic duct fistula: operative technique and physiologic effects in man. *Ann. Surg., 167*:1–8, 1968.
153. Tilney, N. L., Atkinson, J. C., and Murray, J. E.: The immunosuppressive effect of thoracic duct drainage in human kidney transplantation. *Ann. Intern. Med., 72*:59–71, 1970.
154. Turner, M. D.: Organ storage. In Hardy, J. D. (Ed.): *Human Organ Support and Replacement.* Springfield, Ill., Charles C Thomas, 1971.
155. van Rood, J. J.: Tissue typing and organ transplantation. *Lancet, 1*:1142, 1969.
156. van Rood, J. J., and Leewen, A.: Leukocyte grouping. A method and its application. *J. Clin. Invest., 42*:1382, 1963.
157. van Rood, J. J., Leewen, A., Koch, C. T., and Fredricks, E.: HL-A inhibiting activity in serum. In Terasaki, P. I. (Ed.): *Histocompatibility Testing, 1970.* Copenhagen, Munksgaard, 1970.
158. Vidt, D. G.: Selection and preparation of patients for renal transplantation. *Surg. Clin. N. Amer., 51*:1111, 1971.
159. Walsh, A.: Some practical problems in kidney transplantation. *Transplant Proc., 1*:78, 1969.
160. Warshofsky, F.: *The Rebuilt Man. The Story of Spare-Parts Surgery.* New York, Thomas Y. Crowell, 1965.
161. Watson, D. W., and Johnson, A. G.: The clinical use of immunosuppression. *Med. Clin. N. Amer., 53*:1225–1240, 1969.
162. Weil, R., Simmons, R. L., Tallent, M. B., Lillehei, R. C., Kjellstrand, C. M., and Najarian, J. S.: Prevention of urological complication after kidney transplantation. *Ann. Surg., 174*:154, 1971.
163. Williams, G. M., Hume, D. M., Hudson, R. P., Jr., Morris, P. J., Kano, K., and Milgrom, F.: Hyperacute renal homograft rejection in man. *New Eng. J. Med., 279*:611, 1968.
164. Wilson, R. E.: Immunological modalities in clinical allografting. In Hardy, J. D. (Ed.): *Human Organ Support and Replacement.* Springfield, Ill., Charles C. Thomas, 1971.
165. Wilson, W. P., Stickel, D. L., Hayes, C. P., Jr., and Harris, N. L.: Psychiatric considerations of renal transplantation. *Arch. Intern. Med., 122*:502, 1968.
166. Wonham, V. A., Winn, H. J., and Russell, P. S.: Serotyping and genetic analysis in the selection of related renal allograft donors. *New Eng. J. Med., 284*:509, 1971.

CHAPTER 9

Prevention and Control of Renal Disease

The National Kidney Foundation estimates that approximately 60,000 persons in the United States alone die of renal failure annually. Yet, until recently, renal disease was not considered a threat to the nation's health. The reasons for which renal disease was underestimated in this way are complex. For one thing, renal disease is easy to misdiagnose since the symptoms are insidious and can be partially treated or not treated at all without immediate disaster. Second, renal disease is known as a "great impostor"; its vague early symptoms, such as malaise, fatigue, and anorexia, are easily mistaken or treated lightly. In addition most tests of renal function do not detect disease until approximately three fourths of the parenchyma has been affected.

Today, however, clinicians are more aware of the interrelatedness of major diseases such as cardiovascular and renal diseases, and are striving for early detection and prevention. The past three decades have witnessed an almost revolutionary change in our ability to deal with the problems of acute and chronic renal failure. The development of the artificial kidney, of materials for shunts, and of kidney transplantation are unique and impressive landmarks in the biochemical and technological struggle against human infirmity which characterizes twentieth century medical history. In the early 1960's, both local and federal health officials began to investigate avenues of research and development in the treatment of renal disease. Government sponsored dialysis and transplant programs began to spring up throughout the nation. These programs, along with the independent hospital programs, account for the sharp decrease in the nation's mortality rates for acute and chronic renal failure.

The prohibitive cost of treatment of end-stage renal disease caused federal, state, local, and private organizations to consider carefully programs designed to reduce the tremendous burden of renal disease. Unfortunately, clear-cut public health programs designed to reduce the morbidity and death resulting from renal disease are not available on a large scale; however, tremendous strides have been made.

Hopefully the sophistication and drama that surround these advances in treatment of renal disease will not obscure the long-range goal of prevention.

Reorganization in Medicine

Medicine is gradually reorganizing its delivery of health care to provide more emphasis on detection and prevention. Large medical centers now include clinics for essentially healthy individuals, as well as self-care units for persons undergoing diagnostic tests or recuperating from an illness, general care divisions, and specialized intensive care units. Group practice allows a patient to be evaluated by several doctors and provides more sophisticated diagnostic tools and techniques. Recently a few models have appeared that are intended to show how physicians, nurses, and persons in allied health professions can render comprehensive health care by seeking out those who need and will accept such care. In some instances mobile health units are organized and circulate in much the same way as chest x-ray units, while in other cases storefronts in receptive neighborhoods are used to house the medical team and equipment. There is also increasingly greater interest and energy devoted to health care for the poor. Emphasis in the medical profession on the practice of family medicine is providing more and better trained general and family physicians in the community.

In spite of all these advances in medical practice, health care to prevent and detect disease, particularly renal disease, is neonatal. It remains for the emphasis in medical practice to be oriented toward diagnosis and treatment. Community health planning has a long way to go in narrowing the gap between present capacity for health care and the rapidly approaching needs. New techniques for organization and communication, and training and use of allied health personnel are useless without extensive community health care planning. The various medical centers have not yet eliminated the problem of duplication of costly equipment and facilities such as hemodialysis equipment. Hospitals have not yet met their potential as resources for health care in the community.

Health Teaching

Health teaching is one measure that can be instituted immediately to aid in preventing renal disease. Since urinary tract infections are the most common diseases of the genitourinary system, this is the most likely area in which to begin prevention. Prevention begins with health teaching: health teaching of medical personnel so that they in turn can teach the public. Medical personnel frequently consider urinary tract infections in children to be benign affairs. However, the potentially grave outcome of such a problem cannot be overlooked. Statistics show a considerable increase in infections of the kidney and urinary tract in the past 20 years.

The most frequent infections of the urinary tract are of the nonspecific bacterial type. *Escherichia coli* is a frequent causative agent for nonspecific infections that lead to pyelonephritis. Pyelonephritis is the most common disease of the kidneys and correspondingly accounts for more than half of chronic renal disease. Urinary tract infections occur most frequently in female children between the ages of 4 and 10, pregnant women, and individuals with bladder obstructions. Medical personnel in the clinics, doctors' offices, hospitals, and schools can easily practice preventive medicine by instructing patients in how to avoid infections. Women and little girls can be instructed to wipe themselves from front to back after urinating or defecating to prevent *E. coli* contamination. In well-baby clinics or pediatricians' offices mothers of infant girls can be instructed to clean the child well after a bowel movement by wiping in a downward stroke with clean cotton balls that are discarded after each wipe. Nurses in doctors' offices, in hospitals, and in clinics can instruct persons susceptible to urinary tract infections to drink plenty of fluids.

Since acute glomerulonephritis most frequently occurs in children following a streptococcal infection, mothers can be cautioned to seek medical attention for the child whenever an infection is suspected. Parents and teachers can be informed to seek medical examinations for any child complaining of a sore throat. Throat cultures can be done routinely at examination and followed by treatment with antibiotics if necessary. In addition to giving specific information regarding bladder and kidney infections, nurses and doctors in clinics and doctors' offices can encourage parents to bring their school-age children in for regular physical check-ups.

Health education can be conducted indirectly in medical waiting rooms by providing pamphlets, magazines, or slide or film presentations on health. This captive audience is ordinarily highly motivated and receptive to health teaching.

Required health education classes in elementary and secondary schools also aid in imparting vital information to young people. It is, however, important to reach the parents of these children so that there is some follow-through. Lectures by medical personnel at Parent-Teachers Association meetings and community information groups help keep parents informed and motivated.

Hospital employees, particularly nurses, have a tremendous opportunity for health teaching. No one is more interested in his disease and in promoting his own health than the patient himself and his family. Home and follow-up care can be emphasized from the moment the patient is admitted. Planning with the patient for discharge is an ideal way to help insure maximal rehabilitation. The public health nurse and social worker may be excellent resource people in planning for discharge and rehabilitation. Unfortunately, hospital staff members frequently forget that the patient's life extends beyond his hospital stay. Continuing education programs for all medical and paramedical personnel can help keep these people informed on new methods of prevention, detection, and treatment of patients with renal disease.

Research and Study

A tremendous amount of research and study regarding the etiology, classification, treatment and prevention of renal disease is in progress in private and government funded projects. Further research and coordination of efforts are necessary, however, prior to instituting prevention programs for end-stage renal failure, most commonly caused by pyelonephritis and glomerulonephritis.

Relatively little is known about the prevention of pyelonephritis or the natural history of the disease. The symptoms of pyelonephritis are usually mild or absent and the disease is frequently undiagnosed, making it difficult to collect data on a large-scale basis. At present there is a lack of standard criteria for the diagnosis on the basis of clinical, pathological, and bacteriological data, which creates doubt as to the true frequency of the disorder as a cause of death or disability. Until more is known about the underlying causes, natural history, and bacterial response to therapy, and their relationship in chronic pyelonephritis, medicine is limited in its attempts to approach the problem on a large-scale community-wide basis.

Sufficient evidence regarding glomerulonephritis to warrant primary prevention programs is also lacking. Primary and secondary prevention are not yet possible in cases of chronic glomerulonephritis because very little is really known about the etiology of the disease. This is not to say, however, that no preventative measures can be instituted until there is a crystal-clear picture of the diseases.

Detection of Renal Disease

The best mode of prevention at this time is early detection. Early case finding, adequate diagnosis, and treatment to halt the progression of disease and to minimize its destructive effects dominate the present programs. For the future, it is feasible that community diagnostic centers can be established to screen and follow up potential renal disease patients. These centers would include on their staffs pediatricians and internists as well as nephrologists. Laboratory facilities and diagnostic equipment would be necessary. Ideally the groups most frequently affected (including all school children and all pregnant women) would be tested periodically for bacteriuria, albuminuria, hematuria, and kidney stones. At present, the cost of such a clinic is prohibitive; however, with community, state, and federal support, such programs may be possible in the near future.

Control of End-Stage Renal Disease

Approximately 10,000 deaths are prevented annually because of medical treatment for chronic renal failure. Useful and functional lives are achieved for an indefinite period of time with conservative medical management in patients who retain some kidney function. Occasional peritoneal and hemodialysis are useful in supplementing renal function during stressful periods, as in acute infections. More often, however, the slow, unrelenting failure of functioning nephrons that characterizes renal disease results in a progressive decrease of renal function to a point at which life can no longer be supported. Progressive uremia signals the need for more aggressive therapy to prolong useful life for the patient. Chronic glomerulonephritis and chronic pyelonephritis are the most common diagnoses among hemodialysis patients.

Advances in the techniques of hemodialysis and transplantation, the interest of the community, and the increasing survival rates of renal transplants have resulted in pressure from the medical profession and the public to prompt the government, the health insurance industry, hospitals, and members of the medical profession to plan for and prepare to meet the challenge presented by the terminal uremic patient.

End-stage renal disease can be controlled by dialysis and transplantation. At present, many prime candidates for either of these treatments will not be accepted into a program because of the tremendous shortage of equipment and personnel across the country. In addition, the cost of both programs is prohibitive for many patients. The financial burden placed upon the individual patients and families has been somewhat relieved for the majority by the renal amendment to the Medicare bill which became effective in July 1973.

There is a need for parallel dialysis and transplant programs in every community. The patient could then be treated by dialysis until a kidney was available for transplantation. Following transplant, the patient might again require dialysis until adequate function was achieved or, later, during an acute rejection crisis.

Most dialysis and transplant centers are in large private hospitals with private physicians, which places this therapy out of reach of many of the poor patients in the community. Veterans Administration Hospitals throughout the country have large and excellent dialysis-transplant programs available to the medically indigent veteran. However, many community members do not qualify for this program either. Grants and aid for supporting end-stage renal failure patients are very limited. Hence, treatment is not available to all members of the community.

A unique opportunity and a pressing responsibility face the health planner, health administrator, and medical practitioner in developing a community center to provide treatment for all patients with end-stage renal disease. The success or failure of medicine to meet this challenge will depend largely on the local pressure and effort that are directed toward the problem.

Although it is impossible to describe a model for all community dialysis-transplant programs, there are several common elements. First, financial assistance must be identified for the present programs and additional support solicited. The federal government and the states now have a limited number of programs, and health insurance and community fund raising supply the remainder; some patients, however, are not eligible for any of these. The community dialysis-transplant center would be designed to provide funds to all community members on a first-come first-served basis. One solution may be a government-built and community-maintained unit.

In order to insure effective provision and utilization of services, and to avoid duplication of facilities, community-wide planning for new programs and coordination of existing programs are required. Cooperation with hospital planning councils, agencies responsible for the administration of Hill-Burton funds, regional medical programs, and state comprehensive health planning groups must be sought. Assessment of geographical distribution of present facilities and programs would have to be made along with comprehensive planning for future needs.

The authors of this text believe that community dialysis and transplantation programs are not only necessary and possible but are essential to the nation's health while research and further study strive to eliminate renal disease as a health menace.

References

1. Beeson, P. B., and McDermott, W. (Eds.): *Cecil-Loeb Textbook of Medicine.* Thirteenth edition. Philadelphia, W. B. Saunders Co., 1971.
2. Black, D. A. K. (Ed.): *Renal Disease.* Second edition, Philadelphia, F. A. Davis Co., 1967.
3. Brest, A. N., and Moyer, J. H. (Eds.): *Renal Failure.* Philadelphia, J. B. Lippincott Co., 1968.
4. Clark, D. W., and MacMahon, B. (Eds.): *Preventative Medicine.* Boston, Little, Brown and Company, 1967.
5. Darley, W.: Response. Concerns, encouragements, and hopes for comprehensive medicine. *J. Med. Educ., 45*: 493, 1970.
6. Hilleboe, H. E., and Larimore, G. W. (Eds.): *Preventive Medicine: Principles of Prevention in the Occurrence and Progression of Disease.* Second edition. Philadelphia, W. B. Saunders Co. 1965.
7. Hume, D. M.: Kidney transplantation. In Rapaport, F. T., and Dausset, J. (Eds.): *Human Transplantation.* New York, Grune & Stratton, 1968.
8. Kerr, D. N. S.: Chronic renal failure, In Beeson P. B., and McDermott, W. (Eds.): *Cecil-Loeb Textbook of Medicine.* Thirteenth edition, Philadelphia, W. B. Saunders Co., 1971.
9. Kincaid-Smith, P.: Treatment of irreversible renal failure by dialysis and transplantation. In Beeson, P. B., and McDermott, W. (Eds.): *Cecil-Loeb Textbook of Medicine,* Thirteenth edition. Philadelphia, W. B. Saunders Co., 1971.
10. Kolff, W. J.: Artificial organs in the seventies. *Trans. Amer. Soc. Artif. Intern. Organs, 16*:534, 1970.
11. Mannick, J. A., and Egdahl, R. H.: Kidney transplantation. In Strauss, M. B., and Welt, L. G. (Eds.): *Diseases of the Kidney.* Second edition, Boston, Little, Brown and Co., 1971.
12. Merrill, J. P.: The clinical transplant unit. In Rapaport, F. T., and Dausset, J. (Eds.): *Human Transplantation.* New York, Grune & Stratton, 1968.
13. Rapaport, F. T. and Dausset, J. (Eds.): *Human Transplantation.* New York, Grune & Stratton, 1968.
14. Sartwell, P. E. (Ed.): *Preventive Medicine and Public Health.* Ninth edition. New York, Appleton-Century-Crofts, 1965.
15. Schreiner, G. E.: Current problems in the delivery of dialysis and renal transplantation. *Arch. Intern. Med., 123*:558, 1969.
16. Schwarz, K.: *Preventive Medicine in Medical Care.* London, H. K. Lewis and Co., Ltd., 1970.
17. Smillie, W. S.: *Preventive Medicine and Public Health.* New York, The Macmillan Co., 1958.
18. Smillie, W. G., and Kilbourne, E. D.: *Preventive Medicine and Public Health.* Third edition, New York, The Macmillan Co., 1963.
19. Starzl, T. E.: A look ahead at transplantation. *J. Surg. Res, 10*:291, 1970.
20. Surgery Training Committee of the National Institute of General Medical Sciences: *Statistics of Transplantation, 1968.* Washington, D.C., National Institutes of Health, 1968.
21. U.S. Department of Health, Education, and Welfare: *Kidney Disease Prevention and Control.* Washington, D.C., U.S. Government Printing Office, 1969.

APPENDIX A

Normal Laboratory Values for Blood and Urine

Normal Serum or Blood Values

Urea nitrogen, blood		10–20 mg/100 ml
Creatinine, serum		0.7–1.5 mg/100 ml
Uric acid, serum	male	2.5–8.0 mg/100 ml
	female	1.5–6.0 mg/100 ml
Potassium, serum		3.5–5.0 mEq/L
Sodium, serum		136–145 mEq/L
Calcium, serum		4.5–5.5 mEq/L
Magnesium, serum		1.5–2.5 mEq/L
Chloride, serum		96–106 mEq/L
Carbon dioxide content		26–28 mEq/L
Phosphate, inorganic, serum		3.0–4.5 mg/100 ml
Sulfates, inorganic, serum		0.8–1.2 mg/100 ml
pH, arterial, blood		7.35–7.45

Normal Urine Values

Potassium	25–100 mEq/24 hr (varies with intake)
Sodium	130–260 mEq/24 hr (varies with intake)
Calcium	less than 250 mg/24 hr (on usual diet)
Chloride	110–250 mEq/24 hr (varies with intake)
Phosphorus	0.9–1.3 gm/24 hr (varies with intake)
Protein	10–150 mg/24 hr
Osmolality	38–1400 mOsm/kg water
Specific gravity	1.003–1.030
pH	4.6–8.0, average 6.0 (depends on diet)
Red blood cells	0–130,000/24 hr (Addis count)
White blood cells	0–650,000/24 hr (Addis count)
Casts	0–2000/24 hr (Addis count)
Bacteria (clean voided specimen)	less than 100 colonies/ml

APPENDIX B

Drug Dosage in Renal Failure

*Maintenance Dose of Antimicrobials in Renal Failure**

Group 1. Major extrarenal pathways of elimination. Normal dose schedule can be used.

Methicillin	Novobiocin
Cloxacillin	Fusidic acid
Ampicillin	Chloramphenicol
Erythromycin	Sulfadimidine

Group 2. Minor adjustment in dosage is needed. Doses should be spaced more widely than normal, but not more than 24 hours apart. Exact timing is not critical, as there is some extrarenal excretion and/or the drugs are not toxic at moderately elevated blood levels.

Penicillin G	Carbenicillin
Cephalothin	Trimethoprim-sulfamethoxazole
Cephaloridine	Nalidixic acid
Lincomycin	Isoniazid
Clindamycin	

Group 3. Major adjustment is required—doses 24 hours or more apart in severe renal failure.

Tetracycline	Gentamycin†
Oxytetracycline	Vancomycin†
Methacycline	Polymyxin B†
Streptomycin†	Colistin†
Kanamycin†	Amphotericin B†
Cycloserine	Para-amino-salicylate

Group 4. Avoid altogether.

Chlortetracycline
Nitrofurantoin

*From Kerr, D. N. S.: Chronic renal failure. In Beeson, P. B., and McDermott, W.: *Cecil-Loeb Textbook of Medicine.* Thirteenth edition. Philadelphia, W. B. Saunders Co., 1971.

†Daily estimation of blood levels is highly desirable to avoid risk of ototoxicity or nephrotoxicity.

*Additional Information About Doses of Antimicrobials in Renal Failure**

Antimony compounds
  Neostibosan – Definitely decrease dose.
Bacitracin – Definitely decrease dose if it is necessary to give the drug at all; is nephrotoxic.
Chloroguanide – Probably need to decrease dose; a possibility of slowed elimination in uremia exists.
Chloroquine – Give in usual doses for treatment of acute malaria; should not be used for prolonged treatment of malaria except in unusual cases, and then at reduced doses.
Dapsone – Probably need to decrease dose.
Ethambutol – Definitely decrease dose.
Neomycin – Definitely decrease dose; cumulation of the drug produces risk of nephrotoxicity.
Phenazopyridine (Pyridium) – Should not be given to uremic patients; its elimination is impaired in uremia and it is potentially nephrotoxic.
Piperazine (Antepar) – No change in dose necessary.
Pyrvinium (Povan) – No change in dose necessary. Probably a better choice than piperazine for treatment of ascariasis in uremia, as little is absorbed and only one dose is given.
Rifampicin – No change in dose necessary.
Sulfonamides – Probably need to decrease dose for treatment of infections not involving the urinary tract. Proper dosage levels for treatment of urinary tract infection in uremic patients have not been established.
Viomycin – Definitely decrease dose.

*Data from Reidenberg, M. M.: *Renal Function and Drug Action.* Philadelphia, W. B. Saunders Co., 1971.

*Doses of Selected Drugs Other Than Antimicrobials in Renal Failure**

Drug	Probably Need to Decrease Dose	Definitely Decrease Dose	No Change in Dose	Increase Dose	Comments
Acetaminophen (Tylenol)					Best of the nonnarcotic analgesics to use. To decrease exfoliation of renal tubular cells, keep patient well hydrated.
Acetohexamide (Dymelor)					Metabolism and excretion are impaired in some uremic patients.
Allopurinol (Zyloprim)		X			Proper dose in uremia is about 200 mg/day.
Anileridine (Leritine) (see narcotic analgesics and related drugs)					
Aspirin					Should be used with caution in uremic patients. Aspirin can cause GI bleeding, and it impairs platelet function and prolongs bleeding time. The uremic patient already has bleeding tendency and platelet dysfunction. Aspirin causes exfoliation of renal tubular cells.
Atropine and related drugs	X				
Barbital					Should not be used with patients in renal failure, as it accumulates to excessive concentrations. Is an impurity in some preparations of pentobarbital and other barbiturates.
Barbiturates, other than barbital	X				Barbiturate metabolism is normal in uremia, but patients are often sensitive to the drug. Therefore, initial doses of the drug should be low to determine individual sensitivity. Subsequent doses are often somewhat lower than normal.
Bendroflumethiazide (Naturetin)					Drug excreted more slowly and is often ineffective in patients with renal failure. Can cause hypercalcemia.
Benzazoline (Priscoline)	X				

*Data from Reidenberg, M. M.: *Renal Function and Drug Action*. Philadelphia, W. B. Saunders Co., 1971.

Table continued on opposite page.

*Doses of Selected Drugs Other Than Antimicrobials in Renal Failure** (Continued)

Drug	Probably Need to Decrease Dose	Definitely Decrease Dose	No Change in Dose	Increase Dose	Comments
Bishydroxycoumarin (dicumarol) and the oral anticoagulant drugs					In one study, eight out of nine uremic patients required usual doses of dicumarol to increase the prothrombin time to therapeutic levels; one patient required less than the usual dose. But anticoagulation is hazardous because the drug effects are superimposed on the bleeding tendency in uremia; this invalidates the usual "safe" levels of prothrombin time. A safe and effective regimen for anticoagulation in uremia is not yet established.
Buformin		X			
Chlorothiazide (Diuril)					Drug excreted more slowly and is often ineffective in patients with renal failure. Can cause hypercalcemia.
Chlorpropamide (Diabinese)					Excretion slowed in renal failure. Hazardous to patients in renal failure because of risk of prolonged hypoglycemia.
Codeine (see narcotic analgesics and related drugs)					
Compazine (see phenothiazide drugs)					
Diazoxide					If given for a short period of time, no dosage modification required. If repeated doses given, dosage may need to be reduced, as cumulation may occur.
Dichloromethotrexate	X				
Digitoxin		X			
Digoxin		X			See discussion in Chapter 5.
Dimercaprol (BAL)					Should be used with caution in patients with renal failure. (Uremic rats showed normal responses to usual doses.)
Diphenylhydantoin (Dilantin)			X		
Ethacrynic acid (Edecrin)					Tendency to cause ototoxicity.
Ferrioxamine/desferrioxamine					Is excreted in the urine. Renal failure delays excretion and, therefore, effectiveness.

*Data from Reidenberg, M. M.: *Renal Function and Drug Action.* Philadelphia, W. B. Saunders Co., 1971.

Table continued on following page.

Doses of Selected Drugs Other Than Antimicrobials in Renal Failure (Continued)*

Drug	Probably Need to Decrease Dose	Definitely Decrease Dose	No Change in Dose	Increase Dose	Comments
Furosemide (Lasix)					Produces diuresis in patients with GFR greater than 5 ml/min; patients with lower GFR failed to respond. Is ototoxic. Lasix, given in large doses, is the best diuretic for uremic patients at present.
					In general, diuretic therapy is dangerous for the uremic patient: the likelihood of drug intoxication is increased, the likelihood of diuresis is decreased, impairment of existing renal function can occur, and electrolyte imbalance can be produced.
Gold	X				
Guanethidine (Ismelin)	X				
Heroin (see narcotic analgesics and related drugs)					
Hexamethonium and pentamethonium	X				
Idoxuridine	X				
Iodide (I^{131})					I^{131} has decreased rate of excretion in renal failure, which leads to a higher, more prolonged plasma concentration. This can increase the fraction of the dose of I^{131} in the thyroid gland and cause a higher I^{131} uptake test result than usual for any degree of thyroid function.
Lanatoside C		X			
Mannitol					Has prolonged half-life in uremic patients. Is ineffective in producing diuresis in azotemic patients.
Mecamylamine (Inversine)					Adjust dosage to blood pressure response measured with patient standing up. The drug produces postural hypotension, which can cause decreased renal blood flow and further deterioration of renal function.
Meperidine (Pethidine, Demerol) (see narcotic analgesics and related drugs)					

*Data from Reidenberg, M. M.: *Renal Function and Drug Action.* Philadelphia, W. B. Saunders Co., 1971.

Table continued on opposite page.

*Doses of Selected Drugs Other Than Antimicrobials in Renal Failure** (Continued)

Drug	Probably Need to Decrease Dose	Definitely Decrease Dose	No Change in Dose	Increase Dose	Comments
Mercury					Excretion of drug prolonged in uremic patients. Accumulation of mercury can cause further renal damage. Not recommended for uremic patients.
Methadone (Dolophine) (see narcotic analgesics and related drugs)					
Methotrexate		X			
Methyldopa (Aldomet)			X		
Methylglyoxal bis (guanylhydrazone) (Methyl GAG)	X				
Morphine (see narcotic analgesics and related drugs)					
Narcotic analgesics and related drugs					Metabolism of these drugs is normal in uremia. There are no data to suggest that dosage should be decreased in uremia, but many patients are sensitive to them, so initial doses should be lower than normal to determine individual sensitivity.
Neostigmine (Prostigmin)	X				
Ouabain		X			
Penicillamine					The drug is excreted in the urine. Renal failure delays excretion and, therefore, effectiveness.
Pentazocine (Talwin) (see narcotic analgesics and related drugs)					
Phenacetin					Causes exfoliation of renal tubular cells. Is metabolized to acetaminophen, which does not cause nearly as much exfoliation. Therefore, acetaminophen should be used.
Phenergan (see phenothiazide drugs)					
Phenformin (DBI)		X			
Phenothiazide drugs					Give at lowest effective dose and watch for development of side effects, which more commonly occur at higher doses.

*Data from Reidenberg, M. M.: *Renal Function and Drug Action.* Philadelphia, W. B. Saunders Co., 1971.

Table continued on following page.

*Doses of Selected Drugs Other Than Antimicrobials in Renal Failure** (Continued)

Drug	Probably Need to Decrease Dose	Definitely Decrease Dose	No Change in Dose	Increase Dose	Comments
Procainamide (Pronestyl)	X				
Propoxyphene (Darvon) (see narcotic analgesics and related drugs)					
Radiographic contrast media					The patient should not be dehydrated prior to x-ray such as IVP. The purpose of dehydration is to increase the concentration of the dye, but concentrating ability is one of the first functions lost in renal failure. Therefore, dehydration serves no useful purpose. To improve visualization, dialyze patient beforehand, give larger than usual doses of contrast medium, and use laminography to improve definition of faintly visualized kidneys.
Sodium calcium edetate (EDTA)					The drug is excreted in the urine. Renal failure delays its excretion and effectiveness. In addition, the drug is nephrotoxic. Therefore, its use is probably contraindicated in renal failure.
Sparine (see phenothiazide drugs)					
Spironolactone (Aldactone)					Tendency to produce hyperkalemia; therefore, generally not used for uremic patients.
Sulfinpyrazone (Anturane)	X				Half-life is probably prolonged in uremia.
Tetraethylammonium		X			
Thorazine (see phenothiazide drugs)					
Tolbutamide (Orinase)			X		Best choice of oral hypoglycemic agents for uremic patients. May cause hypoglycemia.
Tromethamine (THAM)					This drug depends on renal excretion for its effect of eliminating hydrogen ions from the body. It is, therefore, a poor choice for patients with renal failure.

*Data from Reidenberg, M. M.: *Renal Function and Drug Action.* Philadelphia, W. B. Saunders Co., 1971.

APPENDIX C
Nephrotoxins

Classification of Toxic Nephropathy[*]

CLASS 1. Drugs or their metabolites with a reasonably *direct* effect, producing an identifiable morphologic or persisting functional change in the nephron. Model: bichloride of mercury.

CLASS 2. Compounds producing sensitivity disease identifiable as the *nephrotic* or *nephritic* syndrome in which the initial step may be subtle alteration in the renal cell or alteration of a protein, producing an immune reaction. Model: aminonucleoside nephrosis and nephroallergens producing the nephrotic syndrome.

CLASS 3. Compounds producing sensitivity reactions of the angiitis or vasculitis type involving the kidney as a vascular organ. Model: sulfa sensitivity.

CLASS 4. Compounds that may produce *chronic nephrotoxicity,* when the mechanism extends over a period of months or years and the evidence remains largely epidemiologic or circumstantial. Model: lead nephropathy.

CLASS 5. Compounds that aggravate pre-existing renal disease or predispose to secondary renal disease such as pyelonephritis. Model: diuretics and cathartics predisposing to pyelonephritis via potassium deficiency.

[*]From Schreiner, G. E.: Toxic nephropathy. In Beeson, P. B., and McDermott, W. (Eds.): *Cecil-Loeb Textbook of Medicine.* Thirteenth edition. Philadelphia, W. B. Saunders Co., 1971.

A Partial List of Nephrotoxins[*]

METALS: Mercury (organic and inorganic), bismuth, uranium, cadmium, lead, gold, arsine and arsenic, iron, silver, antimony, copper, and thallium

ORGANIC SOLVENTS: Carbon tetrachloride, tetrachlorethylene, methyl cellosolve, methanol, and miscellaneous solvents

GLYCOLS: Ethylene glycol, ethylene glycol dinitrite, propylene glycol, ethylene dichloride, and diethylene glycol

PHYSICAL AGENTS: Radiation, heat stroke, and electroshock

DIAGNOSTIC AGENTS: Contrast agents in high concentration (pyelography and aortography) and bunamiodyl

THERAPEUTIC AGENTS: *Antimicrobials:* Sulfonamides, penicillin, streptomycin, kanamycin, vancomycin, bacitracin, polymyxin and colistin, neomycin, tetracycline and amphotericin. *Analgesics:* Salicylates, para-aminosalicylate (PAS), ? phenacetin, phenylbutazone, zoxazolamine, phenindione, puromycin, tridione, paradione

OSMOTIC AGENTS: Sucrose, mannitol

INSECTICIDES: Biphenyl, chlorinated hydrocarbons

MISCELLANEOUS CHEMICALS: Carbon monoxide, snake venom, mushroom poison, spider venom, nephroallergens, cresol, beryllium, hemolysins, aniline, and other methemoglobin formers

ABNORMAL CONCENTRATION OF PHYSIOLOGIC SUBSTANCES: Hypercalcemia, hyperuricemia, hypokalemia, hypomagnesemia, etc.

---

*From Schreiner, G. E.: Toxic nephropathy. In Beeson, P. B., and McDermott, W. (Eds.): *Cecil-Loeb Textbook of Medicine.* Thirteenth edition. Philadelphia, W. B. Saunders Co., 1971.

APPENDIX D

Diet in Renal Failure

*40 gm Protein, 500 mg Sodium, 1500 mg Potassium Diet**

Food	Number of Servings	Grams	Protein (gm)	Sodium (mg)	Potassium (mg)	Calories
Milk exchanges	2	240	8	120	180	161
Meat exchanges						
Group A	1	30	7	60	70	188
Group B	1	30	7	25	120	188
Vegetable exchanges						
Group A	2	200	2	18	240	108
Group B	1	100	2	9	230	108
Fruit exchanges						
Group A	1	100	1	2	100	107
Group B	1	100	1	2	145	107
Bread exchanges	4	varies	8	20	200	252
Fat exchanges	4	20	0	200	0	135
Totals			36	456	1285	1354

Beverages, special desserts, and foods from the miscellaneous group are added to increase calories and bring protein, sodium, and potassium to desired amounts.

*Adapted from Mitchell, H. S., Rynbergen, H., Anderson, L. and Dibble, M. V.: *Cooper's Nutrition in Health and Disease.* Fifteenth edition. Philadelphia, J. B. Lippincott Co., 1968.

*Protein, Sodium, and Potassium Restricted Diet Exchange Lists**

MILK EXCHANGES: 1 serving contains 4 gm of protein, 60 mg of sodium, 90 mg of potassium.

Milk	1/2 cup
Light cream	1/2 cup
Heavy cream	3/4 cup
Sour cream	1/2 cup
Half and half	1/2 cup
Ice cream, regular	1/2 cup (1/8 qt)
Sherbet, regular	1 cup (1/4 qt)
Creamed cheese, regular	1 tablespoon

MEAT EXCHANGES: GROUP A. 1 serving contains 7 gm of protein, 60 mg of sodium, 70 mg of potassium.

Egg, prepared any way	1
Cheese, low-sodium	1 ounce
cottage, regular	1/4 cup
Tuna and salmon, canned in water	1/4 cup
Lobster and shrimp, fresh or canned in water	1 ounce
Oysters, fresh	4 in number
Clams, fresh	3 in number

*From Mitchell, H. S., Rynbergen, H., Anderson, L., and Dibble, M. V.: *Cooper's Nutrition in Health and Disease.* Fifteenth edition. Philadelphia, J. B. Lippincott Co., 1968.

Table continued on following page.

*Protein, Sodium, and Potassium Restricted Diet Exchange Lists** (Continued)

MEAT EXCHANGES: GROUP B. 1 serving contains 7 gm of protein, 25 mg of sodium, 120 mg of potassium.

Beef, lamb, liver, rabbit, veal	1 ounce
Chicken, turkey	1 ounce
Fish, fresh water	1 ounce
haddock	1 ounce
halibut	1 ounce
swordfish	1 ounce

VEGETABLE EXCHANGES: GROUP A. 1 serving contains 1 gm of protein, 9 mg of sodium, 120 mg of potassium.

Asparagus	6 spears
Beans, green or wax	1/2 cup
Beets	1/4 cup
Carrots	1/3 cup
Lettuce	2 large leaves
Onions	1 medium
Peas	1/2 cup
Squash, summer, yellow, white	1/2 cup

VEGETABLE EXCHANGES: GROUP B. 1 serving contains 2 gm of protein, 9 mg of sodium, 230 mg of potassium.

Broccoli	1 stalk, 1/2 cup
Brussels sprouts	1/2 cup
Cabbage	1/2 cup
Corn	1/2 cup
Cucumber	8 slices 1/8 in. thick
Eggplant	1/2 cup
Okra	1/2 cup
Potato	1/4 cup
Pumpkin	1/2 cup
Rutabaga	1/2 cup
Squash, acorn, Hubbard	1/2 cup
Tomato	1 small
Tomato juice, low-sodium dietetic	1/2 cup
Turnips	1/3 cup

Vegetables may be fresh, low-sodium dietetic canned, or home-canned if no salt has been added.

Use only frozen vegetables to which no salt or other sodium compound has been added. READ LABELS.

*From Mitchell, H. S., Rynbergen, H., Anderson, L., and Dibble, M. V.: *Cooper's Nutrition in Health and Disease.* Fifteenth edition. Philadelphia, J. B. Lippincott Co., 1968.

Table continued on opposite page.

*Protein, Sodium, and Potassium Restricted Diet Exchange Lists** (Continued)

FRUIT EXCHANGES: GROUP A. 1 serving contains 1 gm of protein, 2 mg of sodium, 100 mg of potassium.

Apple, raw	1
Apple juice	1/2 cup
Applesauce	1/2 cup
Blueberries	1/2 cup
Cherries, Bing and Royal Anne	1/2 cup
Cranberries	1/2 cup
Cranberry juice	1/2 cup
Peaches, canned	1/2 cup
Peach nectar	1/2 cup
Pears, canned	1/2 cup
Pear nectar	1/2 cup

FRUIT EXCHANGES: GROUP B. 1 serving contains 1 gm of protein, 2 mg of sodium, 145 mg of potassium.

Blackberries, fresh or frozen	1/2 cup
Fruit cocktail	1/2 cup
Grapes	1/2 cup
Grape juice	1/2 cup
Grapefruit, raw	1/2 medium fruit
Grapefruit juice	1/2 cup
Grapefruit sections	1/2 cup
Orange, raw	1/2 small fruit
Orange juice	1/3 cup
Peach, raw	1 small fruit
Pear, raw	1 small fruit
Pineapple, canned	1/2 cup
Pineapple juice	1/2 cup
Plums, canned or raw	2 in number
Raspberries, fresh or frozen	1/2 cup
Strawberries, fresh or frozen	1/2 cup
Tangerine	1 medium
Watermelon	1/2 cup

BREAD EXCHANGES: 1 serving contains 2 gm of protein, 5 mg of sodium, 50 mg of potassium.

Low-sodium bread	1 slice
Unsalted cooked cereal	1/2 cup

Cornmeal — Farina
Cream of Rice — Hominy grits
Cream of Wheat — Ralston

May use Instant or Regular. Do not use quick-cooking varieties.

*From Mitchell, H. S., Rynbergen, H., Anderson, L., and Dibble, M. V.: *Cooper's Nutrition in Health and Disease.* Fifteenth edition. Philadelphia, J. B. Lippincott Co., 1968.

Table continued on following page.

*Protein, Sodium, and Potassium Restricted Diet Exchange Lists** (Continued)

Dry cereal		3/4 cup
Puffed Rice	Shredded wheat	
Puffed wheat	Unsalted cornflakes	
Unsalted cooked		1/2 cup
Rice	Noodles	
Macaroni	Spaghetti	
Popcorn, unsalted		1 cup

FAT EXCHANGES: 1 serving contains 0 protein, 50 mg of sodium, 0 potassium.

Butter, salted	1 teaspoon
Margarine, salted	1 teaspoon
Mayonnaise, salted	1 teaspoon

Unsalted butter and margarine and vegetable oil may be used as desired.

BEVERAGES: May be taken as allowed, according to fluid intake.

Ginger ale	Pepsi Cola
Coca Cola	Kool Aids (not orange)

Sodium and potassium content may vary according to local water supply. Juices, milk, ice cream, and sherbet must be counted as fluid in the diet.

DESSERTS: Content varies depending on recipe (see recipes in this appendix).

MISCELLANEOUS: These items may be used as desired to add flavor.

Allspice	Mustard, dry
Caraway	Nutmeg
Cinnamon	Paprika
Curry powder	Pepper
Garlic	Peppermint extract
Garlic powder (not garlic salt)	Sage
Ginger	Syrup, corn
Hard candy	Sugar, white
Honey	Thyme
Jams	Turmeric
Jellies	Vanilla extract
Lollipops	Vinegar
Mace	

Small amounts of the following may be used to season foods:

Celery	Horseradish, fresh
Green pepper	Mushrooms
Onion	

*From Mitchell, H. S., Rynbergen, H., Anderson, L., and Dibble, M. V.: *Cooper's Nutrition in Health and Disease.* Fifteenth edition. Philadelphia, J. B. Lippincott Co., 1968.

*Sample Menu for 40 gm Protein, 500 mg Sodium, 1500 mg Potassium Diet**

Food	Household Measure	Protein (Gm)	Sodium (mg)	Potassium (mg)	Fluids (ml)
Breakfast					
Blueberries	½ cup	1	2	100	...
Shredded wheat	1 biscuit	2	5	50	...
Cream, light	½ cup	4	60	90	120
Coffee, weak	½ cup	...	1	30	120
Sugar, white	1 tablespoon	...	...	...	...
Lunch					
Egg, poached	1	7	60	70	...
Bread, unsalted	1 slice	2	5	50	...
Butter or margarine, salted	1 teaspoon	...	50	...	...
Salad					
Lettuce Asparagus	1 large leaf 3 spears	1	9	120	...
French dressing, unsalted	1 tablespoon	...	...	...	...
Apple pie	⅛ 9-inch pie	2	5	150	...
Ginger ale	8 ounces	...	20	1	240
Dinner					
Beef, ground, cooked in	1 ounce	7	25	120	...
Butter, salted	1 teaspoon	...	50	...	...
Spaghetti, cooked	½ cup	2	5	50	...
Tomato juice, unsalted	½ cup scant	2	9	230	120
Green beans	½ cup	1	9	120	...
Bread, unsalted	1 slice	2	5	50	...
Butter, salted	2 teaspoons	...	100	...	...
Fruit tapioca peach nectar sliced peaches	1 serving	1	2	100	...
Lemonade	8 ounces	...	...	8	240
Evening					
Cream, light, diluted with water	½ cup	4	60	90	120
Cookies	3	1	2	30	...
	Totals	39	484	1459	960

Calories 2089

*Adapted from Mitchell, H. S., Rynbergen, H., Anderson, L., and Dibble, M. V.: *Cooper's Nutrition in Health and Disease.* Fifteenth edition. Philadelphia, J. B. Lippincott Co., 1968.

Recipes Low in Protein, Sodium, and Potassium

FROZEN BUTTER AND SUGAR BALLS*

Ingredients
200 gm sugar
200 gm unsalted butter
1½ tsp vanilla extract and 6 drops peppermint extract or enough lemon juice to flavor the product

Procedure
Cream sugar and butter together, add flavoring, roll into small balls, place in refrigerator until solid.

Contents
No protein, sodium, or potassium; 2250 calories

BUTTER AND SUGAR SOUP*

Ingredients
200 gm sugar
20 gm flour
200 gm unsalted butter
600 ml water
coffee or rum extract

Procedure
Mix sugar and flour together. Add enough water to make a paste. Add the melted butter. Cook 20 minutes in double boiler. Add remainder of water and flavor with coffee or rum extract.
May also be served as pudding. Use less water and serve cold.

Content
No protein, sodium, or potassium; 2300 calories

FRUIT TAPIOCA†

Ingredients
2 cups peach nectar
½ cup water
½ cup sugar
¼ cup tapioca
1 cup peach slices, canned

Procedure
Mix peach nectar, water, sugar, and tapioca in top of double boiler. Cook over water, stirring constantly until mixture thickens slightly, 5 to 8 minutes. Remove from heat and cool. Stir in 1 cup of sliced, canned peaches. A dash of cinnamon or ginger will add flavor. A tablespoon of lemon juice will make the dessert less sweet. Other allowed fruits may be substituted. Yield: 6 servings.

Content
1 serving contains 1 gm protein, 2 mg sodium, and 100 mg potassium.

*From Mitchell, H. S., Rynbergen, H., Anderson, L., and Dibble, M. V.: *Cooper's Nutrition in Health and Disease.* Fifteenth edition. Philadelphia, J. B. Lippincott Co., 1968.

†From Mitchell, M. C., and Smith, J.: Dietary care of the patient with chronic oliguria. *Amer. J. Clin. Nutr., 19*:163–169, 1966.

Recipes continued on opposite page.

Recipes Low in Protein, Sodium, and Potassium (Continued)

Butter Cookies†

Ingredients

1 cup unsalted butter or margarine
1 cup sifted confectioners' sugar
1 teaspoon vanilla extract
2 1/2 cups all-purpose flour

Procedure

Cream butter and confectioners' sugar together. Add vanilla and mix. Sift flour and stir in. Mix thoroughly with hands. Mold into long, smooth roll about 2 inches in diameter. Wrap in wax paper and chill in refrigerator until stiff. With thin, sharp knife, cut into thin, 1/8 to 1/16-inch, slices. Place slices a little apart on ungreased baking sheet. Bake at 400° F until lightly browned. Yield: 6 dozen 2-inch cookies.

Content

3 cookies contain 1 gm protein, 2 mg sodium, and 30 mg potassium.

Pie Crust†

Ingredients

2 cups sifted all-purpose flour
1/2 teaspoon sugar
2/3 cup unsalted shortening
5 to 6 tablespoons ice water

Procedure

Mix flour and sugar. Cut in shortening with two knives or pastry blender. Stir in just enough water to make ingredients adhere together. Pat lightly with hands until dough forms a smooth mixture. Divide in half and roll lightly on floured board, handling as little as possible. If dough is chilled before rolling, it is easier to handle. Yield: makes 9-inch, 2-crust pie.

Apple Pie†

Ingredients

6 medium apples
3/4 cup sugar
2 tablespoons flour
1/4 teaspoon nutmeg
1 tablespoon unsalted butter or margarine
Add up to 1 tablespoon lemon juice or vinegar if apples are very sweet.

Procedure

Mix sugar, flour, and nutmeg. Alternate with layers of peeled, sliced apples in 9-inch pastry-lined pie plate. Dot with butter or margarine and add lemon juice or vinegar if needed. Bake on bottom shelf of oven at 425° F for 15 min. Change to middle shelf and continue baking until apples are tender, about 20 to 30 minutes. Other allowed fruits may be substituted. Yield: 8 servings.

Content

One serving (1/8 pie) contains 2 gm protein, 5 mg sodium, and 150 mg potassium.

---

†From Mitchell, M. C., and Smith, J.: Dietary care of the patient with chronic oliguria. *Amer. J. Clin. Nutr.*, *19*:163–169, 1966.

Recipes continued on following page.

Recipes Low in Protein, Sodium, and Potassium (Continued)

Lemon Pudding‡

Ingredients
- 2/3 cup sugar
- 1/3 cup Resource Baking Mix‡
- 1 cup water
- 1 tsp. grated lemon rind
- 3 tbs. lemon juice
- 1 drop yellow food coloring

Procedure

Blend sugar and Resource in small pan. Add water. Cook over low heat, stirring constantly until mixture comes to a boil. Cook one minute. Remove from heat. Add lemon rind, lemon juice, and food coloring. Cool. Flavor and color levels may be varied according to personal preference. Yield: 3 1/2-cup servings.

Content

Each serving contains 0.2 gm protein, 5 mg sodium, 5 mg potassium, and 219 calories.

Low-Protein Bread‡

Ingredients
- 1 package active dry yeast
- 1 2/3 cup warm water (105 to 115° F)
- 1 bag Resource Baking Mix

Procedure
1. Preheat oven to 425° F. *Generously* grease sides and bottom of loaf pan: 9 × 5 × 3 inches.
2. In large mixer bowl, add 1 2/3 cup warm water and 1 package yeast. Mix slowly a few minutes to dissolve yeast.
3. Add 1 bag Resource Baking Mix. Blend briefly on low speed and then beat on medium speed until smooth and glossy, about 1/2 minute.
4. Pour batter into pan. Let rise uncovered in warm place (100°) until batter in center of pan is just even with edge of pan—about 30 minutes.
5. Immediately place in preheated oven and bake 25 to 30 minutes or until golden brown. After a few minutes, remove from pan. Brush salt-free butter on top of loaf if desired. Cool on wire rack. To store, wrap cooled loaf tightly in plastic wrap or aluminum foil.

Content

One slice (20 slices per loaf) contains 0.2 gm protein, 14 mg sodium, 9 mg potassium, and 100 calories.

---

‡From Doyle Pharmaceutical Co., Highway 100 at West 23 Street, Minneapolis, Minn. 55416.

Recipes continued on opposite page.

Recipes Low in Protein, Sodium, and Potassium (Continued)

Commercial Preparation (Controlyte)

Controlyte is available from Doyle Pharmaceutical Company and is high in calories (1000 calories per 7 oz can), is protein-free, contains 0.01 per cent or less sodium, potassium, phosphorus, and magnesium and is prepared for use by the addition of 240 ml water. Controlyte may be used alone or as a supplement.

The approximate analysis for a 7-oz can of Controlyte added to 1 cup (240 ml) water is as follows:

Volume	370 ml (12.5 fl oz)
Calories	1000
Carbohydrate	143 gm
Protein	0
Fat	48 gm
Sodium	20 mg (0.87 mEq)
Potassium	8 mg (0.20 mEq)
Calcium	4 mg (0.20 mEq)
Phosphorus	2 mg

Protein, Sodium and Potassium Values of Foods

FOODS	AMOUNT	PROTEIN (gm)	SODIUM (mg)	POTASSIUM (mg)
BEVERAGES				
Coca Cola	6 oz	–	2	88
Ginger ale	8 oz	–	18	1
Pepsi Cola	8 oz	–	35	7
Dr. Pepper	10 oz	–	30	5
Diet Dr. Pepper	10 oz.	–	60	5
Diet Pepsi	10 oz	–	20	5
Fresca	10 oz	–	50	5
Tab	10 oz	–	40	5
Seven-Up	10 oz	–	40	5
Orange drink (Sun Crest)	10 oz	–	40	9
Like	10 oz	–	40	5
Coffee, instant, 1 tsp powder w/8 oz water	240 ml (1 cup)	–	1	250
Coffee, decaffeinated, 1 tsp rounded w/8 oz water	240 ml (1 cup)	–	2	60
Coffee, drip	240 ml (1 cup)	–	–	200
Tea, instant, 1 tsp powder w/8 oz water	240 ml (1 cup)	–	–	50
Skim milk	8 oz	8	130	360
Buttermilk (commercial)	8 oz	8	320	340
Whole milk	8 oz	8	120	350
Chocolate milk	8 oz	8	115	360
Kool Aid	8 oz	0	0	0
Rum (1 jigger)	1½ oz	0	0	0
Whiskey (1 jigger)	1½ oz	0	0	0
Gin (1 jigger)	1½ oz	0	0	0
CEREALS AND BREADS				
Bread, rye, American	1 slice	2	120	30
Bread, unsalted	1 slice	2	20	30
Bread, white	1 slice	2	120	30
Bread, whole wheat	1 slice	2	120	60
Crackers, graham	1 square	1	50	25
Crackers, Ritz or Hi-Ho	6 round	2	240	24
Crackers, Saltine	3 squares	1	100	10
Vanilla wafer	6 wafers	1	50	10
Nabisco Sugar Wafer	7 wafers	1	40	10
Puffed Rice	1 cup	1	0	10
Puffed Wheat	1 cup	2	1	40
Shredded Wheat	1 biscuit	2	1	80
Bran Flakes 40%	¾ cup	3	260	
Corn Flakes	¾ cup	2	280	30
Cream of Wheat (Farina)	½ cup	2	1	Trace
Grits	½ cup	2	0	15
Oatmeal	½ cup	2	Trace	70
Rice, white, cooked	½ cup	2	0	20
Noodles, cooked tender	½ cup	3	1	45
Popped popcorn, plain	1 cup	2	Trace	
DAIRY PRODUCTS				
Butter, regular	1 tsp	Trace	50	1
Butter, unsalted	1 tsp	Trace	1	
Cheese, American	1 oz	7	200	20

Table continued on opposite page.

Protein, Sodium and Potassium Values of Foods (Continued)

Foods	Amount	Protein (gm)	Sodium (mg)	Potassium (mg)
Cheese, American, Swiss	1 oz	8	200	30
Cheese, cottage, creamed	1 oz	4	65	20
Cheese, cottage, dry	1 oz	5	90	20
Cheese, process	1 oz	7	320	20
Cream cheese	1 oz	2	70	20
Cream, coffee	1 tbs	.5	5	20
Cream, coffee	2 tbs	1	10	40
Half & Half	2 tbs	1	15	40
Ice cream, vanilla	3 oz	4	55	180
Ice Milk	3 oz	4	60	180
Milk (See Beverages)				
Skim milk powder	1/3 cup	7	105	350
Sherbet (orange)	3 1/2 oz	1	10	20
Egg	1 medium	7	60	60
Egg, white	1 medium	3	45	40
Egg, yolk	1 medium	3	10	20
FRUITS				
Apple, raw	1 medium	0	1	170
Applesauce, sweetened	1/2 cup	0	0	100
Apricots, canned	4 halves	1	1	300
Apricots, dried, cooked	4 halves	1	5	280
Avocado, raw	1/2 pitted	2	5	600
Banana, small	1 (6″)	1	1	370
Banana, medium	1	2	2	560
Cantaloupe, raw	1/4 5″ melon	1	10	250
Cantaloupe, diced	1/2 cup	1	15	300
Blackberries, raw	1 cup	2	1	250
Blackberries, canned	1/2 cup	1	1	140
Blueberries, raw	1 cup	1	1	110
Cherries, red, sour, raw	1/2 cup	1	2	190
Cherries, canned in heavy syrup	1/2 cup	1	1	120
Cherries, sweet, raw	15	1	2	190
Cranberries, raw	1 cup	0	2	80
Dates, pitted	10	2	1	650
Figs, fresh, raw	2 large	1	2	190
Figs, canned in heavy syrup	3 medium	1	2	150
Fruit cocktail	1/2 cup	0	5	170
Grapefruit, raw	1/2 medium	1	1	140
Grapes, raw	22 medium	1	3	160
Lemons, fresh	1 medium	1	2	140
Nectarines, raw	2 medium	1	6	290
Olives, green	2 medium	0	310	5
Olives, ripe, canned	2 large	0	150	5
Olives, ripe, salt cured	3 medium	0	660	5
Orange	1 medium	2	2	300
Orange, segments	1/2 cup	1	1	190
Peaches, raw	1 medium	1	1	200
Peaches, raw, sliced	1 cup	1	2	340
Peaches, canned, heavy syrup	2 halves	0	2	130
Peaches, dried, cooked	3 halves	1	5	300
Peaches, frozen, sliced	2/5 cup	0	2	120
Pears, raw	1/2 pear	1	2	130
Pears, canned, heavy syrup	2 halves	0	1	80
Pineapple, raw	1/2 cup	0	1	100

Table continued on following page.

Protein, Sodium and Potassium Values of Foods (Continued)

Foods	Amount	Protein (gm)	Sodium (mg)	Potassium (mg)
Pineapple, canned, juice packed	1 large slice	0	1	150
Pineapple, canned, heavy syrup	1 large slice	0	1	100
Plums, raw	2 medium	1	2	300
Plums, canned, heavy syrup	3 medium	0	1	140
Prunes, dried, not cooked	3 medium	1	1	200
Prunes, dried, cooked	4 medium	1	4	330
Pumpkin, canned	1/2 cup	1	1	300
Raisins, dried	1 tbs	0	3	80
Raspberries, black, raw	1/2 cup	1	Trace	150
Raspberries, red, raw	1/2 cup	1	Trace	110
Raspberries, canned, WP	1/2 cup	1	1	110
Raspberries, frozen	1/2 cup	1	1	120
Rhubarb, raw, cubed	3/4 cup	1	2	250
Strawberries, raw	10	1	1	160
Strawberries, raw, no stems	1 cup	1	2	250
Strawberries, frozen, sliced	1/2 cup	1	1	140
Tangerine, raw	1 large	1	2	130
Tomato, raw	1 small	1	3	240
Watermelon	1/2 cup	1	1	100
Watermelon, 1 slice 6″ × 1 1/2″		3	6	600
JUICES				
Apple juice	1/2 cup	0	1	120
Apricot Nectar	1/2 cup	0	1	190
Cranberry juice	1/2 cup	0	1	10
Grapefruit juice, fresh	1/2 cup	1	2	200
Grapefruit juice, canned	1/2 cup	1	1	180
Grape juice, bottled	1/2 cup	0	2	140
Grape juice, frozen	1/2 cup	0	1	40
Lemonade, frozen	1/2 cup	0	Trace	20
Orange juice, fresh	1 cup	2	3	500
Orange juice, fresh	1/2 cup	1	2	250
Orange juice, canned	1/2 cup	1	1	250
Orange juice, frozen	1/2 cup	1	1	230
Peach Nectar	1/2 cup	0	2	100
Pear Nectar	1/2 cup	0	2	50
Pineapple juice, canned	1/2 cup	0	1	190
Prune juice	1/2 cup	1	3	280
Tomato juice	1/2 cup	1	240	270
Tomato juice, low sodium	1/2 cup	1	3	280
MEAT, FISH, AND POULTRY				
Beef, roast	1 oz	7	20	110
Canadian bacon	1 oz	7	770	140
Chicken, dark, cooked	1 oz	7	25	100
Chicken, light	1 oz	7	20	120
Crab, boiled in fresh water	1 oz	5		
Crab, canned	1 oz	5	280	30
Codfish, raw, brine dip	1 oz	5	75	120
Codfish, broiled	1 oz	9	30	120
Duck, roast	1 oz	7		
Flounder, baked	1 oz	9	70	180
Frankfurters	1 small	7	540	110
Ham, cured	1 oz	7	260	120

Table continued on opposite page.

Protein, Sodium and Potassium Values of Foods (Continued)

Foods	Amount	Protein (gm)	Sodium (mg)	Potassium (mg)
Ham, fresh	1 oz	7	20	
Haddock, canned	1 oz	7		
Halibut, broiled	1 oz	8	40	160
Lamb, lean, broiled	1 oz	7	20	90
Liver, calf, fried in batter	1 oz	7	45	140
Liver, chicken, stewed	1 oz	7	40	70
Lobster, cooked	1 oz	6	60	50
Oysters (r) Eastern	5–8 medium	8	75	120
Pork, lean, cooked	1 oz	7	20	120
Salmon, canned, pink	1 oz	6	115	110
Salmon, canned, red	1 oz	6	155	100
Salmon, canned (d)	1 oz			
Scallops, fresh, steamed	3 small	7	80	140
Shrimp, raw	3 small	5	40	70
Shrimp, cooked, French fry	3 small	6	55	70
Shrimp, canned	3 small	7		40
Tuna, canned	1/4 cup	7	240	90
Tuna, water packed	1/4 cup	8	15	80
Sardines, canned in oil	2 large or 3 small	6	150	170
Shad, baked	1 oz	7	20	110
Sausage, pork, cooked	1 oz	8	280	80
Sausage, bologna	1 slice	4	390	70
Turkey, light	1 oz	7	25	120
Turkey, dark	1 oz	7	30	120
Veal, roast	1 oz	7	25	150
Bass, average, baked	1 oz	6	20	70
Herring, canned	2–3	6		
Mussels, meat only	2–3	4	85	90
VEGETABLES (All values are for cooked portions)				
Artichoke, fresh bud, base and leaves	1 head	3	30	300
Beans, white	1/2 cup	8	5	420
Beans, red	1/2 cup	9	4	340
Beans, lima, canned, drained	1/2 cup	6	270	260
Beans, lima, fresh	1/2 cup	7	1	420
Beans, lima, dried	1/2 cup	8	2	610
Beans, snap, green, fresh cooked	1 cup	2	5	190
Beans, snap, canned	1/2 cup	1	260	100
Beans, snap, frozen, cut	1/2 cup	2	1	150
Beans, wax, cooked	1 cup	1	3	150
Beans, wax, canned, drained	1/2 cup	1	235	100
Asparagus, frozen	6 spears	3	2	260
Asparagus, canned	6 spears	3	270	190
Beets, red, fresh, raw	2 medium	1	60	340
Beets, cooked, diced	1/2 cup	1	35	170
Beets, canned	1/2 cup	1	195	140
Beet greens	1/2 cup	2	75	330
Broccoli	1 large stick	3	10	270
Broccoli, frozen, cooked	1/2 cup	1	10	160
Brussel sprouts	6–7	4	10	270
Brussel sprouts, frozen	6–7	3	15	300
Cabbage, raw	1 cup	1	20	230
Cabbage, cooked	1/2 cup	1	10	140
Cabbage, red, raw	1 cup	2	25	270

Table continued on following page.

Protein, Sodium and Potassium Values of Foods (Continued)

Foods	Amount	Protein (gm)	Sodium (mg)	Potassium (mg)
Carrots, raw	1 large	1	50	340
Carrots, cooked	1/2 cup	1	25	170
Cauliflower, raw	1/2 cup	2	7	150
Cauliflower, cooked	1/2 cup	1	5	120
Cauliflower, cooked	1 cup	3	10	240
Celery, inner stalk	1 small	0	25	70
Celery, diced	1 cup	1	130	340
Chard, cooked	1/2 cup	2	72	270
Collards, cooked	1/2 cup	3	25	230
Corn, fresh, 4″ ear	1	3	Trace	200
Corn, canned, drained	1/2 cup	2	195	80
Cowpeas, cooked	1/2 cup	7	1	300
Cowpeas, frozen	1/2 cup	6	25	210
Cucumber, pared	1/2 medium	0	3	80
Dandelion greens	1/2 cup	2	40	230
Eggplant, drained	1/2 cup	1	1	150
Kale, cooked	1/2 cup	2	30	150
Mushrooms, canned (Slds and liq.)	1/2 cup	2	400	200
Mustard greens, fresh	1/2 cup	2	20	220
Mustard greens, frozen	1/2 cup	2	10	160
Okra, cooked	8–9 pods	2	2	170
Onion, raw, 1/4″ diameter	1–2	2	10	160
Onion, cooked	1/2 cup	1	7	110
Parsnips, diced	1/2 cup	2	8	380
Lettuce, iceberg	1 1/2 oz	–	5	130
Peas, green	1/2 cup	4	1	150
Peas, canned, drained	1/2 cup	3	160	60
Peas, dried, split	1/2 cup	7	10	270
Peppers, green, empty shell	1 large	1	10	210
Pickle, dill	1 large	1	1428	200
Potatoes, baked w/skin – 1	2 1/2″ diameter	3	4	500
Potatoes, boiled w/o skin – 1	2 1/4″ diameter	2	2	290
Potatoes, boiled in skin	1 medium	2	3	400
Potatoes, French fried	10 pieces	2	3	430
Pumpkin, canned	1/2 cup	1	2	280
Radish, raw, 1″	10 small	1	20	320
Rhubarb, cooked w/sugar	1/2 cup	1	3	210
Rutabagas, cooked	1/2 cup	1	4	170
Sauerkraut, canned	1/2 cup	1	560	110
Soybeans, cooked	1/2 cup	11	2	540
Spinach, fresh, cooked	1/2 cup	3	45	290
Spinach, canned	1/2 cup	2	210	230
Spinach, frozen	1/2 cup	3	50	330
Squash, summer, cooked	1/2 cup	2	1	140
Squash, frozen	1/2 cup	1	1	200
Sweet potatoes, baked in skin	1 large	4	22	540
Sweet potatoes, canned	1 small	2	50	200
Tomatoes, raw	1 small	1	5	240
Tomatoes, raw	1 medium	2	5	370
Tomatoes, cooked, boiled	1/2 cup	1	5	290
Tomatoes, canned	1/2 cup	1	130	220
Tomato catsup	1 tbs	0	180	60
Tomato juice	1/2 cup	1	200	230
Tomato chili sauce	1 tbs	0	230	60
Turnip greens, fresh	1/2 cup	2	30	90

Table continued on opposite page.

Protein, Sodium and Potassium Values of Foods (Continued)

Foods	Amount	Protein (gm)	Sodium (mg)	Potassium (mg)
Turnip greens, frozen	½ cup	3	17	149
Turnips, white	½ cup	1	25	190
LOW Na VEGETABLES				
Asparagus	5–6 spears	3	3	170
Asparagus, white	5–6 spears	2	4	140
Lima beans, drained	½ cup	5	4	200
Snapbeans, drained	½ cup	1	1	60
Carrots, drained	½ cup	1	30	90
Corn, whole kernel drained	½ cup	2	2	60
Green peas, drained	½ cup	3	2	60
Tomatoes, ripe	½ cup	1	3	230
Tomato juice	½ cup	1	3	230
Low Na cheese	1 oz	7	3	60
Low Na peanut butter	1 tbs	5	0	100
LOW Na SOUPS (Campbell)				
Beef vegetable	1 can	5	40	50
Vegetable	1 can	2	25	50
Cream of tomato	1 can	3	25	150
Turkey noodle	1 can	4	40	20
Cellu beef broth	1 pk	0	10	500
Cellu chicken broth	1 pk	1	10	480
REGULAR SOUPS	⅔ cup prepared with water or ⅓ cup condensed			
Beef noodle	"	3	795	70
Chicken noodle	"	3	870	40
Chicken w/rice	"	3	760	80
Green pea	"	7	760	130
Tomato	"	1	810	210
Vegetable	"	3	730	170
Vegetable Beef	"	6	790	130
SALAD DRESSINGS				
French	1 tbs	0	190	10
French Low Calorie	1 tbs	0	110	10
Italian	1 tbs	0	290	20
Mayonnaise	1 tbs	0	80	5
Mayonnaise Low Calorie	1 tbs	0	20	1
Thousand Island	1 tbs	0	100	15
Thousand Island Low Calorie	1 tbs	0	100	15
SWEETS				
Molasses, cane	1 tbs	–	15	300
Dark brown sugar	1 tbs	–	3	30
Hershey–chocolate almond	1 oz	2	10	80
Milk chocolate bar (10c bar)	1 oz	2	30	100
Milk chocolate kisses	1 piece	–	5	20
Milky Way	10c bar	3	160	110
Jelly beans	10 large	Trace	2.8	0
Jelly beans	¼ lb	Trace	13	
Gum drops	¼ lb	–	40	6
Hard candy	30 oz bag	–	30	4
Marshmallows	1	–	4	1

APPENDIX E

Currently Known Dialyzable Poisons*

Barbiturates†
- Barbital
- Phenobarbital
- Amobarbital
- Pentobarbital
- Butabarbital
- Secobarbital
- Cyclobarbital
- Butalbital

Glutethimide†

Depressants, Sedatives and Tranquilizers
- Diphenylhydantoin
- Primidone
- Meprobamate
- Ethchlorvynol†
- Ethinamate
- Methypyrlon
- Diphenhydramine
- Methaqualone
- Heroin
- Gallamine triethiodide
- Paraldehyde
- Chloral hydrate
- Chlordiazepoxide

Antidepressants
- Amphetamine
- Methamphetamine
- Tricyclic secondary amines
- Tricyclic tertiary amines
- Monomine oxidase inhibitors
- Tranylcypromine
- Pargyline
- Phenelzine
- Isocarboxazid

Alcohols
- Ethanol†
- Methanol†
- Isopropanol
- Ethylene glycol

Analgesics
- Acetylsalicylic acid†
- Methylsalicylate†
- Acetophenetidin
- Dextro-propoxyphene
- Paracetamol

Antimicrobials
- Streptomycin
- Kanamycin
- Neomycin
- Bacitracin
- Vancomycin
- Penicillin
- Ampicillin
- Carbenicillin
- Sulfonamides
- Cephalin
- Cephaloridine
- Chloramphenicol
- Tetracycline
- Nitrofurantoin
- Polymyxin
- Isoniazid
- Cycloserine
- Quinine

Metals
- Arsenic
- Copper
- Calcium
- Iron
- Lead
- Lithium
- Magnesium
- Mercury
- Potassium
- Sodium
- Strontium
- Zinc

Halides
- Bromide†
- Chloride†
- Iodide
- Fluoride

Endogenous Toxins
- Ammonia
- Uric acid†
- Tritium†
- Bilirubin
- Lactic acid
- Schizophrenia
- Myasthenia gravis
- Porphyria
- Cystine
- Myocardial Depressant Factor
- Endotoxin
- Uremic Toxin(s)
- Hyperosmolar state†
- Water intoxication

Miscellaneous Substances
- Mannitol
- Thiocyanate†
- Thiols
- Aniline
- Sodium chlorate
- Potassium chlorate
- Eucalyptus oil
- Boric acid
- Potassium dichromate
- Chromic acid
- Digoxin
- Sodium citrate
- Dinitro-ortho-cresol
- Amanita Phalloides
- Carbon tetrachloride
- Ergotamine
- Cyclophosphamide
- 5-Fluorouracil
- Methotrexate
- Camphor
- Trichlorethylene
- Carbon monoxide
- Chlorpropamide
- Peritonitis

*From Schreiner, G. E., and Techan, B. P.: Dialysis of poisons and drugs. Annual review. *Amer. Soc. Artif. Intern. Organs, 17*:513–544, 1971.

†Kinetics of dialysis thoroughly studied and/or clinical experience extensive.

APPENDIX F

Bath Concentrates *(Travenol)*

When one bottle (3.67 liters) of dialysis bath concentrate 100 is diluted to 100 liters of tap water or one bottle of dialysis bath concentrate 120 is diluted to 120 liters, the following compositions result:

Na^+	134.0 mEq/L
K^+	2.6 mEq/L
Ca^{++}	2.5 mEq/L
Mg^{++}	1.5 mEq/L
Cl^-	104.0 mEq/L
Na acetate	36.6 mEq/L
Anhydrous Dextrose USP	2.5 mEq/L

One bottle (3.67 liters of dialysate bath concentrates potassium-free) 100 or 120

Na^+	134.0 mEq/L
Ca^{++}	2.5 mEq/L
Mg^{++}	1.5 mEq/L
Cl^-	101.0 mEq/L
Na acetate	36.6 mEq/L
Anhydrous Dextrose USP	2.5 mEq/L

APPENDIX G

Instructions for Cannula Care

It is important to cleanse your shunt site daily in order to prevent infection and to insure proper functioning of your cannula.

To Clean Shunt

1. Select a clean quiet spot in your house with a table and chair.
2. Gather all your supplies:
   - Sterile gloves
   - Sterile gauze squares
   - Sterile Q tips
   - Cleansing solution
   - Clean Ace bandage
   - Tape or clips
   - Ointment (if needed)
3. Place all supplies within easy reach on the table. Make yourself comfortable and begin.
4. Open 3 packages of gauze squares, being careful not to touch them.
5. Open sterile Q tips, touching the outside wrapper only
6. Saturate one package of gauze squares with cleansing solution. Squeeze ointment onto one dry gauze square.
7. Remove soiled Ace bandage and gauze squares from shunt. Inspect skin for signs of infection—redness, swelling, drainage.
8. Put on sterile gloves.
9. Use saturated gauze squares to cleanse skin around cannula.
10. Use Q tips to cleanse shunt insertion sites on skin.
11. Dry area with sterile gauze.
12. Apply ointment around shunt insertion sites on skin.
13. Place one sterile gauze under shunt and one over it leaving the loop of the shunt visible.
14. Remove gloves.
15. Apply clean Ace bandage and secure.

APPENDIX H

Assessment Tool for Patients with Chronic Uremia

Summary of Medical History

Summary of Social Status

Medical and Nursing Goals

I. Skin
  A. Cleanliness ________
  B. Color
    Pallor ________ Jaundice ________
    Cyanosis ________ Gray-brown ________
  C. Turgor ________
  D. Irregularities
    Pruritus ________ Bruises ________
    Lesions ________ Petechiae ________
    Dryness ________ Crystals ________
    Perspiration ________
II. Body temperature
  Method of measurement ________
  Hypothermia ________
  Hyperthermia ________
  Causes in precipitating factors ________
  ____
III. Body fluids
  A. Weight
    Previous weight ________
    Pre-dialysis ________
      Net gain ________
    Post-dialysis ________
      Net loss ________
  B. Edema
    Slight ________
    Moderate ________
    Pitting ________
      Feet ________ Sacrum ________
      Ankles ________ Abdomen ________
      Legs ________ Periorbital ________
  C. Dehydration
    Slight ________
    Moderate ________
    Severe ________

Summary continued on following page.

D. Total fluid intake daily ____________
Total urine output daily ____________
Vomitus ____________
Diarrhea ____________
Other drainage ____________

IV. Renal system
A. Urinary output
1. Amount
Amount in 24 hr ____________
Amount per voiding ____________
Frequency of voiding ____________
2. Color

Yellow ______	Clear ______
Straw ______	Bloody ______
Pink ______	Cloudy ______
Dark amber ______	Other ______

3. Specific gravity
(N 1.010–1.030) ______
4. Abnormalities
Retention ______
Distention ______
Burning ______
Pain ______
Nocturia ______
Urgency ______
Frequency ______

In urine

Casts ______	Pus ______
RBC's ______	WBC's ______
Bacteria ______	Crystals ______

B. Blood chemistry

	Normal (mg. per 100 ml)	Patient
Urea	10–20	______
Creatinine	0.7–1.5	______
Uric acid	2.5–8.0	______
Potassium	3.5–5.0	______
Sodium	136–145	______
Chloride	96–108	______
Calcium	9–11	______

C. pH of blood
pH 7.35–7.45
CO_2 content 22–30

V. Cardiovascular system
A. Pulses

	Apical	Radial
Rate	______	______
Rhythm	______	______
Volume	______	______
Deficit	______	______

Pericardial friction rub ____________
Pedal pulses ____________

B. Arrhythmias – due to hyperkalemia, hypokalemia, hypoxia, or acidosis.
1. Premature contractions
a. PAC ______ Frequency ______
b. PVC ______ Frequency ______
c. Bigeminy
Atrial ______
Ventricular ______

Summary continued on opposite page.

2. Atrial arrhythmias
   - Atrial tachycardia ________ Rate ________
   - Atrial flutter ________ Rate ________
   - Atrial fibrillation ________ Rate ________
3. Ventricular arrythmias
   - Ventricular tachycardia ________ Rate ________
   - Ventricular flutter ________ Rate ________
   - Ventricular fibrillation ________ Rate ________

VI. Respiratory system

A. General observations

1. Rate ________ Depth ________
2. Interval ________ Odor ________
3. Symmetry of chest expansion ________
4. Breathing
   - Abdominal ________ Mouth ________
   - Chest ________ Nasal ________

B. Difficulties

- Eupnea ________ Cheyne-Stokes ________
- Bradypnea ________ Kussmaul ________
- Tachypnea ________ Apnea ________
- Dyspnea ________ Air hunger ________
  - Bed rest ________ Nasal flare ________
  - Sitting ________ Retraction ________
  - Ambulating ________

C. Cough

- Persistent ________ Hacking ________
- Productive ________ Moist ________
  - Color ________
  - Consistency ________
  - Odor ________
  - Amount ________

D. Lung sounds

- Clear ________ Moist ________
- Rales ________ Wheezes ________

E. Blood gases

- pO_2 ________ O_2 sat ________
- pCO_2 ________

VII. Gastrointestinal system

A. Mouth

- Mucous membranes ________
- Tongue ________
  - Parotitis ________
  - Stomatitis ________
  - Gums ________

B. Appetite

- Anorexia ________
- Nausea ________
- Vomiting ________

C. Diet ________

- Protein ________
- Potassium ________
- Sodium ________
- Fluids ________

D. Difficulties

- Indigestion ________
- Pain ________
- Coffee ground emesis ________
- Diarrhea ________
- Bloody stool ________

Summary continued on following page.

VIII. Musculoskeletal system
- A. Muscles
  - Flaccid ______ Good tone ______
  - Atrophy ______ Cramps ______
- B. Skeletal
  - Osteodystrophy diagnosed by X-ray ______
  - Pathological fractures ______

IX. Endocrine system
- Delayed puberty ______
- Libido ______
- Potency ______
- Ovulation ______
- Amenorrhea ______

X. Nervous system
- A. Mental status
  - Alert ______ Semiconscious ______
  - Drowsy ______ Comatose ______
- B. Orientation to time, place, person ______
- C. Intellectual functioning
  - Level of education ______
  - Ability to recall events
    - Past ______
    - Present ______
  - Ability to compute
    - Ex. subtract from 100 by 7 ______
- D. Sensory disturbances
  - Visual ______
  - Auditory ______
  - Olfactory ______
  - Tactile ______
- E. Motor disturbances
  - Gait ______
  - Tingling ______

XI. Response to illness
- A. Body image disturbances ______
- B. Role disturbance ______
- C. Coping mechanisms
  - Alienation ______
  - Denial ______
  - Projection ______
  - Depression ______
  - Anxiety ______
  - Guilt ______
  - Fear ______
- D. Seen by psychiatrist ______ Date ______

XII. Status of rehabilitation
- A. Work
  - Part-time ______ Unemployed ______
  - Full time ______
- B. Assumes previous responsibilities
  - Partially ______ Totally dependent ______
  - Completely ______
- C. Job retraining
- D. Seen by social worker ______ Date ______

Index

In this index page numbers in *italics* indicate illustrations; those followed by (t) indicate tables.